D0903390

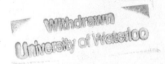

Principles and Practice
of Behavioral Assessment

APPLIED CLINICAL PSYCHOLOGY

Series Editors:

Alan S. Bellack
University of Maryland at Baltimore, Baltimore, Maryland

Michel Hersen
Pacific University, Forest Grove, Oregon

Current volumes in this Series

CONJOINT BEHAVIORAL CONSULTATION
A Procedural Manual
Susan M. Sheridan, Thomas R. Kratochwill, and John R. Bergan

CONTEMPORARY ISSUES IN BEHAVIOR THERAPY
Improving the Human Condition
Edited by Joseph R. Cautela and Waris Ishaq

FUNDAMENTALS OF BEHAVIOR ANALYTIC RESEARCH
Alan Poling, Laura L. Methot, and Mark G. LeSage

HANDBOOK OF RESEARCH METHODS IN HUMAN OPERANT BEHAVIOR
Edited by Kennon A. Lattal and Michael Perone

INTRODUCTION TO SCIENTIFIC PSYCHOLOGY
Henry D. Schlinger, Jr., and Alan Poling

KEY CONCEPTS IN PSYCHOTHERAPY INTEGRATION
Jerold R. Gold

PRINCIPLES AND PRACTICE OF BEHAVIORAL ASSESSMENT
Stephen N. Haynes and William H. O'Brien

PSYCHOLOGICAL ASSESSMENT IN MEDICAL SETTINGS
Ronald H. Rozensky, Jerry J. Sweet, and Steven M. Tovian

THE SCIENTIFIC PRACTICE OF PROFESSIONAL PSYCHOLOGY
Steven J. Trierweiler and George Stricker

SOURCEBOOK OF TREATMENT PROGRAMS FOR SEXUAL OFFENDERS
Edited by William Lamont Marshall, Yolanda M. Fernanadez, Stephen M. Hudson, and Tony Ward

TREATING ADDICTIVE BEHAVIORS, Second Edition
Edited by William R. Miller and Nick Heather

A Continuation Order Plan is available for this series. A continuation order will bring delivery of each new volume immediately upon publication. Volumes are billed only upon actual shipment. For further information please contact the publisher.

Principles and Practice of Behavioral Assessment

Stephen N. Haynes
University of Hawaii at Manoa
Honolulu, Hawaii

and

William Hayes O'Brien
Bowling Green State University
Bowling Green, Ohio

Kluwer Academic / Plenum Publishers
New York, Boston, Dordrecht, London, Moscow

Library of Congress Cataloging-in-Publication Data

Haynes, Stephen N.
    Principles and practice of behavioral assessment / Stephen N. Haynes, William Hayes O'Brien.
      p. cm. -- (Applied clinical psychology)
    Includes bibliographical references and index.
    ISBN 0-306-46221-4
    1. Behavioral assessment. I. O'Brien, William Hayes. II. Title. III. Series.

BF176.5 .H39 1999
150'.287--dc21

                                             99-046705

ISBN: 0-306-46221-4

©2000 Kluwer Academic / Plenum Publishers
233 Spring Street, New York, N.Y. 10013

10 9 8 7 6 5 4 3 2 1

A C.I.P. record for this book is available from the Library of Congress

Printed in the United States of America

To Dorothy, Tamara, Annamarie, Aaron, Liam, and the Lipari-Jordans,
who provide joy and perspective.

Preface

Introduction and Goals of Book

This book presents the concepts and strategies of the behavioral assessment paradigm. Psychological assessment paradigms affect the methods of assessment, the settings in which assessment occurs, the persons from whom assessment data are acquired, how often assessment occurs, and the way assessment information is summarized and integrated. Ultimately, the assessment paradigm affects clinical judgments about clients—judgments about which of a client's multiple problems and treatment goals should be addressed and assumptions about the most likely causes of the client's problems. The assessment paradigm also affects decisions about which treatments would be best for a client and estimates of the effects of treatment.

Behavioral assessment is a psychological assessment paradigm that emphasizes empirically supported, multimethod and multi-informant assessment of specific, observable behaviors and contemporaneous causal variables in the natural environment. The behavioral assessment paradigm stresses the use of well-validated assessment instruments and assumptions that social/environmental, cognitive, and physiological variables are often important sources of behavior variance.

The behavioral assessment paradigm has had a major influence on the field of psychological assessment. It has affected the way research on the causes of behavior disorders is conducted, the way treatment process and outcome are evaluated, and the way treatment decisions are made.

The goal of this book is to present the characteristics and underlying assumptions of the behavioral assessment paradigm and to show how they affect the practice of behavioral assessment. Although all of the concepts and strategies discussed in this book are applicable in research, this book focuses on the use of behavioral assessment to guide clinical judgments.

Principles and Practices of Behavioral Assessment

We emphasize several principles and practices of psychological assessment in this book:

1. The psychological assessment paradigm within which the assessor operates affects the focus and strategies of assessment and the clinical judgments made about the client.

2. Behavioral assessment is composed of a diverse set of assumptions about behavior and its causes, the best strategies for understanding persons with behavior problems, and the best ways to plan and evaluate interventions.

3. Measurement is a central component of a scientific approach to psychological assessment, and the psychometric qualities of obtained measures affect the validity of clinical judgments.

4. The supraordinate characteristics of the behavioral assessment paradigm are the emphases on empiricism and a scholarly approach to psychological assessment.

5. Behavioral assessment is a functional approach to psychological assessment: The applicability and utility of the principles and strategies of behavioral assessment depend on the characteristics of the assessment occasion, particularly on the goals of assessment for that occasion.

6. The validity of clinical judgments can be increased by using multiple validated assessment instruments with multiple informants, applied often.

7. There are many immediate and intermediate goals in clinical assessment, but a supraordinate goal is the development of a behavioral case formulation to guide the focus and methods of intervention.

8. Psychological assessment should have a scholarly, empirical basis. Assessment instruments should be validated for the particular purpose of assessment and the assessor should be knowledgeable of relevant research literature.

9. Time-series assessment strategies can be sensitive to the dynamic time-course of variables.

10. Assessment strategies should include behavioral observation and controlled experimentation.

11. Idiographic assessment strategies are congruent with a functional approach to psychological assessment and are amenable to psychometric evaluation.

12. The most useful level of specificity of variables depends on the goals of an assessment occasion but psychological assessment instruments often provide data that are not sufficiently specific for most behavioral assessment goals.

13. Specific variables promote the use of observational methods, the use of time-series measurement strategies, the measurement of functional relations, and valid clinical judgments.

14. Clients often have multiple, functionally related behavior problems.

15. Behavior problems can vary across situations and time and can have multiple modes, facets, and dimensions.

16. The behavioral assessment paradigm is congruent with a constructional approach to assessment and treatment.

17. Assumptions about causation affect decisions about the best methods of assessment, the variables and functional relations singled out for assessment, the data obtained in the psychological assessment process, and the resultant clinical case formulation.

18. Assessment of causal relations should involve measurement of causal relations in different settings, the use of multiple sources of information, time-series measurement, observation in natural and analog environments, and highly specific measures.

19. A behavior problem can be influenced by multiple causal variables and through multiple causal paths.

20. Environmental variables and reciprocal behavior-environment interactions are particularly important determinants of behavior problems, and learning principles can guide the focus of assessment.

21. In psychological assessment, we are interested in the phase-space functions of behavior problems and causal variables.
22. An empirically informed, broadly focused preintervention assessment is necessary to identify important causal variables and functional relations.
23. Validity coefficients for psychological assessment measures are conditional and help estimate the confidence that can be placed in inferences from those measures. Validity can vary across populations, settings, foci, and goals and is not a generalizable attribute of an assessment instrument.
24. Content validity is an important psychometric evaluative dimensions in behavioral assessment.
25. The functional analysis emphasizes idiographic functional relations relevant to the client's behavior problems.

Organization of Book

This book is divided into three sections. Section I introduces the basic concepts, status, applications, and goals of behavioral assessment. Chapter 1 presents an overview of behavioral assessment. We emphasize a scientific-approach psychological assessment and the role of measurement in clinical judgments, particularly the clinical case formulation. The majority of the chapter previews the underlying assumptions and methods of behavioral assessment that will be treated in greater detail in subsequent chapters. Finally, Chapter 1 briefly discusses the development and historical foundations of behavioral assessment.

In Chapter 2, we discuss the status, applicability, and utility of behavioral assessment. We examine the use of behavioral assessment methods in published treatment outcome studies, circulation of behavioral and nonbehavioral journals, membership in professional organizations, the status of behavioral assessment in graduate training programs, and the use of behavioral assessment methods in clinical practice. In the second section of the chapter we discuss the applicability and utility of behavioral assessment.

In Chapter 3 we define a functional approach to psychological assessment. We also discuss errors in clinical judgments and strategies for reducing them. In Chapter 4 we examine the goals of behavioral assessment and discuss the implications of specific goals for the principles and methods of assessment.

Section II discusses the concepts and assumptions underlying behavioral assessment. In Chapter 5 we emphasize a scholarly, empirically based, hypothesis-testing approach to psychological assessment and the use of time-series measurement strategies. The first sections of Chapter 6 address the rationale underlying nomothetic and idiographic assessment. Later sections of the chapter examine methods of idiographic assessment including Goal Attainment Scaling, advantages and disadvantages of idiographic assessment, and psychometric considerations. Chapter 7 examines the rationale, clinical utility, assets and liabilities, and sources of errors of variables with different degrees of specificity.

Chapter 8 examines assumptions about the nature of behavior problems within a behavioral assessment paradigm. We emphasize several assumptions about behavior problems and the relations between these assumptions and behavioral assessment strategies, particularly the fact that clients often have multiple behavior problems that vary across time and settings.

Chapters 9 and 10 present concepts of causation in behavioral assessment. Chapter 9 introduces concepts of causation: definitions of causal and functional relations, necessary conditions for inferring a causal relation between variables, and limitations of causal inference.

Chapter 10 examines the concepts of causation, most closely associated with the behavioral assessment paradigm, that have been useful in accounting for variance in behavior problems, across persons and time. We discuss the multiple attributes of causal variables, multivariate causality, multiple causal paths and mechanisms, contemporaneous environmental causality, learning principles, reciprocal causation, and setting and contextual events. Implications for these causal models for strategies of assessment are also discussed.

Chapter 11 provides a psychometric framework for evaluating and constructing behavioral assessment instruments, for selecting the best assessment strategy, for interpreting published assessment data, and for drawing inferences from clinical assessment data. We stress construct and content validity, incremental validity and utility, and the conditional nature of psychometric evaluation.

Section III discusses observation and inference in behavioral assessment. Chapter 12 discusses principles and methods of behavioral observation, observation in the natural environment, and observation in analog environments. Chapter 13 reviews assumptions underlying the close assessment–intervention relationship in behavior therapy. Several models of clinical case formulation are reviewed, and the functional analysis is discussed in greater detail.

The Glossary at the end of the book provides definitions for important terms in behavioral assessment and each chapter contains lists of recommended readings.

Caveats

This book is written for readers with differing levels of familiarity with behavioral assessment. However, we have presumed that the reader has some familiarity with basic concepts of psychological assessment, measurement, research design including single-subject designs, and psychometrics. We discuss methods of behavioral assessment throughout the book but we focus on the principles, assumptions, and concepts that underlie those methods.

We recognize and welcome the diversity within the behavioral assessment paradigm. Diversity is necessary for the cybernetic quality and evolution of a paradigm. We have definitive ideas about concepts and strategies of assessment but have tried to acknowledge alternative views. We suggest a careful consideration of, but healthy, scholarly skepticism regarding, the concepts and strategies presented herein. Many concepts and strategies advocated in this book should be considered as hypotheses to be subjected to empirical evaluation. A scholarly skepticism will result in a refined set of concepts and strategies in a behavioral assessment book written 10 years from now.

Acknowledgments

Input on and topics in this book were provided by many graduate students in behavioral assessment courses: Karl Minke, Dan Blaine, Dorothy Chin, Elaine Heiby, and Kelly Vitousek. Chris Chiros and Jennifer McGrath assisted with collecting, codifying, and summarizing data presented in several chapters.

Contents

11. Psychometric Foundations of Behavioral Assessment 199

III. Observation and Inference 223

12. Principles and Strategies of Behavioral Observation 225

I

Introduction to Behavioral Assessment

1

Background, Characteristics, and History

Introduction to Psychological Assessment

Behavioral assessment is one of many psychological assessment paradigms. It is composed of a diverse set of assumptions about behavior and its causes and assumptions about the best strategies for understanding persons with behavior problems, planning interventions, and evaluating the effects of those interventions.

We begin our discussion of behavioral assessment by first defining psychological assessment and emphasizing that measurement is a central component of a scientific approach to psychological assessment. We discuss the important role of measurement in clinical judgments and in the most complex judgment in behavioral assessment—the behavioral case formulation. Next, we discuss the idea of psychological assessment "paradigms," which provide a framework for presenting the behavioral assessment paradigm.

In the major section of this chapter, we preview the underlying assumptions and methods of behavioral assessment. In the last section we discuss the development, sources of influence, and historical foundations of behavioral assessment.

Several ideas are emphasized throughout this chapter:

1. "Psychological assessment" involves the systematic evaluation of a person or persons and includes assumptions, methods, variables, and inferences.
2. Measurement is a central component of a scientific approach to psychological assessment.
3. The psychological assessment paradigm within which the assessor operates affects the variables measured, the strategies of assessment, the information obtained, and clinical judgments about the client.
4. The integration of assessment strategies from different assessment paradigms should be approached cautiously.
5. The behavioral assessment paradigm is composed of an integrated set of assumptions and methods, with an emphasis on empirically supported, multisource, minimally inferential assessment of behaviors, and contemporaneous causal variables in the natural environment.
6. There is considerable overlap between behavioral and nonbehavioral assessment paradigms and within behavioral assessment subparadigms.
7. The supraordinate characteristic of the behavioral assessment paradigm is the emphasis on empiricism and the need for a scientific approach to assessment.
8. The behavioral assessment paradigm has been influenced by generations of behavioral scholars and by research in multiple disciplines.

Psychological Assessment and Measurement

Assessment

Psychological assessment has been defined in many ways (see Box 1-1) but most definitions are congruent with the idea that it is *the systematic evaluation of the behavior of a person or persons* ("behavior" includes motor, verbal, cognitive, and physiological response modes). Psychological assessment is composed of several interrelated conceptual and methodological components, including:

- The methods used to gather information about a person, such as observation and interviews.

Box 1-1
Alternative Definitions of "Psychological Assessment"

The term "psychological assessment" and related constructs such as "psychological testing" have been defined in other ways. These definitions differ in their precision and inclusiveness. Examples include:

(a) The systematic use of a variant of special techniques in order to better understand a given individual, group or social ecology (McReynolds, 1968);

(b) A systematic procedure for comparing the behavior of two or more persons (Cronbach, 1960);

(c) A psychological test is a measurement instrument that has three defining characteristics: 1. A psychological test is a sample of behavior, 2. The sample is obtained under standardized conditions, and 3. There are established rules for scoring, or for obtaining quantitative information from the behavior sample (Murphy & Davidshofer, 1994);

(d) psychological assessment is a complex process of solving problems ... in which psychological tests are often used as one of the methods of collecting relevant data (Maloney & Ward, 1976);

(e) psychological assessment involves four key areas of information (1) the reason for assessment, (2) the raw data, (3) a frame of reference, and (4) interpretation.

(f) psychological assessment is a process of understanding and helping people cope with problems (Walsh & Betz, 1995).

- The setting in which the information is obtained, such as the home, classroom, or clinic.
- The measurement targets, such as a client's problem behaviors, and the variables hypothesized to cause those problem behaviors.
- The informants who provide assessment information, such as a client, spouse, parents and teachers.
- The time-course of measurement—the frequency and duration of measurement.
- Data (measures) and qualitative information derived from an assessment instrument.
- The ways that the assessment data are summarized and analyzed. Assessment data may be summarized as various measures, such as the rates of behavior, conditional probabilities (see Glossary), or as an aggregate scale score from the summation of many questionnaire items.
- The clinical judgments and other inferences based on the information obtained during assessment (e.g., what is the best type of treatment for a client; how successful was a treatment).

These components are important because they affect the information acquired in the psychological assessment of a client.[1] In turn, the information affects clinical judgment about the client, which is the primary outcome of psychological assessment. Ultimately, we engage in psychological assessment to draw inferences about a client, such as estimates of important behavior problems and the causes of these problems.

---

[1]McFall and Townsend (1998) suggested eight layers of scientific model building and testing that are congruent with these components of psychological assessment: Postulates (e.g., assumptions, values), Formal Theoretical Constructions (e.g., hypothesized intervening variables), Referents (reflections of constructs, such as verbal reports of anxiety), Instrumental Methods (e.g., behavioral coding system), Measurement Model, Data Reduction, Data Analysis, and Interpretation and Inference. They suggested that psychological assessment is a form of scientific inquiry: The goal is to draw inferences about an individual based on hypotheses and data.

The assessor's beliefs and values strongly affect the components listed above. For example, the assessor's beliefs about the causes of hyperactive behaviors of children will affect whether he or she examines the classroom environment or limits assessment to cognitive factors (e.g., such as assessment with an intelligence test or continuous performance test) (Vance, 1998).

In summary, many elements of psychological assessment affect the clinical judgments that are the product of the assessment process (see Figure 1-1). As we discuss later, paradigms of psychological assessment differ in their assumptions about behavior and its causes. In turn, different strategies of assessment are preferred. Ultimately, the particular assessment paradigm within which the assessor operates will strongly affect his or her judgments about the client and the treatment that the client receives.

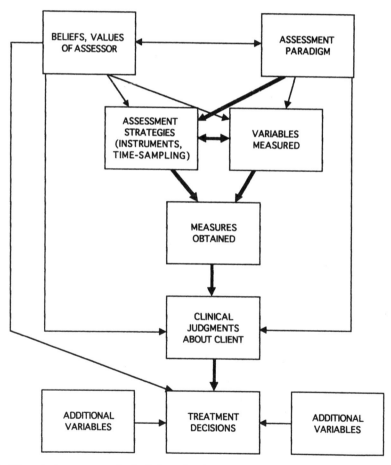

Figure 1-1. The relations among the beliefs and values of the assessor, the psychological assessment paradigm adopted by the assessor, the variables targeted, and the measures obtained in psychological assessment. All components of the psychological assessment process affect clinical judgments about the client and subsequent treatment decisions, which are also affected by other variables (e.g., cooperation from family members, cost of treatment, skills of the therapist).

Measurement

Measurement is a central component of a scientific approach to psychological assessment. Measurement is *the process of assigning a value to an attribute or dimension of a person or variable.* In psychological assessment, we measure many dimensions and modes of behavior, such as the amount of movement by a chronic pain patient and the magnitude of a client's subjective distress during a panic episode. We also measure many dimensions and modes of hypothesized causal variables, such as the intensity and frequency of traumatic life stressors and the probability that a parent will give positive attention when his or her child is doing homework. Sometimes, measurement involves assigning an event to a category, such as when we classify a classroom environment as "demanding" (e.g., when we are observing a classroom environment to identify the precipitants of a child's aggressive behavior), and when we classify a husband's behavior toward his wife as "critical" (e.g., when we are using analogue observation to identify marital communication problems).

Measurement is essential to psychological assessment because it aids clinical judgment. Measurement helps the assessor to predict the client's future behavior, to draw inferences about the causes of the client's behavior problems, to select the best treatment program for the client, and to evaluate the effectiveness of that treatment program. These judgments can be made, and often are made, without the benefit of measurement.

Measurement is the foundation of all sciences, including the behavioral sciences. Advances in the predictive and explanatory power of a science depend on the degree to which the phenomena targeted in that science can accurately be measured. In experimental psychopathology, the accuracy with which the characteristics and dimensions of adult behavior problems can be measured affects the ability to estimate covariance and infer causation. For example, the degree to which childhood trauma contributes to depression cannot be accurately estimated if the magnitude, frequency, and duration of "depression" and "childhood trauma" cannot be measured precisely and validly (Persons & Fresco, 1998). In crosscultural psychology, the degree to which cultural factors are associated with the incidence and characteristics of behavior problems cannot be determined unless we can accurately measure "ethnic identity" as well as the targeted behavior problems (Marsella & Kameoka, 1989).

Another goal of psychological science is prediction—to predict how an individual will behave in different circumstances and settings or to predict the effect of specific events on behavior. The accuracy of predictions is limited by the accuracy with which predictor and predicted variables can be measured. Our ability to predict the likelihood that a client will experience panic attacks in crowded settings (i.e., the conditional probability of panic attacks in crowded settings, relative to all or other settings), the likelihood that a husband will hit his wife when she threatens to leave, and how long a child's tantrum episodes will last depends on the precision with which we can measure panic attacks, marital violence, and tantrums.

It is important to note that different measurement strategies can lead to different estimates and inferences. For example, our estimate of the chance that an antisocial adolescent will steal, lie, destroy property, or provoke fights depends on whether we base our predictions on parent reports, teacher reports, self-reports by the adolescent, direct observation of behavior, or responses to Rorschach cards (Patterson, 1993). We may also reach different estimates depending on which of several parent report instruments we use and with which parent we use them.

Throughout this book we stress that (a) measurement strategies are a central element of clinical judgment, and (b) measurement strategies that are congruent with the behavioral assessment paradigm can be particularly helpful in making valid clinical judgments.

Assessment and Clinical Judgments

In clinical assessment the variables we measure and our assessment strategies affect *clinical judgments*. Measurement can affect judgments about which of a client's multiple behavior problems should be targeted first in treatment, which causal variables for those behavior problems are most important and modifiable, and which treatments would be best for a particular client (see special sections on the assessment-treatment relation in *European Journal of Psychological Assessment*, *14*, 1998; and *Psychological Assessment*, *9*, 1997).

The characteristics of an assessment instrument, particularly its validity and utility, affect the validity of predictions, estimates, and clinical inferences based on obtained measures. The properties of an assessment instrument (more precisely, of the measures derived from them; see Messick, 1993) set upper limits on our ability to use measures obtained from the instrument for clinical judgments.

The validity of clinical judgments also depends on the accuracy (see Glossary) with which we can measure the causal variables. For example, the accuracy with which we can measure potential causal factors for child abuse affects our ability to estimate the probability that a child will be abused by his or her parents. These causal factors might include the type and severity of life stressors experienced by the parents, how the parents think about and cope with those stressors, the parents previous experience with domestic violence, social supports available to the family, substance use, and the skills of the parents in handling difficult child behavior (Hillson & Kuiper, 1994).

Estimates of causal relations are particularly important in behavior therapy because behavioral interventions often attempt to modify the variables hypothesized to cause behavior problems. To understand why some persons but not others experience recurrent distressing thoughts, nightmares, and flashbacks years after a traumatic life event (e.g., sexual assault, natural disasters, severe automobile accidents) we must be able to accurately measure the dimensions of the traumatic events, such as its severity, duration, degree of controllability, and harm. It is also helpful to be able to measure the trauma survivor's behavioral, cognitive, and physiological responses during and immediately following the event. Our understanding of the effects of trauma also depends on how accurately we can measure variables that might moderate the impact of the traumatic event. These moderating variables might include the amount and type of social support available to the person at the time of and immediately following the trauma, social interactions that were occurring during the traumatic event, the person's prior experiences with trauma, the person's belief about his or her role in causing the traumatic event, and the person's physiological and genetic vulnerability.

Measurement strategies can also have an important impact on a client's psychiatric diagnosis. A client's diagnosis can affect whether and for how long he or she is hospitalized and the type of pharmacological and psychological treatment prescribed. A psychiatric diagnosis is based on several lower-order clinical judgments: the assessor's estimate of the presence or absence, severity, and duration of component symptoms. For example, a DSM-IV diagnosis of Attention-Deficit/Hyperactivity Disorder (ADHD) requires that the individual manifest six symptoms of inattention (e.g., careless mistakes in school work, forgetful in daily activities, loses things) or six symptoms of hyperactivity-impulsivity (e.g., fidgets, runs or climbs excessively, talks excessively) for at least six months. The diagnosis also requires "clinically significant impairment" across two or more settings, beginning before the age of seven years (APA, 1994). The accuracy with which the assessor can measure "careless mistakes" and "forgetfulness" and estimate the degree of "impairment" associated with these behaviors can affect the child's diagnosis.

The accuracy with which we measure the component symptoms of an ADHD diagnosis will also have other important consequences, such as whether the client receives medication, placement in a special educational setting, or special instructional programs. The accuracy and validity of the obtained measures of ADHD components will depend on which assessment methods and instruments are used.

Clinical judgments are also affected by the temporal and situational parameters of measurement strategies—how often, for how long, and in what situations we measure the variables of interest. For example, how often and for how long we measure mood and motor activity will affect our estimates about the stability of those behaviors across time and our estimates of the degree to which they are affected by environmental stressors, medication, and behavioral treatment programs. Similarly, our judgments about the causal relations for variables will be affected by the frequency and duration of their measurement.

Integrating Psychological Assessment Data for Clinical Judgments— The Behavioral Case Formulation and Functional Analysis

An important and complex component of psychological assessment is the summarization and integration of assessment data to make clinical judgments (Eels, 1997). The synthesis of assessment data is necessary for all clinical judgments, but is particularly essential in the clinical case formulation. We refer to the summarization and integration of pretreatment behavioral assessment information about a client, as a behavioral clinical case formulation. One type of behavioral case formulation is the **functional analysis**—a synthesis of a client's behavior problems and the variables correlated with and hypothesized to affect those behavior problems (Haynes & O'Brien, 1990; see Chapter 13).

The functional analysis is a hypothesized, working model of the client's problem behaviors, goals, causal variables, and the interrelations among these variables. The treatment program designed for a client is strongly affected not only by assessment data, but also by the inferences that the clinician draws from that data. Different inferences can be drawn from the same data and an erroneous or incomplete functional analysis may increase the chance of treatment failure.

A behavioral case formulation is difficult to derive, in part, because a behavior problem can have a different form and dimension across clients. Furthermore, clients often present with several behavior problems that may affect one another in complex ways. Behavior problems and the components of those problems may also be affected by different causal variables. Additionally, the type and strength of causal variables can differ significantly among clients with the same behavior problem. Finally, most behavior problems are a result of multiple causal variables, which vary in importance, modifiability, and direction of influence across persons.

The behavioral case formulation can also be influenced by the particular assessment instruments used. Each instrument will provide unique data upon which the behavioral case formulation is based. Furthermore, the clinician often must construct a behavioral case formulation with conflicting or insufficient data on important variables.

Summary

The goal of the first section was to introduce psychological assessment, as a context for subsequent discussion of the behavioral assessment paradigm. Psychological assessment is the systematic evaluation of a person's or group of people's behavior. Precise and valid assessment is necessary for the advancement of psychological sciences. Psychological assessment has many components. These include the methods of assessment, the setting and targets of assessment, the sources of information, the time-course of measurement, the data derived and the ways in which they are summarized, and the inferences derived from the assessment process.

Measurement is an important component of psychological assessment. The validity of clinical judgments is limited by the accuracy, precision, and validity of the derived measures. These measures, in turn, depend on the assessment methods, instruments, and strategies used for their collection. One goal of this book is to promote a scientific approach to psychological assessment—the use of assessment methods, instruments, and strategies that provide the most valid and precise measures of the variables that are important for a particular assessment function.

The synthesis of information for clinical judgments is the last and most important component psychological assessment. In behavioral assessment, the summarization and integration of assessment data about a client, a behavioral clinical case formulation, are often called the functional analysis.

Psychological Assessment Paradigms

We now examine the effect of psychological assessment paradigms on assessment strategies and clinical judgments. We noted that information from psychological assessment affects many clinical judgments, such as which assessment methods and instruments are best for a particular client, which behaviors and potential causal variables are the most important targets of assessment, who should be assessed, and how often measures should be obtained. We also noted that decisions about the methods, instruments, and timing of assessment affect the information that will be available to the assessor.

Paradigms as Guides to Psychological Assessment

Definition of Paradigm

Decisions about how to assess a client are guided by the psychological assessment paradigm (see discussions of paradigms by Kuhn, 1970; Krasner, 1992) within which the assessor operates (see Figure 1-1). A **psychological assessment paradigm** is a set of principles, beliefs, values, hypotheses, and methods advocated in an assessment discipline or by its adherents. A psychological assessment paradigm includes beliefs and hypotheses about the relative importance of behavior problems, the most important mode (e.g., physiological vs. cognitive) of behavior problems, the causal variables that affect behavior (e.g., early learning experiences, genetic factors, response contingencies), the mechanisms of causal action (e.g., learning, neurotransmitters, intrapsychic conflict), the importance of assessment to treatment design, and the best methods of obtaining information. It also includes guidelines for deductive and inductive problem solving, decision-making strategies, and how to interpret assessment information (see Box 1-2). Examples of psychological assessment paradigms include behavioral assessment, psychodynamic-projective assessment, personality assessment, intellectual/cognitive assessment, family systems, and neuropsychological assessment.

Box 1-2
Paradigm

The concept of "paradigm," as applied to scientific disciplines (Kuhn, 1970), has been the subject of frequent discourse. The concept of "paradigm" provides a framework from which to view and contrast the assumptions, rules, goals, methods, and accomplishments associated with behavioral assessment. Krasner (1992) suggested that "paradigm" is a more interesting term for "model."

There are several "subparadigms" in behavioral assessment. These subparadigms differ in their emphases on the targets and methods of assessment and in their assumptions about the causes of behavior change. For example, advocates of cognitive-behavioral and behavior-analytic paradigms differ in the role they attribute to unobservable events (e.g., beliefs, expectancies), the relative importance on environmental causal models for behavior problems, and the emphasis placed on direct observation of overt behavior.

Gutting (1980) has edited a book that discusses the concepts of paradigm, scientific revolution, epistemology, theory, and metaphor in the social sciences.

Differences Among Paradigms

Psychological assessment paradigms may differ in their bases for drawing inferences from assessment data. In some assessment paradigms, data obtained in assessment is sometimes interpreted through reference to data obtained from other persons using the same instrument. This is exemplified by the use of norms to estimate a person's relative level of intellectual ability or relative magnitude of social anxiety from their responses to self-report questionnaires. This is an element of a nomothetic approach to assessment (see Chapter 6) and is characteristic of the personality assessment paradigm.

In other paradigms, data obtained in assessment are sometimes interpreted through reference to data from the same client obtained at a different time or situation, or through reference to the client's goals or a criterion. An example is the evaluation of the effects of social contingencies on the observed rates of self-injurious behavior of a developmentally disabled child across several months by systematically manipulating these contingencies in an ABAB (no contingencies/contingencies/no contingencies/contingencies) design. The focus of assessment is the degree to which self-injurious behavior is affected by the contingency, and inferences do not depend on data for self-injurious behaviors in other developmentally disabled individuals. This is an element of an idiographic approach to assessment, characteristic of the behavioral assessment paradigm.

The goals of psychological assessment can also differ across paradigms. Goals of behavioral assessment with a client could include the specification and measurement of behavior problems and goals and of causal and noncausal relations affecting those behavior problems and goals. Goals of assessment with the same client from other paradigms could include diagnosis, the identification of neuropsychological and cognitive deficits, or the identification of personality traits presumed to affect the client's problems in living.

Assessment methods are also guided by the conceptual elements of a paradigm. Within a psychodynamic paradigm, it is assumed that behavior problems often result from unconscious processes and conflicts that may not be directly observable or consciously accessible to the client. Consequently, projective assessment methods, such as the Rorschach, are presumed to be the most effective means of "uncovering" these processes.

There are many psychological assessment paradigms and some assessment methods are congruent with multiple paradigms. The *Handbook of Psychological Assessment* by Goldstein and Hersen (1999) includes chapters on intellectual assessment, achievement testing, neuropsychological assessment, projective assessment, personality assessment, computer-assisted assessment, and behavioral assessment. The *Handbook of Psychological Assessment* by Groth-Marnat (1997) includes chapters on interviewing, behavioral assessment, intellectual assessment, personality assessment, and projective assessment. Sattler's (1988) *Assessment of Children* includes chapters on intellectual assessment, interviewing, neuropsychological assessment, adaptive behavior assessment, and observational methods.

Comparing Psychological Assessment Paradigms

It can be difficult to evaluate the relative merits of different psychological assessment paradigms because they differ in the strategies they presume should govern the evaluation. For example, a demonstration that behavioral assessment methods are superior to projective methods in providing specific data for a behavioral case formulation may not be persuasive to those who adhere to nonbehavioral paradigms. Adherents of a psychodynamic assessment paradigm may not value the molecular-order information that results from behavioral assessment and may fault it for a failure to identify a client's molar traits and underlying intrapsychic mechanisms.

Assessment paradigms can be evaluated on their clinical utility and validity—the degree to which they facilitate specific goals of assessment. For example, assessment methods from different paradigms can be evaluated on the degree to which they predict the future occurrence of important behaviors such as suicide or child abuse. Similarly, different methods can be evaluated on the degree to which they help identify important causal variables and identify the specific effects of treatment. The emphasis on selecting the best assessment strategy for a particular goal of assessment is an element of the functional approach to psychological assessment, that is, the method of assessment should match the function of assessment.

A Conceptual Foundation to Assessment Strategies

The relation between assessment paradigms and strategies, illustrated in Figure 1-1, also means that an assessor should carefully weigh the conceptual implications of implementing any assessment strategy. The use of projective assessment instruments suggests that the assessor embraces a causal model of a behavior problem that emphasizes the primacy of unconscious processes. A projective assessment strategy also deemphasizes the importance of dynamic and conditional characteristics of behavior problems and the identification of specific, minimally inferential, and modifiable behavioral and environmental variables.

It can be useful to integrate strategies from different assessment paradigms. (In 1993, *Behavior Modification, 17*[1], published a series of articles on the integration of behavioral and personality assessment strategies.) However, the integration of assessment strategies from different paradigms is often done in an unsystematic and nonscholarly manner. The selection of conceptually incompatible assessment strategies can reflect a lack of familiarity with their underlying paradigms. Among many questions that should be addressed by an assessor (e.g., Which assessment strategies are best, given the purposes of the assessment?), the assessor should also address the question "What model of behavior problems and their causes underlie this assessment strategy?"

The Characteristics of the Behavioral Assessment Paradigm

The behavioral assessment paradigm includes several sets of assumptions about behavior problems, the probable causes of behavior problems, and the best strategies of assessment. These underlying assumptions and strategies are introduced below and presented in more detail in Section II of this book. The characteristics outlined below differ on two dimensions: The degree to which they distinguish behavioral from nonbehavioral paradigms and the degree to which they are endorsed in various subparadigms of behavioral assessment (see Box 1-2).

As outlined in Table 1-1, behavioral assessment is a psychological assessment paradigm that emphasizes empirically supported, multimethod, and multi-informant assessment of specific, observable behaviors and contemporaneous causal variables in the natural environment. The behavioral assessment paradigm stresses the use of well-validated assessment instruments and assumes that social/environmental and cognitive variables are often important sources of behavior variance. Behavioral assessment is often used to gather data for preintervention assessment (to develop functional analyses of behavior problems), to evaluate treatment effects, and to analyze the conduct of basic and applied behavioral research.

Overlap among and Diversity within Psychological Assessment Paradigms

Overlap Between Behavioral and Nonbehavioral Assessment Paradigms

Most of the characteristics outlined in Table 1-1 are emphasized more in behavioral than in nonbehavioral psychological assessment paradigms. However, the concepts and methods of psychological assessment paradigms partially overlap. Several elements in Table 1-1 are also characteristic of other psychological assessment paradigms, and few perfectly discriminate between behavioral and nonbehavioral assessment paradigms. For example, the use of validated assessment instruments is stressed in personality assessment, and many personality theorists also acknowledge the situation specificity of behavior (Butcher, 1995; Wright & Mischel, 1987). Similarly, many aspects of projective assessment are idiographic, and inferences are often objectively based on an integration of qualitative and quantitative indices (Finch & Belter, 1993; Weiner, 1994). Finally, educational assessment (Linn, 1993) often involves direct, lower-order measures of the behaviors of interest (e.g., measuring reading ability by administering a reading test).

Diversity of Focus, Assumptions, and Methods within the Behavioral Assessment Paradigm

There are also differences among subparadigms subsumed within behavioral assessment in the degree to which they embrace the characteristics outlined in Table 1-1. For example, the behavioral analytic subparadigm emphasizes the clinical utility of individualized, within-person, primarily observational approach to assessment. Alternatively, cognitive-behavioral subparadigms often integrate idiographic and nomothetic assessment strategies when drawing clinical inferences and often use measures from self-report instruments.

The degree of emphasis on social/environmental causal factors (e.g., tangible rewards and verbal response contingencies) also varies across behavioral assessment subparadigms. Environmental response contingencies play a prominent role in behavior analytic causal models (e.g., Van Houten & Axelrod, 1993). Although social/environmental causal factors are incorpo-

Table 1-1
The Characteristics of the Behavioral Assessment Paradigm

Goals of Behavioral Assessment
- To identify, specify, and measure specific problem behaviors and client goals (as opposed to "diagnosis" or the measurement of "latent traits")+*
- To design intervention programs for individual clients+*
- To identify causal variables and functional relations for behavior problems and goals (particularly social/environmental functional relations)+
- To obtain informed consent of clients for assessment and intervention strategies
- To evaluate the outcome and process of intervention programs+
- To acquire clinically important information about a client in a cost-efficient manner
- To derive a behavioral case formulation of an individual client+
- To facilitate basic research in behavior analysis, learning, psychopathology, developmental psychology, and social psychology+
- To implement a functional approach to psychological assessment
- To tie the goals of assessment with the focus, targets, and methods of assessment
- To strengthen and maintain a positive client-assessor relationship
- To select subsequent behavioral assessment strategies (e.g., a funnel approach to assessment, involving increasing more specific and focused assessment)
- To identify variables that moderate causal relations and intervention outcome

Focus and Targets of Behavioral Assessment
- Contemporaneous (as opposed to historical) behaviors and situations and environmental factors (behaviors in the natural environment—next-+)*
- Highly specific, minimally inferential behaviors and variables+*
- Observable behaviors and environmental events (as opposed to intrapsychic events or highly inferential "latent" variables)*
- Behaviors and causal relations as they occur in the natural environment+*
- Functional relations: Behavior-behavior and behavior-environment relations*
- Situational/contextual variables associated with variance in behavior problems*
- Multiple targets in clinical assessment (e.g., main treatment effects, side effects, generalization)+
- Multiple response modes (behavioral, physiological, cognitive)
- Social systems and extended causal relations: A focus on the factors that affect contiguous causal variables for a client's behavior problems

Strategies, Methods, and Inferences
- Critical event sampling (the measurement of functional relations in problematic and high-risk situations)+*
- Time-series measurement strategies as opposed to single-point or prepost "snap shot" measurement)*
- Idiographic, often combined with nomothetic assessment strategies: More often criterion-referenced and within-person (as opposed to norm-referenced) inferences*
- Quantitatively based inferences, supplemented with qualitatively based inferences)
- Direct observation and measurement of behavior in naturalistic or analogue settings*
- An hypothesis testing approach to assessment: Hypotheses are developed during the assessment process, which are evaluated in subsequent assessment+
- The use of multiple methods and informants (e.g., client, staff, parents, teachers, family, spouse), across multiple situations)+
- The use of assessment instruments validated for the specific purposes for which they will be applied+
- Measurement facilitated by instrumentation (e.g., actimeters, ambulatory monitoring, computerized self-monitoring)
- A functional approach to assessment strategies—matching assessment strategies to the goals of assessment and the clinical judgments that are to be derived

Assumptions About the Characteristics of Behavior Problems
- There are between-person differences in the importance of the individual modes and dimensions of a behavior problem+*
- Behavior problems are conditonal and unstable; they can vary systematically across situations, time, states, and contexts+*
- There can be complex interrelations (e.g., noncausal covarying, bidirectional causal) among a client's multiple behavior problems+

Table 1-1 (*Continued*)

Assumptions About the Characteristics of Behavior Problems (*continued*)
- Behavior problems have multiple response modes (motoric, verbal, physiological, cognitive) that sometimes evidence low levels of covariation+
- Behavior problems and their modes have multiple dimensions (onset, duration, magnitude, rate)+
- Clients can have multiple behavior problems

Assumptions About the Causes of Behavior Problems
- The causal relations for a client's behavior problem can differ across situations+*
- Contemporaneous causal relations are often more important and have more clinical utility than original etiological causal relations*
- Learning, especially social/environmental response contingencies and antecedent conditions and stimuli can be particularly important causal factors for behavior problems*
- Multiple causality—Most behavior problems can be the result of different permutations of multiple causal variables+
- Individual differences in causal relations: There can be important between-person differences in the strength of causal relationship of the same behavior problems+
- Reciprocal determinism: A client can effect his or her environment in ways that, in turn, affect the client (i.e., bidirectional causality; reciprocal causation)+
- Extended and noncontemporaneous systems-level variables (family, work, marital, other interpersonal factors) may serve important causal functions
- Causal relations can demonstrate nonlinear (e.g., plateau, critical level) functions
- Moderator and mediator variables (see Glossary) can have important causal functions for a client
- Every causal variable has multiple dimensions (onset, duration, magnitude, rate), which can have different causal effects
- Causal relations can be dynamic: The causes of a client's behavior problem can change across time

+Characteristics endorsed by almost all subparadigms in behavioral assessment.
*Those characteristics that most strongly discriminate between behavioral and nonbehavioral assessment paradigms.
Source: Adapted from Haynes (1998a, 1998b) and influenced by Barrett, Johnston, & Pennypacker (1986); Barrios (1988); Bellack and Hersen (1988); Ciminero (1986); Cone (1988); Hartmann, Roper, & Bradford (1979); Haynes (1978); Kratochwill and Shapiro (1988); Mash and Terdal (1988); Nelson and Hayes (1986); Ollendick and Hersen (1993a); Strosahl and Linehan (1986); and Tryon (1985).

rated in cognitive-behavioral subparadigms, they are sometimes allotted a lower level of importance. In these models "expectancies" regarding contingencies or causal attributions are often presumed to have a stronger impact on behavior problems. Other behavioral assessment subparadigms stress the importance of biological factors (e.g., genetics, neurotransmitter functioning) in the development of many behavior problems.

The Distinctiveness and Dynamic Qualities of the Behavioral Assessment Paradigm

Although each characteristic in Table 1-1 imperfectly differentiates behavioral from nonbehavioral assessment paradigms, behavioral assessment is unique in its adoption of this integrated set of principles, goals, and strategies. It is especially distinctive in the degree to which it emphasizes the primary characteristics identified in Table 1-1—contemporaneous social/environmental causal factors, situational and contextual factors, idiographic time-series assessment, and the measurement of less inferential, lower-order variables.

For example, when specific thoughts and beliefs or cognitive processes (e.g., information processing, selective attention) are invoked to explain the onset or maintenance of behavior problems, they are often integrated in a multivariate causal model that also stresses social/ environmental and contextual elements. To illustrate, Smith (1994) and others have advanced an "expectancy" theory of alcoholism. They view "alcohol expectancies" as the learned contingencies for drinking. Alcoholics have learned, through experiences and observation, that alcohol is associated with the reduction of negative affect, increased social reinforcement and positive feelings, and other positive effects. These learned expectancies then affect future decisions regarding drinking and are triggered by specific situations, such as in the presence of other drinkers. This cognitive-behavioral causal model of alcoholism differs from alternative models that allocate causal primacy to less modifiable and more stable personality traits, "disease," and biological vulnerability factors (see reviews of behavioral and nonbehavioral models of alcoholism in Rychtarik & McGillicuddy, 1998; Nathan, 1993).

The principles and methods of behavioral assessment are also dynamic because they change over time (Haynes, 1999). Recent series on behavioral assessment and personality variables (see *Behavior Modification, 17*, 1992) and behavioral assessment and DSM diagnosis (see *Behavioral Assessment, 10*, 1988; and *Behavioral Assessment, 14*, 1992), and the book on methods of assessment by Hersen and Bellack (1998) illustrate changes in the methods and focus of behavioral assessment. Many advocates of a behavioral assessment paradigm have embraced concepts and methods of assessment that would have been rejected in the 1960s and 1970s.

The behavioral assessment paradigm is especially dynamic in the power and sophistication of its explanatory models. Analyses of complex sequences of behavior (e.g., conditional probabilities; Gottman & Roy, 1990), complex interrelations among many persons (e.g., systems approach; Taylor & Carr, 1992), complex functional relations among causal variables (e.g., functional analytic clinical case models; Haynes, Leisen, & Blaine, 1997), higher-order models of complex behavior-environment interactions (e.g., establishing operations; Michael, 1993), the application of behavioral assessment to clinical decision making (Nezu, Nezu, Friedman, & Haynes, 1997), the increasing integration of behavioral, cognitive, and physiological causal models and treatment (e.g., Gatchel & Blanchard, 1993), and in the technology of assessment (Tryon, 1998) illustrate recent advances in the behavioral assessment paradigm (see review in Haynes, 1999).

The increasing inclusiveness of behavioral assessment methods is a source of concern by some and seen as an asset by others (see discussion of theory, methods, and changes in behavioral assessment by Hartmann, Roper, & Bradford, 1979; Haynes, 1998b; McFall, 1986). The concerns are warranted to the degree that the broadening of the paradigm detracts from its predictive and explanatory power or clinical utility. Does the use of self-report questionnaires detract from the important emphasis on direct observation of behavior? Do models of behavior problems that emphasize cognitive processes detract from an important emphasis on a person's unique learning history and maintaining response contingencies?

New psychological assessment concepts and methods are inevitable and promote the evolution of psychological assessment paradigms. Some innovations will be considered and then discarded and others will be retained because they enhance the accuracy, power, and utility of the assessment paradigm (see Box 1-3).

The power of a psychological assessment paradigm is enhanced if new concepts and methods are evaluated openly but carefully. This can be accomplished by:

- Assuming a Steinbeckian "What if it were so?" attitude toward new ideas.[2]
- Avoiding early rejection of new ideas that seem to contradict existing principles.
- Retaining a strong empirical, hypothesis-testing orientation toward new ideas and methods.

---

[2]In *Log from the Sea of Cortez*, Steinbeck and several friends spent months collecting marine specimens off the coast of western Mexico. At night they retired to their anchored fishing boat and engaged in hours of beer-facilitated discussion of some social and political implications of their findings. One principle of their discussions was that no new idea could immediately be rejected; they were to presume that "it might be true" and then discuss the permutations and ramifications of that idea, before introducing possible limitations.

- Considering the assumptions and underlying models associated with new methods.
- Evaluating the potential contributions of new methods and ideas, rather than their conformity to existing ideas.

Box 1-3
Diversity and Evolution of Psychological Assessment Paradigms

One idea from chaos theory (Briggs & Peat, 1989; Peitgen, Jürgens, & Saupe, 1992) is that diversity may be a necessary condition for the survival and evolution of all systems (including psychological assessment paradigms). Cities without diverse economic bases cannot adapt well to changes in economic forces. Persons with a restricted set of rigidly held ideas or behavioral coping skills cannot adapt well to new situations and challenges. A narrow genetic stock for a particular species may render that species highly susceptible to disease. So, diversity and variance may be necessary conditions for adaptive functioning across systems.

The supraordinate characteristic of the behavioral assessment paradigm is the emphasis on *empiricism*. An empirical assessment paradigm uses carefully designed research strategies, based on defined and measured variables, to answer questions about the validity and utility of assessment strategies, underlying assumptions, and judgments. An empirical approach to assessment encourages the precise and frequent measurement of minimally inferential variables. It encourages the use of multiple validated assessment instruments to estimate sources of variance in behavior.

The dynamic quality of the behavioral assessment paradigm also means that ideas presented in this book are provisional. For example, in Chapter 8, we discuss assumptions about client behavior problems within a behavioral assessment paradigm. We discuss the best level of specificity in clinical assessment, the importance of estimating functional relations among behavior problems, and the multimodal and multidimensional nature of behavior problems. Subsequent research will confirm some of these ideas and suggest that others should be refined or discarded.

Sources of Influence and a Brief History of Behavioral Assessment

Multiple Sources of Influence across Several Decades

The behavioral assessment paradigm reflects multiple sources of influence across several decades. The diversity of these sources reflects the dynamic quality of the paradigm. Krasner (1992), McReynolds (1986), and Nelson (1983) have provided interesting historical overviews of behavioral assessment.

Many conceptual elements of behavioral assessment, such as an emphasis on learning, lower-order, and observable variables, and the functional relations between behavior and environmental events date from Watson, Pavlov, Hull, Guthrie, and Mowrer and have been influenced by the work of Skinner (Alexander & Selesnick, 1966; Kazdin, 1978; Samelson, 1981; Skinner, 1945). Methods of behavioral assessment, such as direct observation of behavior and psychophysiological assessment, also have a long history, dating back to early Greek scholars.

Several methodological and conceptual components of the behavioral assessment paradigm reflect the affiliation with experimental analysis of behavior and other areas of experimental psychology. Major contributors to the development of the behavior therapies and applied behavior analysis in the 1960s, such as Ted Ayllon, Nathan Azrin, Donald Baer, Albert Bandura, Sidney Bijou, A. C. Catania, Hans Eysenck, C. B. Ferster, Cyril Franks, Israel Goldiamond, William Holz, Fred Keller, Leonard Krasner, Ogden Lindsley, Jack Michael, Gerald Patterson, Henry Pennypacker, Todd Risley, Murray Sidman, Arthur Staats, Leonard Ullmann, Roger Ulrich, Montrose Wolf, were well schooled in behavior analysis, learning theory, and experimental psychology. They were exuberant advocates for the transfer of the principles derived from basic human and animal learning research, experimental psychology, and the experimental analysis of behavior, to the analysis and treatment of important personal and social problems.

The experimental psychology and learning background of early contributors continued to influence the scholarly focus and strategies of behavioral assessment through other early contributors and leaders in the field, including Stewart Agras, Joseph Cautela, Hans Eysenck, Marvin Goldfried, Fred Kanfer, Peter Lang, Arnold Lazarus, Joseph Matarazzo, Dan O'Leary, Richard Stuart, Robert Wahler, G. T. Wilson, and Joseph Wolpe.

The conceptual and methodological foundations of the behavioral paradigm were further advanced in the 1970s and 1980s by "second generation" contributors to the field, such as David Barlow, Alan Bellack, Ed Blanchard, Richard Bootzin, Tom Borkovec, John Cone, Ian Evans, Rex Forehand, Sharon Foster, John Gottman, Donald Hartmann, Robert Hawkins, Steven Hayes, Mischel Hersen, Steve Hollon, Neil Jacobson, Alan Kazdin, Phil Kendall, Marsha Linehan, Richard Marlatt, Eric Mash, Richard McFall, Rosemery Nelson-Grey, Thomas Ollendick, and many others.

In the 1990s many early contributors continue to develop and refine the concepts and methods associated with behavioral assessment. They have been joined by hundreds of "third generation" behavioral scientist-practitioners and scholars who are advancing the strategies, applicability, utility, data analytic capabilities, conceptual sophistication, and predictive efficacy of behavioral assessment.

An Historical Emphasis on Functional Relations

The early pioneers in behavioral assessment and behavioral paradigms emphasized a principle that continues to have a major influence on behavioral assessment in applied psychology, education, industrial and organizational psychology, and rehabilitation. It is the principle that important and clinically useful sources of variance for behavior problems are often associated with environmental events, particularly response contingencies. Thousands of studies have found that important sources of variance for behavior are the events that follow it, those naturally occurring or programmed response contingencies.

The enthusiasm for the translation of behavioral principles derived from the experimental laboratories into applied behavior analysis in the natural environment had one unintended drawback. The heuristic emphasis on behavior-environment functional relations was sometimes rendered into a mandate for a univariate model of causality: A presumption that all sources of behavior variance could be explained by an examination of contemporaneous response contingencies or stimulus pairings or a presumption that other sources of variance (e.g., thoughts, physiological mechanisms) might be important but were inaccessible or unmeasurable. Thus, an early error was a failure to recognize that an important element of the behavioral paradigm, the *conditional nature* of behavior and functional relations, also applied to the construct system within which that element was embedded.

Despite occasional overzealousness by some proponents, the emphasis on behavior-behavior and behavior-environment functional relations remains a compelling and clinically useful contribution from early behavioral theorists and researchers, and it is an important focus of behavioral assessment. We can often account for a significant proportion of variance in behavior problems, and we can design methods for changing behavior, by examining the contiguous functional relations relevant to the behavior problem, particularly the events that follow.

Iwata et al. (1994), for example, have repeatedly shown the utility and power of systematic introduction and removal of potential controlling variables in analogue laboratory settings for identifying causal relations for self-injurious behaviors of persons with developmental disabilities. For many of the 156 clients in his 1994 study, Iwata and his coworkers could identify, using interrupted time-series analogue (ABAB) observation designs, whether the self-injurious behavior was more strongly maintained by positive social reinforcement, escape from aversive social or nonsocial situations, or "automatic reinforcement" (e.g., sensory stimulation). The authors suggested that the findings from this method of functional analysis can lead to more powerful treatment programs.

Epistemology and Methods of Assessment

Another important and robust contribution from early developers was an emphasis on a *scientific approach* to psychological assessment: The assumption that the application of scientific methods of analysis of behavior will facilitate our ability to identify and control sources of variance for behavior problems. A scientific approach suggests that we can best explain human behavior problems by using careful observation and measurement of behavior and hypothesized controlling variables (e.g., Bachrach, 1962; Franks, 1969; Krasner & Ullmann, 1965). Also evolving from this emphasis on scientific methods is an emphasis on frequent, multivariate measurement with validated assessment instruments of lower-order, precisely defined variables. Books on single-subject, factorial, and covariance designs by Barlow and Hersen (1984), Kazdin (1998), Kratochwill and Levin (1992), and Sidman (1960) reflect the scientific epistemology of the behavioral assessment paradigm.

Naturalistic and analogue behavioral observation methods have also been affected by early studies in psychology. For example, structured observations played an important role in early research on child development (previously referred to as "genetic" psychology) and social interaction (Bott, 1928; Gesell, 1925; Goodenough, 1928; Parten, 1932). Early developmental psychologists also contributed to principles of time-sampling (e.g., Arrington, 1939). Careful observation and measurement of behavior and the identification of its functional relations with antecedent and consequent environmental stimuli were the hallmark of operant and experimental analysis of behavior. References to observation methods are also found in writings from the Hellenic and Egyptian eras.

As noted above, observation methods have also been influenced by disciplines outside behavioral assessment and behavior therapy. Many advances in the technology for observing, measuring, and analyzing complex sequences of dyadic interactions have come from social psychology (e.g., Vallacher & Nowak, 1994), developmental psychology (Baltes, Reese, & Nesselroade, 1988), ecological psychology (Barker, 1968), education (Boyd & DeVault, 1966), and ethology (Hutt & Hutt, 1970). The statistical analysis of the time-series data, often acquired in behavioral assessment (Suen & Ary, 1989), has been influenced by multiple disciplines (Collins & Horn, 1991). Similarly, many advances in the methods of behavioral assessment follow advances in computer technology and in the technology for ambulatory monitoring (e.g., Tryon, 1998).

Self-report assessment methods, such as questionnaires and interviews, have been adapted from traditional applied psychological disciplines such as educational, developmental, personality, and clinical psychology (see reviews in La Greca, 1990; Haynes & Jensen, 1979). The content and focus of these self-report instruments have sometimes been modified to increase their methodological and conceptual congruence with the behavioral assessment paradigm. Specifically, questionnaires and interviews are congruent with the behavioral assessment paradigm to the degree that they provide measures of precisely defined, nonaggregated, more specific overt behaviors, thoughts, and emotions. A focus on functional relations involving situational and state variables, rather than a focus on describing a behavior, is a particularly important aspect of behavioral self-report methods.

Haynes, Falkin, Sexton-Radek (1989) reviewed behavioral treatment studies and noted a dramatic increase in the use of psychophysiological assessment in the past 30 years. This increase was also noted in their review of treatment studies published in the *Journal of Consulting and Clinical Psychology* and illustrated here in Chapter 2, and may be attributed to an increased focus on physiological components of behavior problems, an increased involvement by behavior therapists in the analysis and treatment of medical-psychological disorders (e.g., cancer, cardiovascular disorders), an increased use of intervention procedures (e.g., relaxation training, desensitization) designed to modify physiological processes, and advances in measurement technology (e.g., ambulatory monitoring and computer technology). The major contributions to psychophysiological assessment technology, including computer-aided data acquisition, data reduction, and statistical analysis, come from basic psychophysiological researchers (e.g., Cacioppo & Tassinary, 1990).

The behavioral assessment paradigm has also been strongly influenced by the methods and foci of behavioral interventions. Although interventions with behavior problems based upon behavioral paradigms occurred in the 1950s and earlier (Kazdin, 1978), extensive applications of behavioral paradigms did not take place until the 1960s (Bachrach, 1962; Bandura, 1969; Ullmann & Krasner, 1965; Ulrich, Stachnik, & Mabry, 1966; Wolpe, 1958). These interventions emphasized the manipulation of the client's interaction with his or her environment. The design of these programs, and the evaluation of their outcome, necessitated the use of assessment procedures that were more direct, less inferential, less static, and more focused on a client's overt behaviors and functional relations than traditional clinical assessment. In particular, traditional assessment methods, such as projective and personality trait-focused questionnaire measures, were not sufficiently specific, molecular, situationally sensitive, or congruent with this new emphasis on environmental and reciprocal determinism.

The evolution of behavioral assessment concepts and methods are mutually dependent. For example, research on stimulus-control, cognitive, and learning factors has influenced the composition of sleep-related questionnaires, interviews, and self-monitoring assessment instruments used with sleep problems (Bootzin et al., 1993) and phobic disorders (Beidel & Morris, 1995). The physiological mechanisms shown to be associated with many behavior problems (Gatchel & Blanchard, 1993) guides the use of psychophysiological assessment in laboratory and clinical settings.

Behavioral assessment methods have also been affected by research on behavior chains and sequences of exchanges in child behavior problems (Voeltz & Evans, 1982), temporally noncontiguous events in marital distress (Margolin, 1981), multiple and interactive causal factors for many behavior problems (Haynes, 1992; Kazdin & Kagan, 1994), extended social systems factors for many behavior problems (Kanfer, 1985), the multiple response modes often characteristic of complex behavior and behavior problems (Lang, 1995), the situational specificity in many behavior problems (McFall, 1982), and the dynamic and nonlinear aspects of behavior problems (Heiby, 1995a, 1995b).

In all of these examples, the development of more powerful causal models depends on the precision with which the variables in the model can be measured. Imprecise, nonspecific measurement hinders the detection of important functional relations and increases the chance that invalid hypotheses will be accepted.

In allied disciplines, assessment methods are very congruent with, but seem to have been developed independently of, the behavioral assessment paradigm. For example "situational tests" (Anastasi & Urbina, 1997) are sometimes used in industrial-organizational personnel selection. In these methods, job candidates are placed in situations that require skills similar to those of the job for which they are applying. An applicant for a supervisor's position may be presented with videotaped scenarios involving a conflict between two supervisees and asked how he or she would solve the conflict. Situational tests are in contrast to traditional assessment strategies that involved the use of personality inventories and intellectual assessment batteries to measure general dispositions and abilities (see Box 1-4).

A continuing impetus for the development of behavioral assessment has been a dissatisfaction with the focus and underlying assumptions of traditional clinical assessment instruments (McFall, 1986; McReynolds, 1986). Projective techniques and global personality trait questionnaires often provide aggregated, imprecise data about highly inferential constructs. For most applications of behavioral assessment, they fail to provide specific data on the events of interest and do not attend to the conditional nature of behavior problems. In addition, traditional assessment instruments often do not provide data on the dynamic characteristics and multiple dimensions and response modes of behavior problems. The aggregated, global nature of many constructs measured in traditional clinical assessment rendered traditional assessment instruments insufficiently sensitive to changes across time or situations and insufficiently amenable to individualized assessment. Often, the constructs measured were permeated with untestable psychodynamic causal connotations with limited clinical utility.

Summary

Psychological assessment is the systematic evaluation of a person's behavior. Psychological assessment has many elements, including the methods used to gather information, the setting in which the information is obtained, the measurement targets and informants, the ways in which the assessment data are summarized, and the time-course of measurement. All components of psychological assessment affect the information acquired and the clinical judgments that depend on that data. A central component of psychological assessment is measurement.

An important component of psychological assessment is the functional analysis—the integration of assessment data about a client—a behavioral clinical case formulation. The functional analysis is a hypothesized, working model of the client's problem behaviors, goals, causal variables, and the interrelations among these variables. It affects the treatment program designed for a client and is strongly affected not only by assessment data, but also by the inferences that the clinician draws from that data.

Box 1-4
An Early Example of Situational Assessment

The Assessment of Men: Selection of Personnel for the Office of Strategic Services, United States Office of Strategic Services (1948) is a fascinating account of the application of a scientific approach to the development and evaluation of situational assessment. During World War II, a group of psychologists and psychiatrists were given the task by the OSS (the precursor of the CIA) of selecting men and women to serve overseas as spies, saboteurs, resistance organizers, and provocateurs. The assessment staff and consultants included Uri Bronfenbrenner, Dwight Chapman, Donald Fiske, Kurt Lewin, Richard S. Lyman, Donald MacKinnon, O.H. Mowrer, and Henry Murray, Charles Thurstone, among others.

Between 1943 and 1945, over 5,000 recruits, in small groups, underwent intensive assessment in one- and three-day periods. Some of the assessment methods were based on "organismic" (Gestalt) principles and involved performance assessment of recruits in analogue situations (interviewer ratings, projective assessment, and self-report questionnaires were also used). Structured assessment situations were developed on a secluded farm 40 miles outside of Washington and on a Pacific beach. All situations were designed to test abilities analogous to those that would be required for success in field operations overseas.

Although the assessment staff were not briefed on the exact nature of the jobs to be performed overseas by the recruits, they generated situations that would test performance in a variety of difficult situations likely to be encountered.

The situational tests included:

1. A Belongings Test—A recruit entered a simulated bedroom in which 26 belongings of a person had been placed. After four minutes, each candidate was interviewed about inferences he or she had drawn about the owner of the belongings.
2. A Terrain Test—A recruit was given a map of a farm with lettered objects. They were allowed to explore the farm and were later tested (without the benefit of notes) on the identity of each lettered object.
3. The Brook—A group of four to seven leaderless recruits was given the task of traversing a steep-sided brook while safely transporting a piece of important equipment. On the bank of the brook were small boards, a barrel, a rock, rope, and pulleys.
4. Stress Interview—Each recruit was subjected to "merciless cross-questioning under disagreeable conditions" with the aim of detecting flaws in a cover story that the recruit had been given only a few minutes to construct.

Observers rated each recruit in every situation on variables such as energy and initiative, effective intelligence, social relations, leadership, and physical ability. At the end of the assessment period the evaluators integrated information from the multiple methods into a profile and description of the assets and liabilities of each recruit.

It is notable that the 1948 book was written with an interest in "improving present methods of diagnosis, assessment and selection" (pg. 3), suggesting that dissatisfaction with traditional assessment methods is at least 50 years old. Also, the authors obtained performance ratings of 1,187 recruits who were sent overseas and presented data on predictive efficacy.

It is notable that many foreign nationals participated in the OSS evaluation and that culturally based biases and errors in evaluation were acknowledged by the authors.

Decisions about the methods, instruments, and timing of psychological assessment affect the type and focus of data that will be collected on a client. Data from different instruments vary in terms of the variables measured, the mode of response upon which they focus (e.g., physiological vs. cognitive), their level of specificity (e.g., molar vs. molecular measures), and their validity. These data, in turn, affect the clinical case formulation, the clinical interventions that a client will receive, and inferences about treatment effectiveness.

A psychological assessment paradigm is a coherent set of principles and methods. Behavioral assessment, one of many paradigms in psychological assessment, emphasizes the use of empirically based multimethod assessment of lower-order, observable behaviors and contemporaneous causal variables. It stresses the use of well-validated assessment instruments and is guided by assumptions that social/environmental and cognitive factors are often important sources of variance in behavior. However, there is considerable overlap in the concepts and methods of psychological assessment paradigms and diversity among subparadigms in behavioral assessment. Because it is based on a scientific epistemology, behavioral assessment is also a dynamic paradigm that changes over time.

The concepts and methods of the behavioral assessment paradigm have been influenced by many sources. Early behavior analysts and experimental psychologists have provided initial guidance. Behavioral assessment also has benefitted from advances in many allied disciplines. The most important contribution from these early developers was an emphasis on empiricism—a presumption that the application of scientific methods in the analysis of behavior will facilitate our ability to identify and control sources of variance for behavior problems.

Suggested Readings

Broadly Focused Discussions of Psychological Assessment

Goldstein, G., & Hersen, M. (Eds.). (1999). *Handbook of psychological assessment.* New York: Elsevier.
Heatherton, T. F. & Weinberger, J. L. (Eds.). (1994). *Can personality change.* Washington, DC: American Psychological Association.
"Research Methods in Psychological Assessment." (1995). *Psychological Assessment, 1* (special issue).

Overviews of Behavioral Assessment

Breen, M. J. & Fiedler, C. R. (Eds.). (1996). *Behavioral approach to assessment of youth with emotional/behavioral disorders—A handbook for school-based practitioners* (pp. 503–582). Austin, TX: PRO-ED.
Gettinger, M., & Kratochwill, T. R. (1987). Behavioral assessment. In C. L. Frame & J. L. Matson (Eds.), *Handbook of assessment in childhood psychopathology applied issues in differential diagnosis and treatment evaluation* (pp. 131–161). New York: Plenum.
Haynes, S. N. (1998). The changing nature of behavioral assessment. In M. Hersen & A. Bellack (Eds.), *Behavioral assessment, A practical handbook* (4th ed., pp. 1–2). Boston: Allyn-Bacon.
Haynes, S. N. (1999). The behavioral assessment of adult disorders. In A. Goldstein & M. Hersen (Eds.), *Handbook of psychological assessment* (3rd ed.). New York: Pergamon.
Hersen, M. & Bellack, A. S. (Eds.). (1998). *Behavioral assessment: A practical handbook* (4th ed.). New York: Pergamon.
Mash, E. J., & Terdal, L. G. (1997). Assessment of child and family disturbance: a behavioral-systems approach. In E. J. Mash & L. G. Terdal (Eds.), *Assessment of childhood disorders* (3rd ed., pp. 3–68). New York: Guilford.
Nelson, R. O., & Hayes, S. C. (1986). The nature of behavioral assessment. In R. O. Nelson & S. C. Hayes (Eds.), *Conceptual foundations of behavioral assessment* (pp. 1–41). New York: Guilford.
O'Brien, W. H., & Haynes, S. N. (1995). Behavioral assessment. In L. Heiden & M. Hersen (Eds.), *Introduction to clinical psychology* (pp. 103–139). New York: Plenum.

Shapiro, E. W., & Kratochwill, T. R. (Eds.). (1988). *Behavioral assessment in schools: Conceptual foundations and practical applications*. New York: Guilford.

Strosahl, K. D., & Linehan, M. M. (1986). Basic issues in behavioral assessment. In A. R. Ciminero, K. S. Calhoun, & H. E. Adams (Eds.), *Handbook of behavioral assessment* (2nd ed., pp. 12–46). New York: John Wiley & Sons.

History and Background of Behavioral Construct Systems (Assessment and Therapy)

The history of American psychology. (1992). *American Psychologist, 47*, 100–334.

Kazdin, A. E. (1978). *History of behavior modification*. Baltimore: University Park Press.

Krasner, L. (1992). The concepts of syndrome and functional analysis: Compatible or incompatible. *Behavioral Assessment, 14*, 307–321.

McReynolds, P. (1986). History of assessment in clinical and educational settings. In R. O. Nelson & S. C. Hayes (Eds.), *Conceptual foundations of behavioral assessment* (pp. 42–80). New York: Guilford.

Paradigms in Psychology and Psychological Assessment

Gutting, G. (Ed.) (1980). *Paradigms and revolutions*. Notre Dame, IN: University of Notre Dame Press.

Kuhn, T. S. (1970). *The structure of scientific revolutions* (2nd ed.). Chicago: University of Chicago Press.

Turner, M. B. (1967). *Philosophy and the science of behavior*. New York: Appleton-Century-Crofts.

2

Current Status and Applications

Introduction

In this chapter we discuss the current status, applicability, and utility of behavioral assessment. We examine the status of the paradigm through several indices: (a) the use of behavioral assessment methods in published treatment outcome studies, (b) circulation of behavioral and nonbehavioral journals, (c) membership in professional organizations, (d) the status of behavioral assessment in graduate training programs, and (e) the use of behavioral assessment methods in clinical practice. In the second section of the chapter we discuss the applicability and utility of behavioral assessment.

We draw several inferences about the applicability and utility of behavioral assessment:

1. The behavioral assessment paradigm is composed of several methods and many instruments, which differ in their applicability and utility across the functions of psychological assessment.
2. Behavioral assessment methods are used more often than projective instruments and personality inventories but less often than narrow-band self-report instruments in treatment outcome research.
3. Behavioral assessment methods are taught less often in graduate training programs than are projective, personality, and intellectual assessment methods, but their rate of inclusion in graduate training programs is increasing.
4. Behavioral assessment methods are applicable across a wide range of clinical populations, target problems, settings, and assessment functions.
5. Behavioral assessment methods are underutilized in psychological science and as aids to clinical judgment.
6. The cost efficiency and clinical utility of behavioral assessment methods are increasing.
7. The applicability and utility of the behavioral assessment paradigm is a function of its conceptual focus, inclusion of multiple methods, and emphasis on specific measurements of variables in natural settings.
8. The applicability and utility of individual methods of behavioral assessment are affected by several variables, including characteristics of the targeted variables, cost and time considerations, characteristics of the client, and congruence between the client and assessment instrument.

The Current Status of Behavioral Assessment

Psychological assessment paradigms differ in their utility, applicability, and their role in contemporary assessment. They differ in how often they are used to aid clinical judgments, such as in the design of intervention programs, and their utility in treatment outcome research. Psychological assessment paradigms also differ in how much they contribute to the development and evaluation of causal models of behavior disorders.

The frequency with which a psychological assessment paradigm is used for a particular assessment goal is influenced by its utility—the degree to which the information it provides assists in attaining that goal. Additionally, an assessment method that efficiently provides useful information, is more likely to be used than one that provides useful information less efficiently. For example, structured interviews can provide information when the goal is psychiatric diagnosis but may be less useful when the goal is treatment outcome evaluation. Similarly, systematic classroom behavioral observations can provide measures of treatment outcome with aggressive children but are less effective and cost-efficient for psychiatric diagnosis.

The frequency with which an assessment method is used is a useful but imperfect measure of its utility. For example, behavioral observation of clients in structured clinic settings (such as in the systematic manipulations of social and nonsocial stimuli to help identify the reinforcers that maintain self-injurious behaviors for a developmentally disabled child using ABAB designs; Iwata et al., 1994) is a powerful but underused clinical assessment method. It may be underused because data are sometimes difficult to reduce and analyze and because many clinicians who work with developmentally disabled persons are unfamiliar with structured analogue observation methods.

The application of an assessment paradigm can be influenced by many factors other than its utility. An assessor may approach behavior problems from a different conceptual framework, the assessor may not be skilled with a particular method, or third-party payers may not reimburse for the costs of an assessment method. Given these caveats, we examine the current status of behavioral assessment paradigm and the changes in its status over time. Data on the role and impact of the behavioral assessment paradigm in clinical, research, and training activities will provide a context for forthcoming discussions of its applicability and utility.

We examine several indicators of the status of the behavioral assessment paradigm: (a) the frequency with which behavioral assessment methods are used in published treatment outcome studies, (b) the strength and growth of professional organizations associated with the behavioral paradigm, (c) the emphasis placed on the assessment paradigm in graduate training programs, (d) the number of journals emphasizing or including the behavioral assessment paradigm, and (e) the use of particular assessment methods by clinicians.

Behavioral Assessment Methods in Treatment Outcome Studies

One measure of the status of a psychological assessment paradigm is the frequency with which its methods are used in treatment outcome studies (see Box 2-1). Table 2-1 presents the percentage of treatment outcome articles published in the *Journal of Consulting and Clinical Psychology* (*JCCP*), in selected years, that used several behavioral and nonbehavioral assessment methods: (a) behavioral observation (in natural and analogue environments; e.g., home, school, institution, clinic role-play), (b) self-monitoring (i.e., frequent recordings by clients of the specified behaviors and events), (c) psychophysiological assessment, (d) projective methods (e.g., Rorschach), and (e) self-report questionnaires. *JCCP* was selected for this evaluation because it is a prestigious, frequently cited, broadly focused treatment research journal sponsored by the American Psychological Association.[1]

An examination of Table 2-1 leads to several conclusions: (a) projective techniques (broad-spectrum personality inventories were not reported in this table) were rarely used as measures of treatment outcome, (b) the most frequently used assessment method was self-report questionnaires of narrowband constructs, such as depression and anxiety, (c) behavioral assessment methods were used in treatment outcome studies significantly more than were projective methods (and personality inventories), and (d) the use of behavioral assessment methods peaked in the mid to late 1970s and 1980s. Importantly, the percentage of treatment outcome articles that used multiple methods of assessment increased steadily from 43% in 1966 to 89% in 1996).

[1]Studies were coded by Kevin Bogan, Laurie Ignacio, Danielle Black, Jeff Stern, Chris Chiros, and Maureen Egan.

Box 2-1
Error in the Measurement of a Latent Variable—A First Example

Data to be presented on the status of behavioral assessment illustrate some limitations of measurement and limitations on the inferences that can be drawn from obtained measures, which are reaffirmed and discussed in greater detail in subsequent chapters: (a) all assessment instruments provide imperfect measures of a construct, and (b) different measures of a construct capture and weight different facets of a construct, and (c) different measures have different sources of error.

The "status of behavioral assessment" is a *latent variable*, which is inferred from observed variables, such as "frequency of application by assessors." Each measure of status has unique sources of error. For example, we presumed that a good measure of the degree to which behavioral assessment methods are used in treatment outcome studies is the frequency of their reported use in the most prestigious psychological treatment research outcome journal—*The Journal of Consulting and Clinical Psychology* (*JCCP*). Data on the use of behavioral assessment instruments in *JCCP* are probably a valid measure of the phenomena of interest but are also affected by other sources of variance, such as the publication policies of different editors, the system we designed to code articles, the years that *JCCP* was sampled, and the bias toward publishing studies with significant outcomes. The impact of measurement errors on estimates of a latent variable can often be reduced by using multiple methods of assessment and multiple validated instruments.

Circulation of Behavioral Journals and Behavioral Articles in General Interest Journals

Table 2-2 illustrates data on the 1992 and 1997 circulations of several behavioral and general interest journals (some data on 1992 were taken from an article by Laties and Mace [1993]). These data indicate that several journals that specialize in behavior therapy and applied and experimental analysis of behavior have a good circulation that has increased since 1992 at a rate similar to that for general psychology and education journals. There are respected journals with a more limited circulation that publish many behavioral articles. These include *Behavior-*

Table 2-1
Percentage of Treatment Outcome Studies Published
in *Journal of Consulting and Clinical Psychology*
that Used Particular Assessment Methods

Year	Number of Studies	Behavioral Observation	Self-Monitoring	Psychophysiology	Projective	Self-Report Questionnaire
1968	9	56	33	0	0	33
1972	23	35	22	0	4	48
1976	34	44	9	18	9	50
1980	21	33	29	14	0	62
1984	37	16	32	16	0	51
1988	21	24	38	10	0	81
1992	21	33	14	9	0	81
1996	28	7	25	25	0	86

Table 2-2
Journal Paid Subscriptions

Journal	Paid Circulation 1992	Paid Circulation 1997	% Change
Behavioral journals			
Behavior Modification	1,322	1,500	13
Behavior Therapy	2,731	3,500	28
Behaviour Research and Therapy	4,300	4,300	0
Journal of Applied Behavior Analysis	4,636	5,500	19
Journal of Behavior Therapy and Experimental Psychiatry	2,000	3,100	55
Average % change			23
Unspecialized journals			
Journal of Applied Psychology	5,647	6,200	10
Journal of Consulting and Clinical Psychology	10,488	12,000	14
Journal of Counseling Psychology	7,454	9,700	30
Psychological Assessment	5,917	6,700	13
Average % change			19

ism, *Journal of Verbal Behavior, Journal of Psychopathology and Behavioral Assessment, School Psychology Review, Journal of Abnormal Child Psychology,* and *The Behavior Analyst.*

As noted in the previous section, some widely distributed journals do not specialize in behavioral assessment, therapy, or theory but publish many articles relevant to the behavioral assessment paradigm. Table 2-3 gives the percentages of behavioral articles (i.e., articles that include behavior therapy procedures, specifically address conceptual issues in behavior therapy, discuss issues in behavioral assessment) in several general interest journals published in 1993. Data in Table 2-3 indicate the degree to which the behavioral assessment and therapy paradigms are represented in general purpose clinical, research, and integrative/review journals.

Table 2-3
Percentage of Behavioral Articles in Several General Interest Journals in 1993

Journal	Primary Focus of Journal	% Behavioral Articles	
		1993	1997
Journal of Consulting and Clinical Psychology	Therapy research and research methods	37%; 43 of 115 articles	32%; 30 of 93 articles
Clinical Psychology Review	Theoretical, assessment and therapy review articles	25%; 5 of 21 articles	38%; 14 of 37 articles
Psychological Assessment	The development, application and validation of assessment instruments	22%; 15 of 68 articles	18%; 6 of 34 articles
*Journal of Abnormal Psychology**	Basic research and theory on abnormal psychology	16%; 12 of 72 articles	17%; 12 of 69 articles

*Data from the *Journal of Abnormal Psychology* represents the percentage of articles that examined models of psychopathology from a perspective congruent with a behavioral paradigm, not the percentage of articles that used behavioral assessment methods. Some articles on psychopathology (e.g., cross-cultural differences in behavior disorders, assessment instrument development, neuropsychological correlates of behavior disorders) used behavioral assessment methods such as teacher ratings, direct observation of participants, and structured interviews.

Behaviorally Oriented Professional Organizations

Figure 2-1 illustrates trends in the membership of the Association for the Advancement of Behavior Therapy (AABT) and selected divisions of APA. From 1971 to 1998 the membership of APA increased 47% and AABT 60%. Division 25 is the Experimental Analysis of Behavior and Division 12 and 38 are broadly focused divisions of clinical and health psychology respectively, which incorporate diverse assessment and treatment paradigms. Divisions 12 and 38 experienced a steady increase in membership until the mid-1990s, while Division 25 membership peaked in the mid-1970s.

Many professional organizations do not have a specific theoretical focus but support activities, such as convention workshops, symposia, and paper presentations that are congruent with a behavioral assessment paradigm. Examples of these organizations include the Society for Behavioral Medicine, Society for Psychotherapy Research, the American Psychological Society, Section III of Division 12 of APA, AERA (American Educational Research Association) regional and state psychological associations, and most organizations focusing on developmental disabilities and rehabilitation.

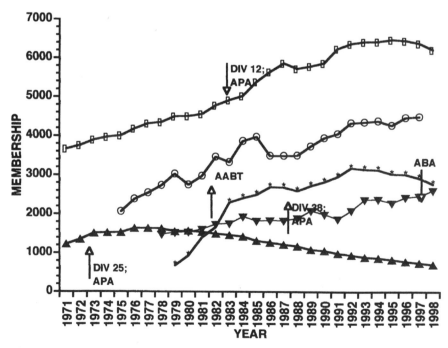

Figure 2-1. Time course of the memberships of the Association for the Advancement of Behavior Therapy (AABT), the Association for Behavior Analysis (ABA), and Clinical Psychology (Division 12), Experimental Analysis of Behavior (Division 25), and Health Psychology (Division 38), divisions of APA.

The Behavioral Assessment Paradigm in Training Programs

Many clinical psychology Ph.D. training programs require courses in behavioral assessment. Piotrowski and Zalewski (1993) reported data on required courses in psychological assessment and on expected changes in required assessment courses, from the training directors of 13 Psy.D. and 67 Ph.D. APA-approved training programs. This sample represented 51% of 158 APA-approved programs. They also compared data from this survey with data from a 1984 study.

Some results of the study by Piotrowski and Zalewski are presented in Table 2-4. These data indicate that behavioral assessment is taught in about one-half of the doctoral training programs in clinical psychology. More important for the expected time-course of training in behavioral assessment, over one-third of the program directors expected an increase in the emphasis on behavioral assessment in the future (45% of the program directors expected a decrease in the emphasis on projective assessment in the future). The proportion of programs that teach behavioral assessment probably has increased since the early 1980s but behavioral assessment was not included as a response option in the 1984 survey.

There was also a difference between the Ph.D. and Psy.D. programs in the expected changes in their emphasis on behavioral assessment: 41% of directors from Ph.D. programs but only 17% of directors from Psy.D. programs expected an increased emphasis on behavioral assessment in the future.

The Behavioral Assessment Paradigm in Clinical Practice

Data from other sources suggest that behavioral assessment is used less frequently than objective personality assessment in clinical settings. For example, Piotrowski and Lubin (1990) reported that in a select sample of 270 members of Division 38 of American Psychological Association (APA) (Health Psychology), the Minnesota Multiphasic Personality Inventory (MMPI) was the most frequently used assessment instrument. Other self-report questionnaires, such as the Beck Depression Inventory, the MacAndrew Alcoholism Scale, and the McGill Pain Questionnaire were also frequently used.

Clinicians who label themselves as behaviorally oriented frequently report using many nonbehavioral assessment strategies. For example, Watkins, Campbell, and McGregor (1990) reported that 80% and 76% of 41 (out of a sample of 630) counseling psychologists who identified themselves as "behavioral" in orientation used the MMPI and Bender Gestalt, respectively, in their practice. Data were based on responses to a list of 22 commonly used

Table 2-4
Percentage of APA-Approved Doctoral Training Programs
that Required Coursework in Various Psychological Assessment Paradigms

Assessment Paradigm	1984	1993	Expected Change		
			Increase	Decrease	No Change
Objective personality assessment	85	89	38	4	58
Projective assessment	79	85	4	45	51
Intellectual assessment	94	94			88
The behavioral assessment	Not surveyed	55	37	7	56

Source: Piotrowski & Zalewski, 1993, 394–405.

"tests," which did not include more specific self-report questionnaires (e.g., pain, depression, state anxiety) or any behavioral assessment methods or instruments. Consequently, it is not possible to determine from these data the relative rate with which behavioral and non-behavioral assessment methods and instruments were used. However, these data are consistent with earlier reports that behaviorally oriented clinicians often use nonbehavioral assessment instruments (Piotrowski & Keller, 1984).

Guevremont and Spiegler (1990) surveyed 988 members of AABT regarding their most frequently used assessment methods. The five most commonly used methods were all self-report strategies: behavioral interviews (90.18%), self-report inventories (63.36%), self-monitoring (55.87%), behavior rating scales (52.83%), behavior checklists (49.70%), and personality inventories (47.76%).

The use of both personality and behavioral assessment strategies by behavioral clinicians is congruent with suggestions by many behavior therapists (e.g., Bellack & Hersen, 1988; Nelson & Hayes, 1986; Russo, 1990) that personality assessment instruments, when conscientiously applied, can facilitate clinical decision making.

While we acknowledge the potential contributions of measures from personality assessment instruments, this book emphasizes a philosophy of *festina lente* (hasten slowly) with regard to such integration. There are many issues associated with the use of aggregated, dispositional, self-report personality trait questionnaires.

Summary of Applications and Cost-Efficiency Considerations

As noted earlier in this chapter, measures of current applications are indirect measures of the status, potential power, and utility of an assessment paradigm. However, data presented in this section suggest that behavioral methods and instruments are frequently incorporated in applied psychological, educational, and social work disciplines and training. Several indices also suggest that the applications of behavioral assessment have increased from the 1960s, although observational methods have evidenced a decrease in treatment outcome studies from the mid-1980s.

Considerations of applicability are relevant to the ***cost-efficiency*** and ***incremental*** utility and validity of an assessment instrument. Briefly, whatever the power of an assessment instrument (the probability that an assessment instrument can detect significant differences between groups, changes across time, or relations between variables), the amount of useful information acquired must warrant the cost of its application.[2] That is, measures derived from an assessment instrument must be incrementally useful and valid, and not prohibitively expensive, to warrant their use: They must provide useful information that is not more easily available from other, less expensive assessment methods.

The cost-efficiency of many behavioral assessment methods are conditional and improving. The cost-efficiency and incremental validity of an assessment instrument varies with the function of assessment, the clinical decisions that will be based on it, the populations and behaviors to which it is applied, and the setting in which the assessment occurs. For example, observations of role-play social interactions in structured clinic situations may be more useful and valid with some clients, target behaviors, and purposes than with others. The applications of an assessment method or instrument can also be influenced by less meritorious factors, such

---

[2]Similar cost-efficiency factors are salient in medical assessment. For example, several studies have questioned the cost-efficiency of mammography for younger women, despite its ability to detect breast tumors in early stages.

as institutionally mandated assessment strategies and reimbursement schedules from third-party payers.

We will try to convince the reader that the cost-efficiency of behavioral assessment methods is often demonstrated, often underestimated, and improving. Behavioral assessment is taught in only 50% of APA-approved clinical psychology training programs. Further, this proportion of programs has only occurred in the past 10 years. Therefore, we can surmise that many clinicians are unfamiliar with the underlying assumptions, conceptual framework, methods, and usefulness of behavioral assessment. Additionally, many behavioral assessment methods, particularly naturalistic and analogue observation assessment, self-monitoring, and psychophysiological assessment are being refined to facilitate their application in clinical assessment situations. Development of computerized self-monitoring, instrument-aided behavioral observation, and ambulatory monitoring of psychophysiological responses illustrate recent advances in the cost-efficiency of behavioral assessment.

The Applicability and Utility of Behavioral Assessment

Psychological assessment paradigms differ in the populations and behavior problems for which they are most amenable, the settings in which they are applicable, the clinical judgments to which they can best contribute, and research questions that they can address. For example, objective personality and projective assessment instruments are frequently used with outpatient and inpatient adults but are less often used for the assessment of children with behavior problems, of persons with severe developmental disabilities, or as measures of family or organizational functioning.

A strength of the behavioral assessment paradigm is its applicability across diverse populations, behavior problems, assessment functions, and settings. Table 2-5 illustrates the diverse applicability of behavioral assessment within these domains. The extended domain of applicability of behavioral assessment is a result of an important characteristic of the paradigm: It is a flexible paradigm that emphasizes strategies and principles of assessment more than specific methods of assessment. The behavioral assessment paradigm is primarily a conceptual approach to clinical and research inferences.

Behavioral assessment also includes many methods of assessment that are differentially useful across diverse populations, behaviors, settings, and goals. It is flexible in that it can provide guidance for how to approach many clinical judgments, and it can also provide the assessor with an array of assessment methods for gathering data relevant to those clinical judgments.

The flexibility of the paradigm extends to many of its conceptual elements. For example, the concept of *reciprocal causation* suggests that a client can affect his or her social environment, which can, in turn, affect the client's behavior problems. The concept of reciprocal causation can guide assessment strategies across a variety of populations, target problems, and assessment goals. For example, for some clients with chronic low-back pain, the rate and type of pain behaviors (e.g., pain complaints) can be influenced by how others respond to them. These responses can, in turn, be affected by the client's responses (Turk & Melzack, 1992). The concept of reciprocal causation also suggests that the assessor should attend to: (a) the interactions between an aggressive adolescent and his or her teachers, parents, and peers (e.g., discipline strategies, punishment contingencies, reinforcement schedules, rules) (Patterson, 1993); (b) the interactions between a maritally distressed client and his or her spouse (O'Leary,

Table 2-5
Illustrations of the Applicability of Behavioral Assessment
Across Populations, Problems, Settings, and Goals

Reference	Population/ Problem	Assessment Setting	Method of Assessment	Goal of Assessment
Bellack et al. (1997)	Clients with a diagnosis of schizophrenia	Psychiatric hospital	Role-play	Functional analysis and treatment outcome
Black & Novaco (1993)	Client with developmental disabilities;	Unstructured natural environment	Self-monitoring	Treatment process and outcome
	Anger	Clinic	Self-report	Perceived consequences
Blanchard et al. (1994)	PTSD (motor vehicle accidents)	Psychophysiology laboratory	Psychophysiological responses to audiotaped scenarios	Research on role of psychophysiological responses in PTSD
Copeland et al. (1995)	Smoking		Questionnaire	Consequences of smoking
Fletcher et al. (1996)	Children with ADHD	Clinic	Observations of parent-child interactions	Clinical research: to identify parent-child interactions
Kern (1991)	Adults with assertion difficulties	Clinic	Role-play	Functional analysis instrument development
Sasso et al. (1992)	Students with autism	Classroom	Observations in the natural environment; experimental functional analysis	Functional analysis of aberrant behavior

1987); and (c) the interactions between a patient with delusions and staff members and other patients (Foxx et al., 1988).

Although reciprocal influences may not be an important causal factor with all clients, the concept suggests that it may be useful for the assessor to focus on person-environment interactions in behavioral observations, self-monitoring, questionnaires, and assessment interviews. Other elements of the behavioral assessment paradigm (delineated in Table 1-1) also broaden its applicability. Assessment strategies (such as the collection of data from multiple sources and methods, time-series assessment) and causal models (such as idiosyncratic and multiple causality) can be useful for many different client populations, behavior problems, causal factors, and assessment settings.

The multiple methods included in the behavioral assessment paradigm also facilitate its applicability. Behavioral observation of dyadic interactions in structured clinic settings can be a useful assessment method for some clients with disturbed marital, family, and peer interactions (Sarwer & Sayer, 1998), but may be less useful for the assessment of some nonsocial anxiety disorders (McGlynn & Rose, 1998). Alternatively, self-monitoring, self-report questionnaires, and psychophysiological assessment methods may be more useful for some clients with anxiety disorders.

The following sections present an overview of the populations, behavior problems, and settings with which behavioral assessment has been applied. More detailed reviews of the applicability of specific behavioral assessment methods can be found in later chapters in this book and in several other books (see Suggested Readings at the end of this chapter).

Applicability to Clinical Populations

The populations with which the behavioral assessment paradigm has been applied vary on several dimensions of individual differences: (a) age, (b) physical impairment, (c) intellectual and cognitive functioning, (d) occupational roles, (e) language abilities, (f) ethnicity, (g) institutional status (e.g., prisoners, inpatients), and (h) educational and economic status. Examples of this diversity in populations include children with learning and cognitive disabilities, males and females with sexual dysfunctions and paraphilias, medical patients with acute and chronic pain, clients reporting depression and anxiety, persons with post-traumatic stress symptoms, persons receiving surgical and other medical treatments, children and adults with headache and sleep disorders, adolescents who are aggressive, delinquent, and abuse drugs, rehabilitation patients with head trauma, psychiatric inpatients with severe social and inferential difficulties, and many others populations.

Applicability to Behavior Problems and Therapy Goals

The behavioral assessment paradigm has been applied with a wide array of behavior problems. The list of targeted problems includes most behavior problems listed in DSM-IV, most symptoms that contribute to DSM-IV diagnoses, and most "mental health" problems covered in child and adult abnormal psychology texts. Behavioral assessment has been used across dimensions of: (a) severity of behavioral disturbance and impairment (e.g., persons with mild to severe self-injurious or mood disturbances), (b) response mode (e.g., physiological, behavioral, cognitive), (c) chronicity of behavior problems (e.g., patients with acute and chronic pain), (d) overt/covert nature of behavior problems (e.g., conduct disorders, depressed mood), (e) behavior problem parameters (e.g., onset, magnitude, recurrence), and (f) social vs. individual systems (e.g., a problem classroom vs. a problem child in the classroom).

Behavioral assessment has also been used to help achieve treatment goals. Examples of treatment goals include enhanced interpersonal comfort, satisfaction, and skills, decreased self-injurious behaviors, better school performance, the development of goal attainment strategies, and the reduction of goal conflicts. Other therapy goals include enhanced quality of life, increased marital, family, and sexual satisfaction, improved physical health, the development of anger management strategies, enhanced teaching and parenting effectiveness, and better self-help skills. A focus on therapy goals is one component of a ***constructional approach*** to behavioral assessment (Evans, 1993a).

Applicability to Settings

Behavioral assessment is also unique in the diversity of settings in which it has been applied. Behavioral assessment strategies have been used in the home, workplace, classroom, inpatient psychiatric unit, restaurant, hospital, dental office, hospital emergency room, cancer treatment waiting room, playground, community center, automobile, military training center, prison, school lunchrooms, crisis intervention center, substance abuse treatment center, outpatient psychiatric treatment center, surgery room, birthing center, transitional houses, homes for developmentally disabled adults and children, and shopping centers.

Applicability in Applied and Basic Research

As illustrated in Table 2-2 behavioral assessment methods are frequently used in published treatment outcome studies. Behavioral assessment methods have been applied for a variety of purposes in treatment outcome research: (a) to select, screen, and diagnose participants for treatment outcome studies, (b) to measure dependent variables before, during, and following treatment, (c) to measure therapy process variables, (d) to measure variables that may moderate or predict treatment compliance, outcome, or maintenance, and (e) to measure independent variables in treatment.

An exemplar of the use of behavioral assessment in therapy process research is the work by Chamberlain and associates (1984) and by Stoolmiller and associates (1993). These researchers developed the Therapy Process Coding System to measure client resistance during therapy sessions with the parents of aggressive adolescents. They hypothesized that "client resistance" for successful cases would first increase and then decrease. Behaviors representing the construct of "resistance" included confrontative, challenging, blaming, defensive, side-tracking, and contradictory comments by parents. They found that changes in client resistance predicted treatment outcome in the manner predicted. Furthermore, client resistance could be operationalized, identified, and measured reliably by external observers across sessions. It is notable that favorable treatment outcome was associated more strongly with the phase-space (see Chapter 5) of resistance behaviors than with low levels of resistance. Clients who demonstrated a particular nonlinear function—an increase followed by a decrease in resistance behaviors—were more likely to have maintained treatment gains at follow-up than clients who maintained low levels of resistance behaviors across treatment sessions.

This research illustrates the power, utility, and flexibility of the behavioral assessment paradigm. The direct measurement of precisely defined, observable, minimally inferential variables, in a time-series assessment strategy, can provide valid, richly detailed, and clinically useful data. In contrast, trait-based, molar, self-report questionnaires on "client resistance" or personality questionnaires on the likelihood of therapy termination often provide less specific, less clinically useful, and more inferential measures.

Although this book focuses on the clinical applications of the behavioral assessment paradigm, behavioral assessment methods are also widely used in behavioral neuroscience, behavior analysis, experimental psychopathology, and other basic research disciplines. For example, direct observation has been used in thousands of studies in learning, psychopharmacology, behavior genetics, ecological psychology, social and developmental psychology, and the experimental analysis of behavior. Reviews of assessment methods in some of these disciplines can be found in Brewer and Crano (1994), Kail and Wickes-Nelson (1993), and McGuigan (1990).

Caveats

The Differential Applicability of the Conceptual Elements of Behavioral Assessment

The behavioral assessment paradigm offers guiding principles for the assessor. The paradigm suggests that examination of particular variables and functional relations, using particular strategies and methods, will often result in powerful and clinically useful case conceptualizations and clinical judgments.

Although they have been widely applied, the conceptual elements of the behavioral assessment paradigm differ in the degree to which they are useful across populations, behavior problems, and setting domains. For example, there is convincing evidence that *social response contingencies*, such as the immediate responses of parents and teachers to children's behavior can significantly affect the rate of self-injurious behavior in individuals with developmental disabilities (e.g., Iwata et al., 1994). However, there is little evidence that social response contingencies play an important role in the onset of migraine headache, asthma episodes, or cardiovascular disorders (Gatchel & Blanchard, 1993). It is illogical to presume that response contingencies, despite thousands of studies supporting their powerful effects on behavior, are an important causal factor for all behavior problems or for all persons with the same behavior problem, or in all settings. Research on causal factors with self-injurious behavior illustrates this latter point. In many studies, the self-injurious behaviors of about 20 to 35% of the persons studied were unaffected by manipulation of response contingencies (Iwata et al., 1994).

Social response contingencies are often important causal factors for behavior problems and can be used to weaken maladaptive behaviors and to strengthen alternative behaviors. The assessor's mandate is to use the conceptual elements of the behavioral assessment paradigm to guide the assessment focus—for example, to presume that response contingencies may be an important causal variable for a client's behavior problems and goals. This presumption will guide the assessor toward a careful assessment of response contingencies that will frequently, but not invariably, lead to a more powerful and clinically useful behavioral case formulation.

Differential Applicability of the Methods of Behavioral Assessment

A similar caveat applies to the applicability of specific behavioral assessment methods. For example, behavioral observation in analogue settings can be a powerful method of assessing social interactions of psychiatric inpatients and other adults with interpersonal difficulties (e.g., Kern, 1991). However, analogue observation may be less useful in the assessment of some persons with mood or sleep problems. For some persons and for some behavior problems, self-monitoring, behavioral interviews, and ambulatory psychophysiological assessment methods may provide data that are more clinically useful than analogue observation.

As we noted previously, the multiple methods and instruments of behavioral assessment paradigm are two of its strengths. However, each method and instrument is differentially applicable and useful across behavior problems, goals, populations, and settings. Different clients, assessment settings, and assessment goals will require different methods of assessment. For example, the assessment of social response contingencies might best be approached with analogue observation when the focus is on parent or staff-child interactions of high frequency behaviors (Iwata et al., 1994), with a questionnaire when the focus is on parental responses to a child's headache (Budd et al., 1993), and self-monitoring when the focus is on how a client responds to his or her spouse (Halford, Sanders, & Behrens, 1994). The decisions about the best method depend on the characteristics of the client's behavior, assessment setting, goals of assessment, and available resources.

Specifically, the applicability and utility of individual methods of behavioral assessment are affected by several variables:

- *Developmental level of the client.* For example, Ollendick and Hersen (1993b) noted that cognitive abilities affect the applicability of self-monitoring with children; very young children (e.g., less than six years) may not be able to accurately track their behaviors.
- *Cognitive functioning.* Data from self-monitoring, interviewing, and questionnaire

assessment methods can also be affected by medication, neurological diseases, attention dysfunctions, and acquired head trauma (e.g., Maisto, McKay, & Connors, 1990; Walitzer & Connors, 1994).

- *Reactive effects of the assessment method.* When applied to some behavior problems, clients, or in some assessment settings, assessment instruments can change the variables being measured or affect the social interactions. For example, Haynes and Horn (1982) reviewed studies that showed that behavioral observation sometimes modifies the occurrence of many behaviors.
- *Availability of, and cooperation from, persons in the client's social environment.* Many behavioral assessment methods involve cooperation by clients' spouses, teachers, supervising staff members, family members, and other persons. For example, accurate participant observation of the behavior of psychiatric inpatients by hospital staff requires the consent and cooperation of the staff members (Anderson, Vaulx-Smith, & Keshavan, 1994).
- *Characteristics of the target behaviors and causal variables.* Some behavior problems and causal variables are more amenable to measurement with some methods than with others. Important characteristics include: (a) whether the variable is currently occurring, (b) the frequency of the variable, and (c) the setting in which the variable occurs. For example, early traumatic life experiences can be assessed most easily through behavioral interviews. Also, some important social contingencies can be observed by others but not readily reported by clients (e.g., a parent may not understand how his or her behavior is reinforcing the oppositional behavior of a teenager).
- *The congruence between the targeted variables and the variables targeted by an assessment instrument.* Assessment instruments differ in the degree to which they provide data on the variables of primary interest in a specific assessment occasion. For example, if an assessor is interested in identifying situations that trigger a client's anxiety reactions, anxiety inventories that emphasize state or trait measurement would be less useful than self-monitoring or self-report instruments that provide information about anxiety-eliciting situations.
- *Costs of an assessment method and resources of the assessor.* As we noted earlier in this chapter, some behavioral assessment methods, such as observation in the natural environment and ambulatory monitoring of psychophysiological responses, are prohibitively expensive to administer and score. For example, the use of a few trained observers to collect data on family interactions in a client's home may require scores of hours for observer training, coding, and data analysis. The expense of some assessment methods may explain their more frequent use in well-funded clinical research settings associated with universities and medical schools than in less well-supported clinical settings.
- *Constraints and contingencies on the assessor.* Sometimes assessment strategies are dictated by contingencies operating on the assessor. For example, a comprehensive behavioral case formulation of self-injurious behavior (to determine if the self-injurious behaviors are affected by social reinforcement, termination of demands, etc.) using systematic manipulation of possible functional variables in a clinic office is difficult in some outpatient clinic situations where the assessors are allotted a limited amount of time with the clients or where such methods are not reimbursed.

Summary

The behavioral assessment paradigm is applicable to diverse populations, behavior problems, goals, and settings. This broad applicability is a result of the diversity of methods encompassed by the paradigm and is also a result of broadly applicable concepts and assumptions. These conceptual foundations can guide assessment strategies for specific populations, behavior problems, and assessment goals. They can also guide the assessor when he or she is confronted with novel or unusual assessment questions and challenges.

A number of factors affect the applicability of behavioral assessment methods. These include the developmental level of the client, cognitive functioning, reactive effects of the assessment, cooperation from the client's social environment, the nature of the target behaviors and causal variables, the variables targeted by a specific assessment instrument, reactive effects of assessment, time constraints, and costs of assessment.

Summary

This chapter examined the status and phase-state of behavioral assessment. Although inferential errors in equating application with utility were noted, the application and role of behavioral assessment in research, clinical practice, and training were surveyed. Several conclusions were offered: (a) behavioral assessment strategies are frequently used in treatment outcome research and in clinical practice, (b) the use of, and training in, behavioral assessment has increased across several decades, (c) the behavioral assessment paradigm is well represented in professional organizations, and membership in organizations with a behavioral orientation has been increasing at a rate similar to that of general interest professional organizations, (d) behavioral assessment is taught in about half of the graduate training programs, and this proportion is projected to increase, and (e) the behavioral paradigm may contribute more to the development of treatment procedures and to treatment outcome evaluation than to basic psychopathology research or to the development of causal models for behavior disorders.

The behavioral assessment paradigm is broadly applicable across populations, behavior problems, and settings. This applicability is a result of its emphasis on strategies and principles of assessment, rather than specific methods of assessment. Because of this emphasis, the behavioral assessment paradigm includes an array of methods of assessment, some of which can be applied in most clinical and research situations. Rather than prescribing a specific method of acquiring data, the behavioral assessment paradigm suggests principles and general strategies to assist the assessor in deriving clinical judgments.

Several caveats were offered regarding the applicability of behavioral assessment. The most evident is that conceptual and methodological elements of the paradigm are differentially useful across populations, behaviors, goals, and settings. However, the paradigm suggests that clinical judgments will often be strengthened by the examination of particular variables and functional relationships, using particular strategies and methods.

The applicability of the specific methods of behavioral assessment is influenced by the developmental level of the client, the client's level of cognitive functioning, the reactive effects of the assessment method, the availability of and cooperation from persons in the client's social environment, the nature of the target behaviors and causal variables, the congruence between the targeted variables and the variables obtained with an assessment instrument, costs of an assessment method and resources of the assessor, and time constraints.

Suggested Readings

Barrios, B. A. (1988). On the changing nature of behavioral assessment. In A. S. Bellack & M. Hersen (Eds.), *Behavioral assessment: A practical handbook* (3rd ed., pp. 3–41). New York: Pergamon.

Haynes, S. N. (1998). The changing nature of behavioral assessment. In M. Hersen & A. Bellack (Eds.), *Behavioral assessment: A practical guide* (4th ed., pp. 1–21). Boston: Allyn & Bacon.

Hersen, M., & Bellack, A. S. (Eds.). (1998). *Behavioral assessment: A practical handbook* (4th ed.). Boston: Allyn & Bacon.

Mash, E. J., & Terdal, L. G. (Eds.). (1997). *Assessment of childhood disorders* (3rd ed.) New York: Guilford.

Ollendick, T. H., & Hersen, M. (Eds.). (1993). *Handbook of child and adolescent assessment*. Boston: Allyn & Bacon.

Shapiro, E. W., & Kratochwill, T. W. (Eds.). (1988). *Behavioral assessment in schools: Conceptual foundations and practical applications*. New York: Guilford.

3

Functional Psychological Assessment and Clinical Judgment

Introduction

An important goal of psychological assessment is to increase the validity of clinical judgments. Judgments about a client's behavior problems, factors that contribute to those problems, and the best strategies of intervention with a client should be more valid when based on accurate information from psychological assessment.

It is also important to note that the types of clinical judgments (e.g., the identification of a client's behavior problems, or clinical case formulation) can vary across assessment occasions, clients, settings, and the stages of the assessment-treatment process. Consequently, the role and strategies of psychological assessment also vary across these domains.

Congruent with this "conditional" view of psychological assessment, behavioral assessment is a *functional approach* to psychological assessment. That is, the applicability and utility of principles and methods of assessment vary as a function of the many characteristics of an assessment occasion (see Box 3-1).

In the first part of this chapter we define a functional approach to psychological assessment. We then review several types of clinical judgments and describe how they are affected by

---

Box 3-1
Alternative Definitions of Functional Assessment

The term "functional assessment" has a long history and different meanings in other assessment paradigms (Boring, 1957; Rust & Golombok, 1989). "Functional assessment" in neuropsychology, rehabilitation, personnel selection, and education is often used to refer to the assessment of a person's skills or level of functioning.

For example, "functional assessment" in neuropsychology often involves the identification of specific cognitive, verbal, and motor deficits and capabilities of a client following a head trauma, stroke, or spinal cord damage. Used in this manner, "functional assessment" could more accurately be described as the "assessment of functioning."

To illustrate, Milton et al. (1991) discussed the importance to rehabilitation efforts of assessing integration, critical thinking, visual processing, and conversational processing skills of adolescents following traumatic brain injury. Applegate, Blass, John, and Williams (1990) discussed the assessment of physical functioning, cognitive functioning, "emotional status," and social activities in older patients in order to guide intervention efforts. In an article on "Functional Assessment in Rehabilitation" Wallace (1986) reviewed 11 structured interviews on the social living skills of chronically mentally ill persons.

Similarly, in personnel assessment, if a particular job requires a high degree of mechanical aptitude or supervisory skills, a "functional" approach to assessment would emphasize direct tests of mechanical aptitude and supervisory skills, rather than indirect measures of these skills through measurement of "general intelligence" or "extraversion."

In contrast, Cattell and Johnson (1986) identified "functional psychological testing" as a movement in psychological assessment characterized by the examination of trait structures and state change using dynamic mathematical models with psychometrically validated instruments.

"Functional assessment" is used by some behavior analysts to refer to the process of estimating functional relations for behavior problems through methods other than systematic observation of behavior in controlled (e.g., ABAB) situations. For example, Sisson and Taylor (1993) defined functional assessment as the identification of the antecedent and consequent events that occasion and maintain a target response, and used the term "experimental behavioral case formulation" for controlled observation methods.

data from behavioral assessment. In the latter sections, we discuss errors in clinical judgments and strategies for reducing them.

We emphasize several points about functional assessment and clinical judgment:

1. The applicability and utility of the methods, principles, and strategies of behavioral assessment are influenced by characteristics of an assessment occasion, particularly the goals of assessment.
2. The applicability of psychometric dimensions of evaluation and sources of measurement error vary across the goals and methods of assessment.
3. Assessment strategies should be matched to the goals of each assessment occasion.
4. A clinical judgment is a prediction, inference, or decision that has important implications for a client.
5. There are many sources of errors in clinical judgments.
6. The use of multiple validated assessment instruments and multiple informants can often decrease measurement and judgment errors and increase the validity of clinical judgments.
7. Research on clinical judgment is increasing but lags behind research on psychological assessment instruments.
8. Clinicians often use oversimplification strategies when required to make clinical judgments in the context of complex arrays of assessment information about a client.
9. The reliability and validity of clinical judgments can be enhanced with quantitatively aided decision-making strategies and quantitative criteria.

Behavioral Assessment as Functional Psychological Assessment

As we noted in Chapter 2, and will again discuss in Chapter 4, the applicability and utility of methods and principles of the behavioral assessment paradigm are affected by the function of the assessment. Although some principles (e.g., an empirical approach to assessment and an emphasis on the use of minimally inferential constructs) are applicable across all assessment occasions, the applicability of many principles is influenced by the specific goals of the assessment. For example, the importance of time-series assessment strategies is increased when the goal of assessment is treatment outcome evaluation.

An important characteristic of the behavioral assessment paradigm is its functional character. The functional character of behavioral assessment has implications for assessment methods, instruments, and strategies; psychometric evaluation, and the inferences derived from obtained measures. Consequently, it has implications for clinical case formulation, treatment design, and treatment outcome evaluation.

The goal of each assessment occasion also affects the applicability and utility of behavioral assessment methods and instruments (Silverman & Kurtines, 1996). Behavioral observation is more useful when the goal of assessment is to evaluate interactions between family members than when the goal is to identify a client's catastrophic thoughts during a panic episode. In the same way, the assessment goal influences the best way to aggregate data, the applicability of various psychometric principles to obtained measures, the time- and behavior-sampling strategies used in measurement, and the variables targeted in the assessment. Figure 3-1 illustrates the relations among the goals, principles, and methods of psychological assessment.

Later, we discuss a functional approach to psychometrics. For example, one goal of psychological assessment can be the identification and measurement of covert variables for a

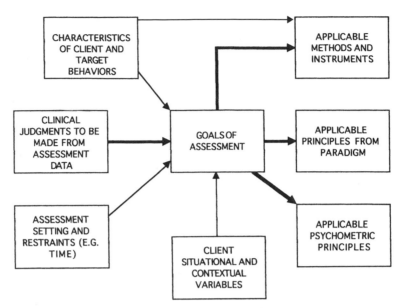

Figure 3-1. A functional model of psychological assessment: The best methods and applicable principles of assessment depend on the goals of assessment for a particular assessment occasion.

depressed client, such as the magnitude of "feelings of sadness" and "frequency of negative thoughts about the future" as measures of treatment outcome. In this case, important psychometric dimensions are the validity and bias of self-reports of unobservable variables. We may use several measures of these constructs to tap different aspects of them. Then, we may be interested in the degree of shared variance among multiple measures of these constructs.

The relative importance of diagnostic "hits" and "misses" can also vary, depending on the goals of assessment. For example, if a goal of assessment in a marital and family treatment center is to identify women who are in a physically violent relationship (e.g., O'Leary, Vivian, & Malone, 1992) highly structured and focused interviews may be most useful. Furthermore, the *sensitivity* of the interviews (the proportion of women in a violent relationship who are accurately identified by the interview) may be more important than *specificity* (the proportion of women who are not in a violent relationship who are accurately identified). Sensitivity is particularly important if the goal of assessment is to identify candidates for more detailed assessments and when the goal is to identify important behaviors such as aggression, suicide, risky behaviors, and self-injurious behaviors.

Behavioral observation elicits different evaluative dimensions. A frequent goal in the clinical assessment of children with behavior problems is to identify interactions between a parent and child that maintain the child's behavior problems (see reviews in Mash & Terdal, 1997a; Ollendick & Hersen, 1993a). Clinical observations of parent-child interactions during structured play activities may be a particularly useful method of approaching this goal. In these analogue observation assessment settings, reactive effects associated with the method, observer accuracy and interobserver agreement, situation-specificity of the interactions, and generalizability of the obtained measures and inferences to the natural environment, and time-sampling parameters are important considerations. A number of conceptual elements of the behavioral assessment paradigm, such as reciprocal causality and the dynamic qualities of the observed behaviors, are also more important in observations of interactions than in the measurement of covert events.

As these examples illustrate, there are several characteristics of a functional approach to psychological assessment.

- The variables selected for measurement, and the methods used to measure them, should be appropriate for the goals of assessment and for the characteristics of the client. For example, if the goal of assessment is to evaluate the outcome of a treatment program for a client with bulimic behavior patterns, assessment should target the important components of this eating disorder, such as weight, bingeing and purging frequency, and self-ideal body image discrepancies (Foreyt & McGavin, 1989; Schlundt, Johnson & Jarrell, 1986). If the goal of assessment is to develop a clinical case formulation of this client, assessment targets should also include hypothesized causal relations for purging.[1] Daily self-monitoring, client interviews, family interviews, and eating-related questionnaires might be congruent with these goals.
- Analogously, the utility of an assessment method (i.e., of the measures derived from an instrument) varies across assessment occasions. A method can be useful for some clinical judgments and not others.
- The applicability of psychometric evaluative dimensions varies across assessment methods, instruments, and the characteristics of a particular assessment occasion. For example, temporal consistency of obtained measures helps estimate the validity of a questionnaire measure of a latent personality trait. It is less helpful, however, in estimating validity of behavioral observation measures, where stability across time or situations is not presumed.
- Data on the psychometric characteristics of an assessment instrument should be interpreted in the context of the goals and the characteristics of the assessment occasion. The psychometric characteristics of measures are conditional—they depend on the assessment purpose, the characteristics of the sample, and on other aspects of the assessment situation.
- Sampling strategies should be congruent with the goals and conditions of each assessment occasion. For example, in observing the behaviors of aggressive children in a classroom, several participant sampling methods could be used, depending on the purpose of the assessment. An observer could monitor the behaviors of the most aggressive children, all of the children, or a randomly selected subset of children. Whether the observer monitored the responses of the teacher would depend on the utility of information on teacher-delivered response contingencies. Similarly, the number of hours and days that observation occurs and the duration of the observation intervals (i.e., the time sampling strategies) should depend on the specific behaviors that are observed and their dimensions of interest (e.g., duration, rate).
- Assessment instruments should be selected that provide the least inferential measures of the variables. In a less functional approach to evaluating treatment outcome for a client with an eating disorder, an assessor might obtain measures of "locus of control," or "self-esteem" because these constructs are correlated with eating disorders and might be expected to change as a result of treatment. However, although these variables can

---

[1]A focus on specific bulimia-related variables does not preclude the measurement of other variables. Inferences about the effectiveness of a treatment for bulimia would be influenced, for example, by its effects on the use of other substances by the client and its effects on interpersonal relationships, both of which would be important assessment targets and reflect the "systems" emphasis of behavioral assessment.

provide some information, they are insufficiently specific to draw inferences about a client's eating behaviors that could be used for a clinical case formulation, for the design of an intervention program, or for the evaluation of specific treatment effects.

- Given the points raised above, it should be evident that the utility of an assessment instrument is variable and conditional. Most carefully developed and validated psychological assessment instruments can provide useful information for some assessment purposes, clients, and settings. They can also answer some assessment questions and contribute to some clinical judgments. For example, a questionnaire on "introversion/extraversion" may be insufficiently specific to be useful for generating a clinical case formulation or evaluating the specific effects of a social skills intervention program. It lacks the degree of precision regarding situations, responses, and functional relations that is desirable for those purposes. However, it may be useful when the goal of assessment is to screen a large sample for dispositions or to detect longitudinal changes in general attitudes and expectancies regarding social interactions.

- The utility of an assessment instrument is a dimension on which an assessment instrument can be evaluated. Assessment instruments can vary in the degree to which data derived from the instrument is congruent with the function of the assessment.

- Specific variables, functional relations, and measures are often more useful than global, less specific measures, as aids to clinical judgments. More specific measures can often provide more useful information regarding a client's behavior problems and causal variables.

- Standardized clinical assessment batteries should be augmented by assessment strategies that are congruent with the characteristics of specific clients. Standardized batteries can provide information on the characteristics and treatment responses of groups of clients but may not provide specific information on clients' idiosyncratic problems and causal variables.

- Intermediate clinical judgments should contribute to ultimate clinical judgments. Both authors of this book have attended clinical staff meetings that involved prolonged and intensive debate about the diagnosis of a client, when diagnosis was irrelevant to selecting the best treatment strategies for that client. An example would be attempting to differentiate between Asperger's and Autistic diagnoses for a client. Differential diagnosis would have no impact on which social skills, self-help, and educational training strategies would be of most help for this client.

In sum, the assessor should carefully specify the precise goal of each assessment occasion and each clinical judgment and how assessment data could contribute those judgments. Is the goal of assessment to identify persons who are at risk for a problem from a large sample? To provide validation evidence for an assessment instrument? To identify situations that occasion and contingencies that maintain a behavior problem? A careful specification of clinical judgments and matching assessment strategies to those judgments are essential elements of a functional approach to psychological assessment.

Summary

Many judgments are made in the clinical assessment contexts, and the supraordinate goal of psychological assessment is to increase their validity. The specific goals of assessment for each assessment occasion affect the applicability and utility of assessment methods and instruments, as well as the underlying conceptual and psychometric elements. Consequently, the applicability and utility of each element of the behavioral assessment paradigm depends on the goals of a particular assessment occasion. The next section discusses more specifically the role of behavioral assessment in clinical judgments. Chapter 4 discusses the specific functions of behavioral assessment.

Clinical Judgments and the Role of Behavioral Assessment

Clinical Judgments

A *clinical judgment* is prediction, inference, or decision about the behavior of a client. Clinical judgments are usually influenced by qualitative and quantitative assessment information about a client or the services that the client should receive. Clinical judgments can include a psychiatric diagnosis applied to a client's behavior problems, the behaviors identified as being problematic for a client, and estimates of the magnitude of covariance among behavior problems. Clinical judgments can also include hypotheses about the causal relations affecting a client's behavior problems, a client's assets, the best treatment strategy for a client, and the variables that are likely to affect treatment outcome.

Clinical judgments have important consequences for clients. For example, estimates of the risk of suicide or physical violence by a client can affect whether the client is hospitalized and which medication dosage the client receives. Estimates of the importance of marital distress for a client's depressed behaviors can affect whether the client's spouse is included in the assessment-treatment program. Additionally, clinicians estimate of the effects of a client's treatment program can influence whether the program is modified. One clinical judgment that can strongly influence decisions about hospitalization and financial support for treatment is a psychiatric diagnosis (Costello, 1993; Hodges & Cools, 1990; see the miniseries "Behavioral Assessment in the DSM Era" in *Behavioral Assessment, 14*, 1992, 293–386).

As these examples illustrate, lower-order clinical judgments often influence subsequent higher-order judgments about a clinical case formulation and the best intervention program for a client. For example, on the basis of pretreatment assessment of marital communication patterns with a distressed couple (e.g., through analogue observations of problem solving, spouse reports of communication problems), a clinician may estimate the potential effects of marital communication training—the estimated magnitude of effects associated with enhanced problem-solving skills. In order to begin a communication training program for the couple, lower-order clinical judgments would be necessary, such as: (a) what specific communication behaviors impede satisfactory communication: should communication training focus on promoting positive assertive responses, increasing "listening" skills, or decreasing escalations, and (b) are beliefs and expectancies involved: should communication training precede or follow a focus on cognitive factors.

As we have noted many times, the primary purpose of psychological assessment is to provide information that increases the validity of clinical judgments. A basic proposition of the behavioral assessment paradigm is that the validity of clinical judgments will be strengthened to the degree that they are based on measures and strategies that are valid for the particular client, for the particular assessment context, and for the particular judgment that is to be made.

We further suggest that the validity of clinical judgments will often be strengthened to the degree that the assessor applies the basic tenets of the behavioral assessment paradigm:

Clinical judgments are most likely to be valid when they are based on highly specific and multimodal, multidimensional measures obtained from multiple informants across multiple situations using multimethod assessment strategies.

Many judgments are made in clinical assessment settings. Although principles of assessment are relevant to judgments such as diagnosis and treatment outcome evaluation, this book focuses on clinical case formulation (especially the functional analysis) and the design of intervention programs for clients. As a prelude to our discussion of the clinical case formulation in Chapter 13, Table 3-1 lists several clinical judgments about a client that are fundamental to the design of behavioral intervention programs.

Although the judgments outlined in Table 3-1 contribute to treatment decisions in many therapy paradigms, they are particularly important in behavioral interventions because behavioral interventions are more often individually tailored to match the characteristics of the individual client. For example, hypotheses about the causal variables that affect a client's problem behaviors and goals and the relative importance of a client's behavior problems often have an important impact on the design of intervention programs (Haynes, 1992).

In a behavioral assessment paradigm, interventions may vary across clients with similar behavior problems if the clients differ in the causal variables relevant to and functional relations among those behavior problems. Different intervention strategies might be recommended for two clients with similar depressive behaviors if the depressive behaviors were judged to be a function of automatic negative thoughts and deficient coping skills in response to a very stressful work situation for one client and a function of marital distress for the other client (see Rehm et al., 1994). When clients have multiple behavior problems, judgments about the relative importance of each problem, and the types of functional relations (e.g., causal, correlational) with other behavior problems, can also affect decisions about where to initially focus treatment efforts.

Clinical judgments have been the subject of numerous studies and are reviewed in many books and articles (see Suggested Readings at the end of this chapter). Baysean decision analysis and other statistical and cognitive models have been profitably applied to the analysis of clinical judgment. However, an extensive discussion of these methods is beyond the domain of this book. The goal of the following section is to outline some sources of error in clinical judgments and to suggest strategies for reducing judgment.

Research on Clinical Judgment in Behavior Therapy

Despite the centrality of clinical judgment to the design of behavioral intervention programs, clinical judgment and decision making in behavior therapy have been the subject of few

Table 3-1

Some Clinical Judgments that Affect the Design of Behavioral Intervention Programs

1. The best assessment strategies to use with a client
2. The identification and specification of a client's behavior problems and goals
3. The form and strength of relations among a client's multiple behavior problems and goals
4. The identification of the causal variables that affect a client's behavior problems and goals
5. The identification of variables that moderate a client's behavior problems and goals
6. The client's cognitive, physical, and social-environmental resources and deficits
7. The integration of multiple clinical judgments into a functional analytic case conceptualization

scholarly publications and fewer data-based articles. Hundreds of studies focus on the validity, accuracy, and sources of error in behavioral assessment methods and instruments. Many scholarly articles have championed the importance of clinical judgment. However, fewer empirical studies have evaluated the clinical judgment process or the validity and sources of error in clinical judgments.

Fortunately, research on clinical judgment is growing. Analogue studies have examined the reliability of clinical judgments among students and trainees (e.g., Felton & Nelson, 1984; Persons, Mooney, & Padesky, 1995). Several miniseries relevant to clinical judgment have been published in the 1980s and 1990s. For example, a special series on the selection of target behaviors in behavior therapy was published in 1985 in *Behavioral Assessment* and *Psychological Assessment* has published several series on the role of assessment in treatment decisions (see Suggested Readings at the end of this chapter).

Special series have also addressed the relation between psychiatric diagnosis and behavioral assessment. A series on "Behavioral Assessment and the DSM-III-R" was published in 1988 in *Behavioral Assessment* (Volume 10[1]) and included articles on DSM and depression, diagnosis of childhood disorders, problems with implementing a diagnostic strategy with complex causal models, and the integration of psychiatric diagnosis in behavioral assessment. A series on "Behavioral Assessment in the DSM Era" was published in 1992 in *Behavioral Assessment* (Volume 14[314]) and included articles on the relations among DSM-IV, syndromes, situational factors, and behavioral assessment. Some of the best reviews of clinical judgment research are presented in an edited book by Garb (1998), and in a special section edited by Garb in *Psychological Assessment* (2000, Volume 12[1]).

A series titled "Clinical Applications of Psychological Assessment" was published in 1993 in *Psychological Assessment* (Volume 5[3]). This series included articles on the identification of psychotherapy failure, constructional perspectives in clinical assessment, the identification of causal relations for treatment planning, client goal systems in clinical assessment, and identifying and selecting target behaviors in clinical assessment. *Psychological Assessment* (Volume 9[4]) published, in 1997, another series on assessment-treatment relations. This series included articles on functional analysis, personality assessment, and projective assessment contributions to treatment design.

Behavior Therapy (Volume 25[4]) published a miniseries in 1994, "Research Contributions to Clinical Assessment." Articles in this series addressed clinical implications of assessment research, the clinical utility of assessment instruments, the integration of assessment and treatment, and the functions of assessment. Individual articles covered these issues in reference to substance use, insomnia, panic disorder, obsessive-compulsive disorders, and binge eating.

We have found four books that address clinical decision making particularly well (e.g., Kanfer & Schefft, 1988; Nezu & Nezu, 1989; Turk & Salovey, 1988; and Garb, 1998). Additionally, several articles or chapters (e.g., Arkes, 1981; Dumont & Lecomte, 1987; Kanfer & Grimm, 1980; Kleinmuntz, 1990; Lanyon & Lanyon, 1976; Russo, Hamada & Marques, 1988) discuss clinical judgments. However, most books on behavioral or psychological assessment and therapy (e.g., Bellack & Hersen, 1988, 1998; Groth-Marnat, 1997; Haynes, 1978; Haynes & Wilson, 1979; La Greca, 1990; Mash & Barkley, 1989; Mash & Terdall, 1997b; Turner, Calhoun, & Adams, 1992) devote only a few pages to clinical judgments in behavior therapy.

Judgments of the degree of change associated with clinical interventions have also been the subject of numerous articles. The measurement procedures, statistical analyses, criteria, and the rationale for judging the clinical significance of treatment outcome has been set forth, applied, and discussed in numerous articles (for example, see the nine articles in the miniseries in *Behavioral Assessment*, "Defining Clinically Significant Change," *10*, 1988, pp. 131–223; see discussions in Maruish, 1994).

In sum, although many series and book chapters have been published on the topic, clinical judgment has not been addressed with the degree of empirical rigor applied to other components of the behavioral assessment and therapy paradigms. First, there are few empirically based guidelines for making clinical judgments from assessment data. There are no validated procedures for making the clinical judgments outlined in Table 3-1. There are no validated methods for ranking the importance of a client's multiple behavior problems and goals. There are also no broadly applicable methods for estimating the strength and direction of causal relations affecting a behavior problem, or for estimating the operation and strength of mediating and moderating variables (an exception may be the excellent work with self-injurious behaviors; Iwata et al., 1994). Most importantly, methods have not been developed for integrating data obtained from multiple sources into a clinical case formulation.

We note the dearth of research on clinical judgment to reemphasize a caveat introduced in the Preface of this book: Readers should assume an orientation of "optimistic skepticism" about recommendations regarding clinical judgment offered in this chapter. Our advocacy of strategies for arriving at valid clinical judgments should be considered to be hypotheses, subject to refinement through empirical evaluation.

Biases and Errors in Clinical Judgment

The dearth of empirically supported guidelines for clinical judgment encourages simplified, intuitive, and biased decision-making strategies. Several authors (Dumont & Lecomte, 1987; Kanfer & Schefft, 1988; Kleinmuntz, 1990) have remarked that the absence of empirically based guidelines for clinical judgments increases the probability of and degree to which clinical judgments are affected by the biases of the clinician. The dearth of validated guidelines also decreases the degree to which judgments are affected by the characteristics of the client. Rather than reflecting assessment-based information on the client, judgments are more likely to reflect the clinician's personal preferences, biases, idiosyncratic inferential strategies, and other predispositions. In effect, clinical judgments about a client can often be predicted more accurately from knowledge of the clinician than from knowledge of the client.

Table 3-2 outlines some sources of error in clinical judgments. Intuition, values, training, theoretical orientation, and biases inevitably influence clinical judgments. It is logical to assume that a clinician's recent training experiences will affect his or her clinical judgments. Training experiences are designed to promote particular assessment strategies and treatment models. A well-conducted three-day workshop on cognitive assessment and intervention strategies would probably increase the chance that participants would use those strategies with their clients (see Box 3-2). It is probably unavoidable that clinicians' intuitions and biases would affect clinical judgment because of the inherent complexity of these judgments (see Box 3-3). Clinical assessment situations often require that the clinician make judgments based on incomplete, inconsistent, and complex arrays of assessment data. The complexity of data sets often exceeds a clinician's integrative abilities, and there is currently little help in organizing these data. Many promising computer-based and statistically based decision-making algorithms have been developed (see reviews in Garb, 1998), and models for clinical decision making have been proposed (see Chapter 13) but these have not been validated or widely applied.

To further complicate decision making, the variables upon which clinical case formulations and treatment decisions are based can change over time. The behavior problems of a client

Table 3-2

Interrelated Sources of Error in Clinical Judgment (with a Focus on Pretreatment Judgments)

Errors and deficiencies associated with the assessment strategy

1. A failure to measure important behavior problems and causal variables for a client
2. A failure to focus on important facets of behavior problems and causal variables (e.g., focusing on cognitive but not behavioral facets of depression)
3. A failure to measure dynamic variables frequently across time or situations (basing judgments of a dynamic variable on a single measure)
4. Obtaining invalid data (e.g., use of assessment instruments that are not validated for the population or assessment goal for which they are applied)
5. Obtaining trivial information (e.g., data on unimporant variables can diminish the impact of data on important variables)
6. Failure to obtain information that is situationally specific or that reflects the conditional nature of behavior problems
7. A failure to use multiple sources of information (e.g., multiple informants, multiple instruments)
8. Use of a limited set of narrowly focused assessment instruments (e.g., monomethod)

Problems with the integration of conflicting data

1. A failure to reconcile or evaluate conflicting data collected from different informants, instruments, or assessment occasions

Making invalid judgments from valid measures

1. Overemphasizing data that confirms the clinician's a priori hypotheses
2. Misestimating conditional probabilities and covariance between variables (not detecting important functional relations; covariation misestimation [Arkes, 1981]; overestimating or underestimating the correlation between variables)
3. Construction of a clinical case formulation that is inconsistent with obtained information
4. Overestimating the likelihood of low probability events (e.g., not attending to local base rates of a diagnostic category when making diagnostic judgments)
5. Bounded rationality: Errors associated with the difficulties in integrating complex arrays of data (Nezu & Nezu, 1989)

Errors associated with the clinician's biases

1. Selective attention and unwarranted importance ascribed to some variables because of the clinician's recent training experiences, workshops, and clinical experiences (e.g., the "availability heuristic")
2. An overemphasis of "internal" causes and making circular causal attributions (e.g., attributing causal properties to "intrapsychic conflicts," personality dispositions, or diagnostic categories)
3. Judgments excessively and too quickly affected by initial impressions of the client (premature judgments about a client's problems, causal variables, best treatment approaches; "anchoring heuristic")
4. Judgments excessively affected by diagnostic information (insufficient recognition of the important differences among persons with the same diagnosis)
5. Inflexibility of judgments (e.g., judgments held too rigidly in the face of contradictory data)
6. Univariate and causal models (e.g., presuming that a specific behavior problem has a specific cause; a failure to consider multiple causal factor and causal mechanisms and a failure to consider differences in causality among persons with the same behavior problems; "oversimplification")
7. Premature schema referral (e.g., assuming that a person with some depressive behaviors will exhibit all behaviors associated with the depression syndrome; a "representative heuristic")
8. Causal presuppositions (assuming that an adult with significant interpersonal difficulties experienced an abusive childhood environment)
9. Minimax principle (judgments are based on minimizing the worst outcome [Elstein, 1988])
10. Judgments that are inappropriately influenced by the age, sex, sexual orientation, disability status, and ethnicity of the client
11. Confusing salience with utility (an excessive focus on important but unmodifiable variables, such as early trauma)
12. Overconfidence in the validity of one's judgments

Based on Dumont & Lecomte, 1987; Einhorn, 1988; Elstein, 1988; Garb, 1998 Groth-Marnat, 1997; Haynes, 1992; Kanfer & Schefft, 1988; Kleinmuntz, 1990; Nezu & Nezu, 1989; Tallent, 1992; Turk & Salovey, 1989; Weist, Finney, & Ollendick, 1992)

Box 3-2
Professional Training and Clinical Judgment

Professional training workshops promote a particular orientation to assessment and treatment. However, professional training does not necessarily enhance the validity of assessment, case formulations, and treatment decisions of participants. Some professional training workshops are not conducted within a hypothesis-testing, scholarly ambience, but assume an advocacy ambience. Workshops can strengthen a scholarly approach to the discipline to the degree that they also acknowledge areas of needed research and limitations on inferences that can be drawn.

Training workshops, practitioners' guidebooks, and clinical seminars probably increase judgment biases to the degree that they (a) are not empirically based, (b) function to "promote" rather than "examine" a strategy, (c) do not stress caveats and limitations associated with a strategy, and (d) do not emphasize a hypothesis-testing orientation to assessment and treatment.

can change in magnitude, frequency, and importance; the social contingencies and antecedent stimuli that affect a behavior problem can change; new behavior problems can be identified during the assessment-treatment process, unexpected and abrupt changes can occur in the client's environment, and a client's treatment goals can change during the assessment-treatment process.

In summary, there are many possible errors in clinical judgment. Some judgment errors result from mistakes in the original assessment strategies. Other judgment errors result from difficulties inherent in integrating complex arrays of assessment data. Errors can also be attributed to the clinician's biases. All types of errors can be reduced with an adherence to the basic principles of the behavioral assessment paradigm—more thoughtful, empirically based assessment strategies and a more systematic approach to integrating assessment data.

Oversimplification Strategies and Clinical Judgments

Ideally, clinical judgments are guided by careful integration of valid measures from carefully designed assessment strategies. However, there are few empirically supported

Box 3-3
Bias in Clinical Judgment

Bias refers to a systematic, nonrandom error in clinical judgments. Similar to the concept of "bias" in statistics (Vogt, 1993), a biased judgment reliably differs from an expected judgment. One may overestimate the magnitude of depression or aggression in female compared to male clients, or underestimate the intellectual functioning in older compared to younger adults.

A *source of bias* is the variable associated with this systematic deviation. Clinical judgments should covary most strongly with the relevant characteristics of the client. Judgments are biased when they covary to an unwarranted degree with irrelevant characteristics, the age, sex, or ethnicity of the client, or a priori causal models of the assessor. Biases are probably unavoidable in most clinical judgments but can be reduced if the assessor has identified potential sources of bias and attempts to moderate those dispositions.

methods available to the clinician for organizing multivariate assessment data to facilitate valid clinical judgments. Consequently, when confronted with complex, incomplete, or inconsistent assessment data it is logical for clinicians to use *oversimplification strategies*. With oversimplification strategies clinical judgments are rendered without integrating the available assessment data. To facilitate the judgments, the clinician discards part of the available data and bases clinical judgments on a subset of data. Unfortunately, oversimplification strategies increase the chance of biased or erroneous judgments.

Dumont and Lecomte (1987), Garb (1998), Kleinmuntz (1990), Nezu and Nezu (1988), and Table 3-2 describe many oversimplification strategies. Examples of oversimplification strategies that may limit the validity of clinical judgments include basing judgments on a single salient feature of a client, deriving causal inferences about a client's behavior problems based on a priori beliefs, presuming that there is an invariant single cause for a behavior disorder, basing treatment plans only on a client's diagnosis, and drawing clinical inferences prematurely and from initial impressions.

Many oversimplification strategies are in response to the *bounded rationality* of clinicians. The idea of "bounded rationality" suggests that clinicians are limited in the complexity of information that they can effectively synthesize. Because of memory and information processing limitations (Kareken & Williams, 1994), it is difficult for most clinicians to weight and integrate hundreds of bits of assessment data to derive the complex clinical case formulations that guide treatment decisions. To overcome these deficiencies, clinicians often reduce the amount of information upon which decisions are based; they select a small subset of data (e.g., psychiatric diagnosis) or use arbitrarily invoked decision-making rules.

There are many examples of oversimplification strategies in clinical judgment. One common strategy is to expose all clients with a particular behavior problem to the same treatment protocol, such as exposing all distressed couples to dyadic communication training, or assigning all depressed patients to cognitive therapy for automatic negative thoughts. This "prescriptive" treatment strategy (e.g., Acierno, Hersen, & Van Hasselt, 1998; Hersen & Ammerman, 1994) reduces the necessity of integrating, in the examples noted, observation and self-report data on dyadic communication patterns, of determining the causal role of communication difficulties, of identifying the specific communication difficulties of each couple prior to treatment, and of examining the causal relation between automatic negative thoughts and depressed mood. The oversimplification strategy of assigning all persons with a similar behavior problem to the same treatment protocol presumes that a classification of a client into a behavior problem category is sufficient to determine the most appropriate treatment strategy.

Another oversimplification strategy is to presume that a behavior problem is invariably associated with a single cause, such as presuming that depressed mood is always a function of irrational beliefs or dysfunctions in neurotransmitter systems. Presuming that all clients with depressed mood have irrationally negative beliefs about themselves and that these beliefs trigger depressed moods is an oversimplification because it limits the amount of information that must be collected and integrated. This presumption decreases the importance of information on social interactions, and other cognitive, biological, and learning factors. Univariate causal models also make it unnecessary to integrate assessment data on multiple variables into a clinical case formulation to design an individualized intervention program.

Assessment strategies can also be oversimplified by relying on a limited array of sources of information. An example would be the use of a standardized "battery" with every client (e.g., an intake interview, WAIS, and MMPI). This strategy limits the amount and type of information that the assessor must integrate to make a judgment.

Other examples of oversimplification strategies include: presuming that a self-injurious behavior of a child with developmental disabilities is maintained by positive or negative reinforcement (without testing the validity of that presumption); placing a psychiatric inpatient on a medication regime solely on the basis of a diagnosis; presuming (without supporting evidence) that an adult client's history of neglect by his or her parents is an important cause of the client's social difficulties.

Oversimplification strategies are attractive. First, they limit the amount of data that the clinician must integrate. This can help address the difficulties with integrating large amounts of information. However, reducing the amount of information can increase bias in clinical judgments because those judgments can be swayed to an inappropriate degree to a few sources of information.

Second, judgments can be generated more quickly, more reliably, and with greater confidence (remember not to confuse reliability with validity). The increasing use of oversimplification strategies by a clinician across time may partially account for the finding that clinical experience often increases the confidence in but not the validity of clinical judgments (Kareken & Williams, 1994; see general discussion Garb, 1998; Kleinmuntz, 1990; Nezu & Nezu, 1989). For example, Kleinmuntz (1990) noted that increased confidence in clinical decisions is associated with subjectively overweighting the importance of confirming, and underweighting the importance of disconfirming, evidence. Additionally, incorrect decisions are less likely to be detected by clinicians when limited data are collected (see Box 3-4).

Finally, oversimplification strategies are enticing because they promise more cost-efficient clinical judgments. Examples of enticements to oversimplification strategies in clinical judgment often appear in ads in the APA *Monitor*. For example, there are many ads for short questionnaires that help the assessor quickly estimate intellectual functioning, children's behavior problems, make child custody recommendations, or generate "quick" treatment plans.

Box 3-4
Colinearity of Obtained Measures and Clinical Judgment

Two measures are *colinear* to the degree that they are highly correlated. The use of assessment instruments that provide colinear measures (e.g., measures that are correlated above .8 or .9) fail to increase the validity of clinical judgment in several ways. First, the use of colinear measures reduces the amount of new information that a measure contributes to clinical judgment because much of the information obtained from one instrument is redundant with information obtained from the other. Therefore, the *cost-effectiveness* of an assessment strategy is reduced if instruments with highly correlated measures are used. In this case one instrument could be omitted without significantly reducing the amount of information acquired.

The instruments used in assessment should be those that measure important variables in the most valid and efficient manner. This can most easily be accomplished by careful selection of instruments that incrementally contribute to clinical judgments. Collecting additional measures on a client is useful only to the degree that they help estimate important variables and relations and do so better than extant measures.

Colinearity is most often a problem with monomethod assessment strategies focused on a narrow range of variables. Two self-report measures of depressed mood are more likely to be colinear (if based on the same model of depression) than are measures derived from different methods and from different informants.

Whatever their potential assets, most oversimplification strategies can decrease the validity of clinical judgments. Validity impairment occurs because any source of error in the measures upon which decisions are based are undetected and unmoderated by other measures. There may be an "illusion of enhanced validity" because judgments can be made more reliably when they are based on a more limited array of data. However, errors in the measures and inferences cannot easily be detected without collecting additional measures that can potentially conflict with the available data set.

Increasing the Validity of Clinical Judgments

Although intuitive judgments, biases, and oversimplified assessment strategies are unavoidable in many assessment situations, the validity of clinical judgments can often be strengthened by conducting assessment congruent with the principles of the behavioral assessment paradigm. The strategies for increasing the validity of clinical judgments differ across various goals and settings of assessment. The recommended strategies encompass the methodological components of the behavioral assessment paradigm, which are discussed throughout this book. For example, we suggest that clinical judgments are more likely to be valid when based on multiple and minimally inferential measures of well-specified behaviors and events.

In brief, we suggest that the validity of clinical judgments can be enhanced with the following strategies:

- *Use multiple methods of assessment, with multiple informants*: Multimethod and multi-informant assessment can help reduce the impact of systematic measurement error associated with a particular measurement method and informant. However, the use of multiple sources of information also involves risks. Clinicians should remember that the magnitude of agreement between different types of judges (e.g., parents, teachers, spouses, children) are often low to moderate. Furthermore, differences between informants may reflect true differences in the targeted phenomena or error by one or more informant. It is often difficult to appropriately assign weights to data from conflicting sources or to know if differential weighting is warranted.
- *Use a broadly focused and systems-level multivariate assessment strategy*: To increase the content validity of judgments, measure as many important behavior problems, causal variables, and moderating variables as feasible.
- *Use assessment instruments* validated for the target, population, and goal for which they will be applied.
- *Use a time-series assessment strategy*: Frequent measurement over time allows the assessor to track changes in important dependent and independent variables and in functional relations and strengthens inferences about dynamic phenomena.
- *Use direct, minimally inferential measures of the phenomena of interest*.
- *Use clearly defined criteria for judgments*: Precisely define the criteria for treatment success and termination.
- *Use clearly delineated procedures for judgments*: Precisely define the rules under which assessment data will be collected and criteria will be applied.
- *Use the empirical literature to guide assessment strategies*: Knowledge of the scholarly literature on assessment instruments and targeted behavior problems and causal vari-

ables increase the chance that valid instruments will be used to measure all important variables.

- *Avoid quick judgments*. Reflect on obtained measures, extant literature, assessment goals, possible sources of error.
- *Regard judgments as modifiable, conditional hypotheses, and refrain from unwarranted overconfidence in clinical judgments*. Clinical judgments are always conditional and they can change across time and situations.
- *Assume the role of a theoretical Theseus when examining data*:[2] Avoid selective weighting of data to conform to a particular theoretical model.
- *Examine the costs and benefits associated with judgment errors*: Often errors in one direction (e.g., including or excluding someone in a particular treatment group) will have different costs and benefits than errors in the other direction.
- *Keep data on the accuracy or treatment utility of your clinical judgments*: This provides feedback about the validity of judgments and increases the chance that a clinician will make increasingly valid decisions with time.
- *Discuss clinical judgments with colleagues and supervisors to obtain feedback and alternative viewpoints*: Be humble and flexible in your judgments and remain open to feedback from others.
- *Use quantitative procedures and experiments* to test hypotheses whenever possible.

Quantitative Aids to Clinical Judgment

The reliability and validity of clinical judgments can sometimes be enhanced through quantitatively aided decision-making strategies and quantitative criteria (see Table 3-3). One example of a quantitative approach to clinical judgment is the use of quantitative criteria or formulae to draw inferences about the *"clinical significance"* of treatment effects (de Beurs et al., 1994; Jacobson & Truax, 1991; Nietzel & Trull, 1988; Tingey, Lambert, Burlingame, & Hansen, 1996). For example, Michelson (1986) judged the level of functioning of clients with agoraphobia, before and after treatment, from: (a) the degree of behavioral performance and magnitude of self-reported distress during a behavioral avoidance test, (b) clinician ratings (on a five-point scale) of functioning, and (c) client self-rating of phobia severity, anxiety, and associated avoidance behaviors. He also used multiple informants and multiple methods to derive data for these estimates. Such a clearly specified, quantitatively based approach to clinical judgment reduces the chance that judgments about treatment success will be influenced by superfluous or erroneous phenomena or clinician biases; it enhances the reliability of clinical judgments across time, clinicians, and clients.

Another example of a quantitative approach to clinical inference is the use of *time-series regression analysis* to estimate causal relations. For example, in a study by Hazlett and Haynes (1992), 11 patients with a chronic pain disorder monitored their sleep patterns, pain symptoms, and stressors daily for 60 days. After correcting for autocorrelation in data sets, time-lagged regression analyses indicated that the magnitude of pain symptoms was significantly correlated with daily stress levels for four patients. These quantitatively based causal inferences could be helpful in designing treatment programs. With additional assessment data supporting hypothe-

---

[2]In Greek mythology, Theseus was the slayer of Polypemon (known as Procrustes) who stretched or amputated protruding parts of unwary travelers so that they fit his bed. The clinician should imprecate against the tendency to selectively attend to data that confirm and selectively disregard data that disconfirm his or her theories. (Unfortunately for this analogy, Theseus resorted to the same treatment of Polypemon.)

Table 3-3
Quantitatively Aided Strategies for Clinical Judgment

Strategy	Description	Representative References
Quantitatively based judgments of clinical significance of treatment outcome	Judgments of the clinical significance of a treatment are based on distributions of scores from functional and dysfunctional groups, standard deviations of change, impact ratings	Jacobson & Truax, 1992 Tingley et al., 1996
Functional analytic clinical case models	Estimates of the effects of modifying causal variables for a client's behavior problems	Haynes, Leisen, & Blaine, 1997
Predictive power/ sensitivity	Estimates the probability that a client with a particular score has a particular disorder and the probability of accurately identifying clients with a particular disorder	Kraemer, 1992
Shared variance estimates	Estimates of shared variance (obtainable from multiple assessment strategies) to help identify important functional relations	Haynes, Richard, & Kubany, 1995
Use of norms	Use of empirically derived norms to describe the level of functioning and degree of impairment of a client	Garb, 1998
Use of base rates	Use of information about the expected probability of an event or problem to estimate its likelihood with a client	Garb, 1998
Statistical decision-making rules	Use of linear and nonlinear combinations of measures to estimate an event (usually a diagnostic category)	Wiggins, 1973
Use of cut scores	Use of predetermined scores from an assessment instrument as the basis for judgments about a person	Dwyer, 1996

sized stress-pain relations, stress management training might be suggested for some patients and not for others.

All quantitative approaches to clinical judgments have the same purpose—to increase the validity of clinical judgments. However, all quantitative approaches to clinical judgment have subjective elements. For example, inferences of clinically significant treatment change are subjectively based: They have been inferred partially from a post-treatment client score of "1" or "2" on a nine-point self-report scale of symptom severity (Michelson et al., 1990) or a change in symptom indices of two standard deviations in a positive direction (Jacobson & Revenstorf, 1988). The magnitude of covariation that suggests a "strong" relation varies across studies and acceptable levels of sensitivity, and specificity in diagnostic applications of assessment instruments vary across diagnosticians, settings, and disorders. These criteria seem reasonable yet alternative criteria seem equally reasonable and result in reliable, valid, accurate, yet different, judgments.

The role of subjective judgment is reduced (except in the original selection of assessment instruments) in statistical prediction models, which are constructed backward. These begin with an available data set and establish parameters that result in the best predictions of data (Einhorn, 1988). For example, variables that predict the best outcome for a particular treatment can be selected through discriminant function or logistic regression analyses. If replicated, results from these studies can be used to help select those for whom a particular treatment might be most effective (see Box 3-5).

As with all aspects of assessment, the utility of quantification in clinical judgment is conditional. The clinician will be faced with many situations in which quick judgments are

---

Box 3-5
Clinical versus Statistical Prediction

Paul Meehl's book, *Clinical vs. Statistical Prediction: A Theoretical Analysis and Review of the Evidence*, advanced a thesis that statistical formulae were often more accurate than clinicians in predicting future and past behavior. His contention generated considerable and sometimes intense debate. However, his inferences were quite conditional in that he also addressed conditions in which clinical judgments might be aided by statistical methods and the types of research that might help identify the clinical judgment process and strategies for strengthening its validity. These issues have also been discussed by Tallent (1992) and by Meehl (1986).

---

necessary and data to aid clinical judgment will not be available. Many judgments are made within treatment sessions, such as an estimate of the probability that a patient will harm him- or herself or others, or a change in treatment plan because of some unintended effects. In other circumstances decisions regarding the magnitude of treatment outcome, the strength of causal relations, and diagnosis can be made more thoughtfully, but must be made without data such as norms, time-series regression coefficients, or conditional probability data analyses that would provide quantitative basis for the decisions. At other times, the unique characteristics of a particular client may suggest that the formulae be overridden.

Problems in the use of quantitative aids to clinical judgments were illustrated by Dwyer (1996). Although "cut scores" (e.g., an a priori designation of a score indicative of a diagnosis or indicative of significant change) were used to increase the reliability of clinical judgments, the original selection of a cut score entails a judgment that must depend on other measures. Furthermore, Dwyer noted that cut scores impose a dichotomy on nondichotomous measures and always result in some clients being misclassified.

Given these caveats, the most important contribution of quantitative aids to clinical judgment is that they reduce one major source of error: Quantitative aids reduce clinician biases and inconsistencies across judges and across time for a particular judge. The results of formulae do not vary with the clinician's recent training or clinical experiences, variable weights do not differ across assessment situations, the results do not reflect the biases of individual clinicians, and formulae can be applied with data sets that are too complex for intuitive analysis.

Summary

Behavioral assessment is a functional approach to psychological assessment—the methods, instruments, strategies, focus, and product of behavioral assessment are determined by the function of each assessment occasion. In functional psychological assessment the questions addressed on each assessment occasion determine the variables measured, the methods and instruments used to measure them, and the sampling strategies employed. A functional approach also emphasizes direct measures of minimally inferential variables.

Clinical judgments are predictions, inferences, or decisions about a client. They are inferences that affect the evaluation or treatment of a client or other services that the client will receive. Data from psychological assessment provide information to enhance the soundness of clinical judgments. Clinical judgments are particularly important when they affect the type of intervention designed for a client and the specific elements of that intervention. Hypotheses about the causal variables that affect a client's problem behaviors and goals are particularly important determinants of intervention program design.

There are few empirically based guidelines for making data-based clinical judgments and almost no guidelines for designing intervention programs. The dearth of guidelines has encouraged the use of purely intuitive approaches to clinical judgment. There are many sources of error in clinical judgment: errors in the original selection of assessment strategies, conflicting assessment data, inferential errors from valid data, and errors associated with the clinician's biases. In addition, different assessment instruments may provide conflicting data and clinicians must often make important clinical judgments with insufficient or invalid data. Furthermore, a client's behavior problems and the matrix of causal relations can change.

Clinicians often cope with large and complex arrays of data by using oversimplification strategies. All oversimplification strategies, such as adoption of univariate causal models or tying treatment directly to diagnosis, address the bounded rationality of the clinician. To overcome limitations in reasoning abilities, clinicians limit the amount of information available for judgments or use decision-making rules that depend on only a small part of the available data. Although they can enhance reliability and sometimes validity of clinical judgments, many oversimplification strategies can enhance bias in clinical judgment.

The validity of clinical judgments can be enhanced by adopting an assessment strategy that involves the measurement of multiple variables, using multiple methods, from multiple sources. Validity of clinical judgments can also be enhanced using a time-series assessment strategy along with direct, validated measures. It is also helpful to use clearly defined criteria and procedures for judgments. Finally, clinicians should remain flexible in their hypotheses, seek consultation often, and maintain data on their clinical judgments.

One way to increase the reliability, accuracy, validity, and utility of clinical judgments is to use quantitative methods and criteria. This is designed to increase the degree to which clinical judgments are reliable across time and to which clinicians are accurate and valid.

Suggested Readings

Books and Articles on Clinical Judgment and Decision Making

Dawes, R. M., Faust, D., & Meehl, P. E. (1989). Clinical versus actuarial judgment. *Science, 243*, 1668–1673.

Garb, H. N. (1998). *Studying the clinician—Judgment research and psychological assessment.* Washington, DC: American Psychological Association.

Goldstein, W. M., & Hogarth, R. M. (Eds.). (1997). *Research on judgement and decision making: Currents, connections, and controversies.* New York: Cambridge University Press.

Kleinmuntz, B. (1990). Why we still use our heads instead of formulas: Toward an integrative approach. *Psychological Bulletin, 107*, 296–310.

Kraemer, H. C. (1992). *Evaluating medical tests—Objective and quantitative guidelines.* Beverly Hills, CA: Sage.

Mellers, B. A., Schwartz, A., & Cooke, A. D. J. (1998). Judgment and decision making. *Annual review of psychology, 49* (pp. 447–477). Palo Alto, CA: Annual Reviews.

Nezu, A. M., & Nezu, C. M. (1989). *Clinical decision making in behavior therapy: A problem-solving perspective.* Champaign, IL: Research Press

Turk, D. C., & Salovey, P. (Eds.). (1988). *Reasoning, inference, and judgment in clinical psychology.* New York: Free Press.

Special Series on Clinical Judgment and Decision Making

"Behavioral Assessment in the DSM Era"; A special series published in *Behavioral Assessment, 14(3–4)*, 1992.

"Clinical Applications of Psychological Assessment"; A special series published in *Psychological Assessment, 5(3)*, 1993.

"Selection of Target Behaviors"; A special series published in *Behavioral Assessment, 10(1)*, 1998.

"Research Contributions to Clinical Assessment"; A miniseries published in *Behavior Therapy, 25(4)*, 1994.

"Treatment Implications of Psychological Assessment"; A special section published in *Psychological Assessment, 9(4)*, 1997.

"The Use of Computers for Making Judgments and Decisions"; A special section edited by Howard Garb, published in *Psychological Assessment, 12(1)*, 2000.

4

Goals

Introduction

In Chapter 3 we discussed the conditional utility of the elements of the behavioral assessment paradigm: Behavioral assessment is a functional approach to assessment in that the utility of each element of the paradigm varies across assessment occasions. Utility is affected by many aspects of an assessment occasion, but it is particularly affected by the goals of the assessment.

The convergence of goals, principles, and methods of behavioral assessment exemplifies a functional approach to psychological assessment. The flexibility of the behavioral assessment paradigm means that it is applicable across a broad range of populations, behavior problems, settings, and goals. In particular, the paradigm helps the assessor to select the methods, strategies, and principles that are best suited for the particular goals of an assessment occasion.

In this chapter we examine the goals of behavioral assessment—the clinical and empirical judgments aided by information from behavioral assessment. We also discuss the relations among the goals, principles, and methods of assessment. Finally, we consider further the limitations of behavioral assessment. (Chapters by Barrios [1988] and Mash and Terdal [1997a] also provide overviews of the goals of behavioral assessment.)

We emphasize several points about the goals of behavioral assessment:

1. The goals of behavioral assessment at each assessment occasion influence the applicable principles of assessment and best strategies for assessment.
2. There are many immediate and intermediate goals in clinical assessment but a supraordinate goal is the development of a clinical case formulation to guide intervention foci and strategies.
3. The goals of behavioral assessment include the selection of a content-valid assessment strategy—a strategy in which the measures obtained are relevant and representative for the goals of assessment and the characteristics of the client.
4. The content validity of an assessment strategy will be strengthened to the degree that assessment instruments and methods validly sample all variables and relations relevant to the clinical judgments that must be made.
5. The assessor must decide if information from previous assessments and assistance from other professionals are needed.
6. An important goal in preintervention behavioral assessment is the development of a clinical case formulation, a functional analysis. This includes many intermediate goals involving the specification of behavior problems, treatment goals, causal variables, and functional relations.
7. The design of an intervention program is an important goal that is influenced by the functional analysis and other client, therapist, and environmental variables.
8. Clinical assessment is an ongoing process that continues during intervention.
9. Judgments about treatment effects are facilitated by the measurement of immediate and intermediate outcomes.
10. Client adherence, cooperation, and resistance include behaviors that help or impede the therapy process and are important assessment targets.
11. Client satisfaction can affect adherence to intervention programs.
12. Clinicians are often required to provide a psychiatric diagnosis, and behavioral assessment strategies can increase the reliability of those judgments.
13. Clients should be knowledgeable about all assessment strategies and goals.
14. Additional assessment targets are the client's knowledge, social environment, important life events, and cognitive abilities.

An Overview of the Goals of Behavioral Assessment

By "goal" of an assessment occasion, we are referring to the clinical judgments that are to be informed by the assessment information. There are many goals that correspond to the judgments outlined in Table 3-1, but the ultimate goal of many assessment occasions is to provide information that is useful for the design or evaluation of intervention programs. However, there are also immediate or intermediate goals, such as the identification of a client's behavior problems, or the identification of causal variables relevant to a client's behavior problems.

The goals of assessment are *dynamic*—they can change across assessment occasions for one client and can differ between clients. For example, the goal of assessment may be to provide information that will help the clinician estimate the risk that a client will harm him- or herself. In turn, this estimate can help the clinician decide if restrictions on the client's behavior are warranted. In another instance, the goal of assessment may be to identify automatic negative thoughts that trigger a client's depressed mood in response to a distressing environmental event. Finally, a clinician may want to estimate the degree to which a child's disruptive classroom behavior is affected by response-contingent attention from teachers. Each of these goals are elements in a chain that approach the ultimate goal of the assessment—each provides information helpful in the selection of the best intervention strategy for the client (see Box 4-1).

These examples reiterate our earlier comments about the reciprocal relations among assessment goals, principles, and methods. Behavioral observation in the natural environment and time-series measurement are more important when the goal of assessment is to detect environmental contingencies for disruptive classroom behavior. Structured behavioral observation is less important when the goal of assessment is to estimate the risk of suicide. Similarly, the measurement of multiple response modes is important when the goal of assessment is to develop a clinical case formulation for a client's persistent sleep difficulties following a trauma.

Box 4-1
Task Analysis as a Goal in Psychological Assessment

In Chapter 3 we promoted a functional approach to assessment, one component of which is an emphasis on direct assessment of behavior. **Task analysis** (sometimes called task decomposition) is an example of such an approach.

Assessment specialists in personnel selection, educational psychology, neuropsychology, and developmental disabilities often use a task analysis to identify chains of specific skills and processes necessary to successfully perform a task. Following a decomposition of the task, assessment methods are selected to evaluate a client's performance on those components.

In behavior analysis (Martin & Pear, 1996) the task of toothbrushing for a child with developmental disabilities might be decomposed into components such as holding a toothbrush, placing toothpaste on the brush, and the appropriate hand movements. Assessment would focus on the child's performance of the individual components to decide at what point in the chain intervention was needed.

Personnel selection often involves the measurement of specific abilities necessary for a particular job, rather than the measurement of global traits (Cascio, 1991; Murphy & Cleveland, 1995).

Educational measurement specialists (e.g., Ebel & Frisbie, 1991) often identify specific educational objectives and then select assessment instruments to measure the degree to which students attained those objectives.

It is less important when the goal of assessment is to develop a clinical case formulation for a child's feeding problems.

On some assessment occasions, the goals and methods of behavioral assessment remain consistent across clients. For example, the effects of a social skills training program on a psychiatric unit can be evaluated with the same set of assessment instruments (e.g., staff members' participant observation of delusional speech, measures of cognitive/intellectual functioning) for all patients. Similarly, the strengths and deficits in social skills of children in a classroom for students with developmental disabilities can be evaluated with a standard assessment battery. In these assessment contexts, the methods are similar across assessment occasions because the goals are similar.

Table 4-1 outlines some important goals of behavioral assessment, many of which correspond to the functions of behavioral assessment introduced in Chapter 2. These goals reflect clinical judgments that must be made by psychologists, social workers, educators, psychiatrists, psychiatric nurses, and other behavioral health specialists, and are discussed in greater detail in subsequent sections of this chapter.

Table 4-1

An Overview of the Outcome Goals of Behavioral Assessment

1. Supraordinate Goal: To increase the validity of clinical judgments.
2. Selection of Assessment Strategies (e.g., one goal of initial intake interviews is the selection of analogue observation situations and time-sampling measurement strategies, and questionnaires to be used in subsequent assessment occasions).
3. Determine if Consultation and Referral Are Appropriate (e.g., to determine if consultation with a pediatrician is appropriate in the assessment of a family who is experiencing behavior problems with their medically fragile child).
4. Development of a Clinical Case Formulation
    A. The identification of behavior problems and their interrelations.
    B. The identification of causal variables and their interrelations.
5. Design of Intervention Programs
    A. The identification of client intervention goals and strengths.
    B. The identification of variables that moderate intervention effects (e.g., client social support, strengths, limitations, additional life stressors).
    C. Assessment of client knowledge about goals, problems, interventions.
    D. Evaluation of medical complications that might affect intervention process or outcome.
    E. Potential side effects of intervention.
    F. Acceptability of an intervention to the client.
    G. Time and financial constraints of the client and therapist.
6. Intervention Process Evaluation
    A. Evaluation of intervention adherence, cooperations, and satisfaction.
    B. Evaluation of client-therapist interaction and rapport.
7. Intervention Outcome Evaluation (immediate, intermediate, and ultimate intervention goals)
8. Diagnosis (although diagnosis is de-emphasized, behavioral assessment strategies can be used to increase the validity of information upon which diagnosis is based).
9. Predicting Behavior (e.g., to estimate the risk that a client will harm himself or herself)
10. Informed Consent (to inform clients and other participants about the strategies, goals, and rationale for assessment).
11. Nonclinical Goals
    A. Theory development (e.g., evaluating learning models for behavior problems).
    B. Assessment instrument development and evaluation.
    C. Development and testing causal models of behavioral disorders.

Specific Goals of Behavioral Assessment

The Supraordinate Goal of Behavioral Assessment: To Increase the Validity of Clinical Judgments

As we emphasized in Chapter 3, the supraordinate goal of behavioral assessment is to increase the validity of clinical judgments, particularly judgments about the clinical case formulation and intervention effects. These are the higher-order goals of most assessment occasions and provide a context for the more specific immediate and intermediate goals discussed in this chapter.

In Chapter 3 we also noted that the validity of clinical judgments can be strengthened through several strategies: (a) the specification and measurement, to the greatest extent possible, of all behaviors, variables, and functional relations relevant for a client; (b) the reduction of measurement error and bias; (c) the use of valid and applicable assessment instruments; (d) an emphasis on the assessment of behavior and contemporaneous causal variables in the natural environment; and (e) the adoption of a scholarly, empirically guided, hypothesis-testing approach to psychological assessment. These can be regarded as "methodological goals" that help the assessor achieve several outcome goals, as outlined in Table 4-1. In the following sections we discuss several outcome goals of behavioral assessment.

The Selection of an Assessment Strategy

Early in the clinical assessment process, usually before the end of the first assessment session, the clinician must select the assessment strategies (e.g., the specific assessment instruments) that are most likely to provide valid information, efficiently, on the variables and functional relations potentially relevant to the client's behavior problems. For example, with a client seeking assistance for marital difficulties, the clinician must decide if the spouse should be involved in the assessment process—perhaps, to participate in a conjoint marital interview and analogue communication assessment to help identify problem-solving difficulties or goal conflicts. With this client the assessor would also decide if other problems (e.g., depressed mood, increased use of alcohol) are functionally related to marital distress and should be assessed. Also, the assessor would decide if self-monitoring (e.g., of positive exchanges with the spouse) and marital questionnaires might provide useful information (see overview of marital assessment in Floyd, Haynes, & Kelly, 1997; O'Leary, 1987).

Decisions regarding the assessment strategy to use with a client can affect the clinician's subsequent clinical judgments because these early decisions affect the information upon which the clinician's subsequent judgments will be based. If dyadic exchanges have not been observed in a structured assessment situation, a clinician is less likely to recommend communication training with a couple even though they are experiencing communication problems.

Content Validity of an Assessment Strategy

The validity of clinical inferences is affected by the **content validity** of the assessment strategy. The concept of "content validity" is most often applied to the development and initial evaluation of assessment instruments. It is *the degree to which elements of an assessment instrument are relevant to and representative of the targeted construct* (Haynes, Richard, & Kubany, 1995; see Glossary). In reference to an assessment strategy, content validity refers to the degree to which the measures obtained are relevant and representative for the goals of assessment and the characteristics of the client.

In the example of a client with marital problems, content validity of the assessment strategy would be limited to the degree that the assessor failed to assess marital communication patterns, or failed to determine if there were cooccurring behavior problems, such as depressed mood or substance use. With these omissions, the information obtained would not tap the range of problems and causal variables relevant to that client. Similarly, the inclusion of instruments that provided information not relevant to the client or the goals of assessment (e.g., information from projective assessment on intrapsychic defense mechanisms) would also compromise the content validity of the assessment strategy.

The stress on the content validity of an assessment strategy reemphasizes the functional and conditional nature of the behavioral assessment. Assessment instruments vary across clients and assessment goals in the degree to which they provide relevant and appropriate information. Thus, an instrument may strengthen or weaken content validity of an assessment strategy, depending on the conditions of the assessment (see Box 4-2).

Because the supraordinate goal of clinical assessment is to enhance the validity of clinical judgments, it is important to select the assessment instruments that provide the most valid measure of the targeted variables and to apply these instruments at appropriate intervals and situations. For example, if the ultimate goal of assessment is to design an intervention program for an adolescent exhibiting severe oppositional and antisocial behaviors, assessment information based only on the self-report of the adolescent would have a low degree of content validity. Self-report measures are important assessment methods but because of potential bias, they are unlikely to adequately sample the domain of adolescent antisocial behaviors and potential causal variables. The adolescent may provide biased data and important functional relations may escape detection. Additionally, important behavior problems (e.g., stealing, lying, excessive use of alcohol, discomfort in social situations) and some important causal relations (e.g., peer approval) may not accurately be reported. The content validity of the assessment could be enhanced if the adolescent self-reports were augmented with parent reports, teacher reports, record review, and role-play assessment.

In another example, an assessment strategy for developing a clinical case formulation for a client with PTSD that omitted measures of trauma-related guilt or avoidance behaviors (Wilson & Keane, 1997) would have limited content validity because recent research has documented the importance of these variables as symptoms of, and maintaining variables for, PTSD among some persons. In these examples, the assessment strategies would be insufficient

---

Box 4-2
Assessment Instruments Differ in the Degree
to Which They Measure Different Facets of a Targeted Construct

One reason that assessment instruments must be carefully selected to match the goal of assessment for each occasion is that the measures from different assessment instruments that purport to measure the same construct have different meanings. For example, different "depression" self-report questionnaires provide measures that differ in the degree to which they reflect cognitive, mood, psychophysiological, and behavioral response modes of depression. Additionally, the aggregated scores from these instruments (i.e., scale scores, total score) often differ in the facets of depression that they most strongly reflect.

to gather valid data on variables and relations that were important for drawing clinical inferences about the causes and treatment of a client's behavior problems.

To summarize, the content validity of an assessment strategy can be compromised in several ways:

- Invalid assessment instruments can be used, in which case the information derived is not relevant to, and may undermine, clinical judgments.
- Validated assessment instruments can be applied inappropriately (e.g., using measures from a questionnaire validated only as a general screening instrument to help develop a clinical case formulation of a depressed client).
- Data relevant to important settings may not be acquired (e.g., interpersonal problems at school vs. home).
- Potentially important variables may not be measured.

Table 4-2 outlines several ways to increase the content validity of a clinical assessment strategy. These recommendations should be familiar to the reader: Many overlap with the factors discussed in the first three chapters that influence the validity of clinical judgments.

Standardized assessment strategies are sometimes used when the goal of assessment is consistent across clients. For example, one goal of assessment at a center serving children with developmental disabilities may be to evaluate the effects of a social reinforcement program for strengthening self-help behaviors. Standardized assessment protocols in such settings can be useful and have a high degree of content validity if they facilitate inferences about causal models and intervention effects for groups of clients with similar problems or intervention goals.

However, even in settings where the goals of assessment are the same and clients are similar on important dimensions, the most content-valid assessment strategy may differ across clients. Therefore, individualized assessment strategies may be necessary for many clients.

Table 4-2
Increasing the Content Validity of an Assessment Strategy

1. Use valid assessment instruments. (Assessment instruments should be validated for the population, situation, and purpose for which it is being applied.)
2. Use assessment instruments that are congruent with the goals of assessment. (Assessment instruments should specifically measure those behaviors and variables that are most important and provide information of greatest use for the clinical judgments that must be made.)
3. Measure all hypothesized important dependent and independent variables. (e.g., main behavior problems, intervention adherence, positive alternatives to negative target behaviors, potential intervention side effects, intervention goals.)
4. Measure the most important dimensions of the behavior problems and causal variables (e.g., frequency, intensity, duration of variables).
5. Measure important facets of behavior problems and causal variables (e.g., cognitive, behavioral, emotional, psychophysiological facets of anxiety disorders).
6. Use multiple methods of assessment.
7. Gather data from multiple informants (e.g., parents, staff, siblings, spouses, teachers, family members).
8. Use instruments that are sensitive to the dynamic aspects of behavior problems and causal variables.
9. Measure behavior in relevant settings (e.g., home and school settings when assessing an aggressive child; different social situations with assessing a socially anxious adult).
10. Let the research literature guide assessment decisions. (Prior research can help select which variables to measure and which assessment instruments to use.)

For example, assessment strategies may differ across clients as a function of the characteristics of the client's behavior problems, of the client's social environment, and of cooccurring behavior problems. Parent observations of a child in the home may be a valid and useful source of data on a child who lives at home and when there are cooperative parents who have the time to monitor their children's behavior. Analogue observations of the child in a clinic or reports from staff may be more useful and valid when the child is embedded in a chaotic home, institutional, or foster-care environment. As we will discuss in Chapter 6, the content validity of an assessment strategy can sometimes be strengthened by using both standardized and individualized strategies.

A "Funnel" Approach to Selecting an Assessment Strategy

A "funnel" approach may be most helpful in selecting assessment methods and targets with a client (e.g., Hawkins, 1986; Mash & Hunsley, 1990; Ollendick & Hersen, 1993b). The assessment process begins with broadly focused assessment instruments to scan the array of possible behavior problems, causal variables, and other important variables. Assessment methods at this early stage might include problem-survey questionnaires and broadly focused structured interviews. As the clinician forms hypotheses about the client's most important behavior problems, more focused instruments are selected to specify and quantify each problem (books by Hersen and Bellack 1988 and Corcoran and Fischer, 1987; present general behavior problems survey instruments). Finally, causal variables and functional relations are identified and specified for each problem.

A case presented in Floyd, Haynes, and Kelly (1997) illustrates a funnel approach to assessment. Nancy, a 36-year-old professional woman, was self-referred and initially interviewed in an unstructured format. One goal of the initial interview was to identify an array of concerns, goals, and behavior problems. Although she reported episodes of depressed mood, marital distress, and excessive alcohol use, a particularly important concern was the increasing frequency and severity of her ritualistic self-injury. A semi-structured interview then focused on further specifying her self-injurious behaviors and possible causal factors. She had been lightly cutting her arms with razor blades several times per month, for about 10 years but the rate and intensity of self-cutting had been increasing in recent months. The cutting had been described as superficial and painless, usually 10 to 15 minor cuts across her forearms, until recently when her cuts were deeper and more frequently inflicted (average 2 to 4 times per week). Important social and emotional consequences (e.g., attention, reduction of negative mood) and precipitating situations (e.g., interpersonal conflict) were identified.

Marital assessment was indicated when she reported that marital arguments were a frequent trigger for self-injury episodes, and that the quality of her marriage was another concern. The assessment strategy then evolved to a more specific focus on the marital relationship, using structured interviews and questionnaires with her and her husband. Significant communication and problem-solving difficulties were identified and hypothesized to serve as moderator variables for her self-injury. Assessment then focused even more narrowly on dyadic problem-solving communication abilities, using structure analogue communication exercises, specific communication questionnaires, and self-monitoring of problem-solving interactions at home.

In summary, the strategies used in the assessment of a client affect the information obtained and subsequent clinical judgments. The content validity of an assessment strategy is the degree to which the measures obtained are relevant and representative for the judgments that are to be made. The content validity of an assessment strategy will be strengthened to the degree that assessment instruments and methods validly sample all variables and relations relevant to the clinical judgments that must be made and 10 strategies were presented for increasing the content validity. A "funnel" approach may be helpful in selecting the most appropriate assessment methods and targets with a client.

Determining the Need for Assessment Consultation and Referral

Two goals early in the assessment process are (a) to determine if information from previous assessments is needed, and (b) to determine if assistance will be needed from other professionals.

Obtaining Prior Assessment Records

Information from previous assessments can sometimes aid in the development of a clinical case formulation. Information may be available from school records, hospital records, and the records of previous clinical assessors and therapists. Records from prior assessments can be particularly helpful in identifying behavior problems, the time-course of the behavior problem, possible triggering and maintaining factors, and variables that might moderate intervention outcome.

There are many sources of error in historical assessment information, and inferences from them should be drawn cautiously. To illustrate, psychiatric hospital records can be very useful to a case formulation, but the bases of some information and observations upon which inferences in the records are based may be unclear. Also, important events may not be noted when hospital staff members are busy or when their interpretation of the same behaviors differ. Many historical records also fail to describe functional relations—they describe behavior problems but fail to describe the situations in which they occur, contextual factors, chains of events, or response contingencies.

The integration of historical information with contemporary assessment information can aid clinical judgments, but the degree to which judgments are influenced by the historical information should depend on the validity and relevance of the information.

Historical assessment data should be interpreted in the context of:

- The characteristics of the assessors (e.g., training, supervision, familiarity with the client).
- The context of the assessment (e.g., frequency of assessment, situation in which assessment occurs).
- The methods of assessment (e.g., whether a diagnosis was based on unstructured interview or a structured and previously validated structured clinical interview, whether judgments about a client's behavior change were based on time samples or staff conferences).
- The reliability of inferences across multiple sources (e.g., confidence is increased in inferences from historical data when there is a concurrence among independent assessors or across assessment occasions, acknowledging that written records are sometimes influenced by prior written records).
- How long ago the information was obtained (consider the dynamic aspects of behavior problems and causal variables—is the information still applicable?).
- The state of the client when assessment occurred (e.g., medication state, time since a trauma).

The assessor should apply the same psychometric standards when drawing inferences from historical information that are applied to information from contemporaneous assessment. A primary concern is that clinical judgments will be adversely influenced by errors in prior assessments.

Seeking Consultation

Consultation with and referral to other professionals are often important components of psychological assessment. Most behavior problems can be the product of multiple causal paths involving multiple response systems and modalities. Consequently, referral and consultation with other professionals are mandated in cases where important determinants may be involved with a client's behavior problems that exceed the domain of competence of the assessor.

Failure to adopt a multidisciplinary approach can impair intervention outcome for some clients and adversely affect their health. Consider the consequences of a failure to seek consultation when assessing a child with genetically influenced severe developmental disabilities that include feeding and physical mobility problems. Consultation with other professionals is also necessary preceding interventions, such as diet or exercise programs, that may interact adversely with existing medical conditions.

Physical/medical examinations by qualified professionals are an important component of assessment for many behavior problems and disorders. Medical consultation is indicated for client with schizophrenic symptoms (Anderson, Vaulx-Smith, & Keshavan, 1994), erectile difficulties (Wincze & Carey, 1991), hypertension (McCann, 1987), headaches (Diamond & Dalessio, 1992), chronic pain (Turk & Melzack, 1992), sleep difficulties (Morin, 1993), developmental disabilities (Marcus & Schopler, 1993), and many other disorders that often have important medical components (see Gatchel & Blanchard, 1993).

Professionals vary in their degree of expertise across disorders. Consultations and referrals should occur only to professionals experienced with the targeted behavior problems. For example, sex therapists and researchers have often noted that many physicians are unfamiliar with current tests for possible neuroendocrine and peripheral circulatory and neurological causal factors for erectile dysfunction (see discussions in Wincze & Carey, 1991). In sum, select your consultants carefully!

Supplementary assessment data from other professionals can aid clinical judgments in many ways. For example, the evaluation of the severity, time-course, and response to a behavioral intervention of a client with rheumatoid arthritis can be aided with data on erythrocyte sedimentation rate and C-reactive protein (measures of rheumatoid disease activity) (Kraaimaat, Brons, Greenen, & Bijlsma, 1995). Without these data, the assessor must rely on client self-report measures of pain and mobility (see reviews of pain assessment in Turk & Melzack, 1992), which can also covary with social demands and social contingencies. Similarly, the effectiveness of behavioral intervention of localized tenderness and sensitivity to pressure or fibromyalgia patients can be evaluated with Dolorimeter measurements (Merskey & Spear, 1964). The specification of a client's sleep problems and the possible role of sleep apnea can be aided with polysomnography (see review in Riedel & Lichstein, 1994).

As indicated in Table 4-3, we recommend that the assessor seek consultation with other professionals any time information from the other professional would increase the validity of the clinical judgments. This incremental contribution is particularly likely when there is a behavior problem, potential causal or moderating variable, or source of individual difference (e.g., ethnicity, age, sexual orientation, sex) outside the assessor's training and expertise.

Consultation decisions are aided by a scholarly approach to psychological assessment. To

Table 4-3

Common Indications for Referral and Consultation During Preintervention Behavioral Assessment

1. The client has *medical conditions* that may contribute to his or her behavior problems or be affected by behavioral interventions.
2. *Medications* taken by the client may contribute to a client's behavior problems, affect assessment results, or affect the outcome of behavioral interventions.
3. The client has *neuropsychological dysfunctions* that may affect the design of intervention strategies.
4. The client has special *communication problems*.
5. The client has *learning difficulties* that may affect the design of intervention strategies.
6. There are other sources of *individual differences* (e.g., ethnicity, sexual orientation, religion, physical disability, sex, age) with which the assessor has had limited experience.
7. *Prior assessments* are available on variables targeted in or related to the current assessment.
8. Information is needed about a child's *developmental level* relative to other children.
9. The assessor is unfamiliar with *information from prior assessments* (e.g., the interpretation of serum analysis).
10. The client has *rare or severe behavior problems* with which the assessor has little experience.

know when to seek consultation, the assessor must (a) be familiar with the biomedical, psychological, and sociocultural literature pertinent to the client's behavior problems; (b) identify clients for whom biomedical or other factors outside the typical domain of psychological assessment are important; (c) understand possible interactions among multiple biological, psychological, and sociological variables; (d) identify medical and other professionals who are competent to conduct supplementary assessments; and (e) competently interpret the results of adjunctive assessments, with the aid of the consulting professional.

Consultation with other professionals is congruent with the ethical standards of most professional mental health organizations. It is also congruent with the scholarly, individualized, client-focused, and professionally respectful approach to clinical assessment advocated within the behavioral assessment paradigm. However, we repeat an important caveat in the use of information from other professionals: Data from other sources should be carefully scrutinized and evaluated with the same degree of skepticism and rigor applied to data collected by the behavioral assessor. Daily logs in hospital records can be completed by paraprofessionals who are unfamiliar with the client, unfamiliar with the client's intervention program, and untrained in basic observation and recording skills. All medical tests are amenable to measurement and inferential errors and are sometimes conducted in laboratories that have an unacceptable rate of error or contamination. The results from "standardized" assessment instruments (e.g., personality or cognitive-intellectual assessments) are sometimes compromised because they are administered in an unstandardized manner, in a shortened form, or by untrained persons. Consequently, the assessor should consider the degree of confidence that can be placed in the adjunctive data before forming clinical judgments based on that data.

The Development of a Clinical Case Formulation

A defining characteristic of the behavioral assessment paradigm and an important product of behavioral assessment is the ***clinical case formulation***. There are several strategies for developing a clinical case formulation. We focus on the functional analysis—*the identification of important, controllable, causal functional relations applicable to a specified set of target behaviors for an individual client* (Haynes & O'Brien, 1990). The functional analysis, like the models for clinical case conceptualizations of Persons (1989) and Nezu and Nezu (1989) and

Linehan (1993), is an integration of many clinical judgments. It emphasizes the specification of problem behaviors and intervention goals and the identification of important functional relations relevant to those problems and goals.

The importance of the clinical case formulation derives from its effect on intervention decisions. Behavioral interventions are often designed on the basis of hypothesized functional relations because the interventions are implemented to modify the variables that control the behavior problems or affect goal attainment. The clinical case formulation affects the clinician's decisions about which intervention strategies will be used with a client and the variables upon which those intervention strategies will focus.

We briefly introduced the clinical case formulation in Chapter 1, and it is the main focus of Chapter 13. As a primer, we introduce below some basic concepts of the functional analysis:

- The functional analysis is *idiographic*. A functional analysis reflects the estimated functional relations relevant for an individual client, and we cannot assume that the estimated functional relations are generalizable across clients with the same behavior problems.
- The functional analysis emphasizes *relations among causal variables and behavior problems*.
- Only some variables functionally related to a target behavior are *clinically useful*; only some will be *important*, *controllable*, and *causal*.
- A functional analysis can reflect a *constructional approach* to therapy. That is, a functional analysis can focus on functional relations relevant to intervention goals of a client, as well as the behavior problems of the client.
- A functional analysis usually involves *multiple response modes and multiple response dimensions*.
- A functional analysis is *a hypothesized model* of a client. It is a "best clinical judgment" based upon data available to the assessor.
- A functional analysis is *dynamic* and is likely to change over time, because changes can occur in behavior problems and causal variables or the assessor could acquire new information about the client.
- A functional analysis is *conditional*. A functional analysis may be valid for a client in some situations and client states and not in others.

In the following sections, we describe more specifically goals of behavioral assessment that are components of the functional analysis.

The Specification of Client Behavior Problems

The functional analysis centers on functional relations relevant to a client's behavior problems (sometimes called "target behaviors") (Hawkins, 1986), intervention goals, or alternatives to behavior problems. Consequently, the specification of a client's behavior problems is a major, and a deceptively complex, goal of behavioral assessment.

It can be difficult to identify and specify a client's behavior problems. Clients often seek psychological services for poorly defined concerns. Referrals of clients from family members or other professionals and staff can be equally ambiguous (e.g., consultation may be requested for a student who is not showing a "sense of responsibility," or a child who "gets frustrated easily"). The task of the assessor is to identify behavior problems with a degree of specificity that enables their measurement and facilitates clinical judgment about the best intervention strategy. Behavior problem specification may require the use of multiple assessment instruments and multiple sources of information.

The task of specifying a client's target behaviors is complicated in other ways as well: (a) the importance, components, and characteristics of behavior problems can change over time, (b) there may be conflicting information about behavior problems, and (c) many clients have multiple behavior problems. Despite these difficulties, behavior problem identification is usually the initial step in the clinical assessment process (see Chapter 8).

The Identification of Functional Response Classes

A *functional response class* is a group of different behaviors that have a similar relation with a controlling event. That is, a response class is composed of different behaviors that similarly affect the environment, are similarly influenced by the same antecedent events, or are similarly affected by the same contingencies. A critical characteristic of a functional response class is that the individual behaviors subsumed within it covary. For example, there are many different ways for a child to attract the attention of peers in a classroom (e.g., answering teacher questions, clothes selections, teasing other students); of injuring oneself (e.g., head banging, striking oneself with a fist); or of initiating intimate social interactions. Behaviors in these response classes may have different forms but they have similar effects.

Functional response classes can suggest positive alternatives to behavior problems. They help answer the question, "Are there better ways to achieve the effects of the undesirable behavior?" For example, Mark Durand (e.g., Durand & Carr, 1991) hypothesized that self-injurious behaviors sometimes have communicative functions and that self-injury may be reduced if the alternative methods of communicating are taught.

Second, functional response classes can help the assessor estimate difficult-to-assess behaviors. Because different behaviors in the response class covary, easy-to-assess behaviors can sometimes be used as estimates of difficult-to-assess behaviors. For example, we may not be able to directly observe (or collect other valid measures on) the effects of a parent training program on an adolescent's stealing. However, we may be able to measure change in correlated and observable behaviors, such as oppositional behaviors or verbal aggression.

The Specification of Client Goals and Resources

The identification of functional response classes is congruent with another important goal of behavioral assessment—the identification of positive intervention goals. Although we often discuss behavioral assessment in terms of identifying client behavior problems and their causes, behavioral assessment and intervention often assume a *constructional approach*. In a constructional approach to assessment, the goals of assessment are to identify the client's resources and strengths and, in particular, to identify and specify positive intervention goals. This is in contrast to a psychopathological or "positive symptom" orientation, which emphasizes identification of functional relations relevant to the reduction of behavior problems. For example, we may approach a client who is a psychiatric inpatient in terms of reducing his paranoid delusions. Alternatively, we may adopt a constructional approach and focus our assessment and intervention efforts on increasing valid appraisal or hypothesis testing with his social environment (see Table 4-4).

For most clients, intervention strategies involve both the reduction of undesirable behaviors and the initiation and strengthening of desirable behaviors (see discussion of constructional approaches in Evans, 1993a). Goals of intervention may be the reduction of elevated

Table 4-4
Elements of a Constructional Approach to Assessment

1. The identification and measurement of a client's *behavioral skills, strengths, and assets* (e.g., social skills, cognitive abilities, areas of expertise, self-management skills).
2. The identification of *resources in the client's social environment* (e.g., supportive family members, spouse, teachers, and friends who could help in therapy).
3. The identification of *positive alternatives to undesirable behaviors* (e.g., social communication alternatives to self-injurious behaviors).
4. The identification of other *positive intervention goals* (e.g., enhanced marital communication, more friendships, better sleep).
5. Measurement of goal attainment (e.g., use of Goal Attainment Scaling).
6. The identification of *reinforcing events and situations* (e.g., interests such as music, hobbies, physical activities).
7. The design of *positive intervention strategies* to help the client attain positive goals (rather than an intervention strategy to decrease behavior problems).

serum cholesterol levels, a reduction in alcohol intake, or fewer panic episodes. These may be necessary outcomes for effective intervention. However, these outcomes can often be facilitated by focusing on positive intervention goals, such as strengthening healthier eating habits, more effective coping strategies in stressful conditions, and more positive coping thoughts during panic episodes.

There are many advantages to a constructional emphasis in assessment. First, positive intervention goals may be more acceptable and elicit less discomfort for some clients and social agents (e.g., parents, staff). For example, a focus on communication skills may be more acceptable to parents of a child with developmental disabilities than would be a focus on reducing self-injurious behaviors. Second, a focus on the acquisition of positive behaviors, rather than the reduction in behavior problems, encourages the use of positive (e.g. response contingent positive reinforcement) rather than aversive (e.g., punishment, time-out) intervention procedures.

Third, a constructional approach can offer an alternative to the difficulties of measuring low-frequency behavior problems because a constructional approach can focus on the acquisition of higher-frequency alternative behaviors. Fourth, a constructional approach may alleviate some undesirable causal attribution problems (i.e., blame) associated with a behavior problem focus. For example, assessment can focus on ways to help a parent develop positive parenting skills, rather than focus on how the parent's behavior serves to maintain the child's behavior problems. Finally, a constructional approach reduces the importance of psychiatric diagnoses and labels and promotes individualized interventions.

The Specification of the Causal Variables and Causal Relations Relevant to a Client's Behavior Problems and Goals

Causal variables and relations are also an important component of the functional analysis and will be discussed in Chapters 9 and 10. Hypotheses about the causal relations applicable to a client's behavior problems and intervention goals affect decisions about assessment strategies, the focus of intervention, and relapse prevention. Causal hypotheses are particularly important because behavioral interventions are often designed to modify the presumed causes of a client's behavior problems.

For example, a client who was experiencing impairment in daily living because of chronic pain (Banks & Kerns, 1996; Hatch, 1993) might be taught how to use attentional focusing or positive self-statements if assessment results suggested that the client's thoughts about his or her pain strongly influenced the amount of subjective discomfort or the degree to which the pain disrupted the client's life. Alternatively, the intervention program for the same client might target sleeping difficulties or the responses of family members to pain complaints if preintervention assessment suggested an important pain-maintenance role for these variables.

Causal relations for a client's behavior problems or goals are difficult to specify. Causal effects can often be delayed in time, can change over time, can occur through multiple paths, and may not be accessible through client self-report or other efficient assessment methods. Acknowledging these difficulties, causal relations remain a cardinal component of the functional analysis and an important determinant of the focus of intervention.

The Design of Intervention Programs

One of the most important goals of behavioral assessment is to provide information to guide the selection of an intervention strategy. As discussed in Chapter 1, the importance of preintervention assessment for the design of intervention programs differs across assessment/ therapy paradigms and depends on several factors. First, the importance of assessment for intervention decisions depends on the degree to which the characteristics and determinants of behavior problems are presumed to vary across classes of behavior disorders and to vary across persons within a behavior problem class. For example, the importance of preintervention assessment will covary with the degree to which persons with a diagnosis of Major Depressive Disorder (DSM-IV) differ in the causes and symptoms associated with depression and the degree to which the symptoms and causes of depression are presumed to differ from the symptoms and causes of other behavior problems.

Second, the importance of preintervention assessment covaries with assumptions about the mechanisms of intervention effects. For example, if the primary mechanism of change in therapy is assumed to be "a supportive patient-therapist relationship" or "accessing the inner deeper experiencing," preintervention assessment would have a limited effect on the intervention method.

Finally, the importance of preintervention assessment in a paradigm covaries with the diversity of intervention strategies that are available for a particular behavior problem. If all patients received the same type of intervention (as in standardized intervention protocols), a preintervention clinical case formulation may be useful for some purposes (e.g., to gather baseline data for evaluating intervention outcome) but would have little effect on decisions regarding the general intervention approach.

As we have noted, the behavioral assessment and therapy paradigms recognize multiple possible causal factors for behavior problems, and between-person differences in the causes of behavior problems, include a large array of intervention strategies, and acknowledge multiple mechanisms of intervention effects. Consequently, preintervention assessment plays a central role in the assessment-intervention process.

Although the clinical case formulation is the primary determinant of behavioral intervention design, intervention decisions are also influenced by other factors, which are important foci of preintervention assessment. These include:

- The social supports available to the client for behavior change.
- The resources, skills, and abilities of the client (e.g., cognitive functioning, physical abilities).

- Limitations of the client (e.g., communicative and learning disabilities, physical limitations).
- The client's goals.
- The relative cost-effectiveness of interventions.
- The side-effects of an intervention.
- The acceptability of the interventions to the client.
- Time and financial constraints.
- Other moderators of intervention outcome, such as situational factors, medical complications, and concurrent life stressors.

The Evaluation of Intervention Process and Outcome

A principal tenet of the behavioral assessment paradigm is that clinical assessment is an ongoing process. Assessment continues during intervention although the focus and methods of assessment can change across time. Common assessment targets during the intervention are outlined in Table 4-5. Time-series assessment (i.e., frequent and regular measurement of variables) ideally continues throughout the treatment process for several reasons. First, elements of the functional analysis (e.g., the importance of behavior problems, the most important causal variables) can change across time and as a result of intervention. The changes can reflect more valid clinical judgments or true changes in variables and functional relations: (a) estimates of functional relations can change as additional information is acquired, and (b) causal variables and causal relations relevant to behavior problems can change over time. The identification of such changes have important implications for intervention foci because

Table 4-5
Common Targets in the Assessment of Intervention Process and Outcome

Variables	Description
Treatment Outcome Variables	
Ultimate outcome variables	The outcome variables (e.g., self-injury, marital satisfaction, academic achievement) upon which intervention effectivenss is ultimately judged
Immediate and intermediate	Those variables whose changes precede change in the ultimate outcome variables (e.g., when an increase in problem-solving skills precedes an increase in relationship satisfaction)
Goal attainment	Similar to "ultimate outcome variables" above, the degree to which goals specified in intervention are approximated
Potential side effects of intervention	Effects of the intervention other than those for which it was initiated (e.g., unintended cardiovascular effects of an exercise program)
Variables that Moderate Intervention Outcome	
Independent variables in the intervention process	Those variables, usually client behaviors, that affect the outcome variables (e.g., a parent's use of appropriate response contingencies with a child with oppositional behaviors)
Client adherence/ compliance to intervention	The degree to which the client emits behaviors that are selected for change (e.g., practices relaxation, initiates positive conversations, takes medication, attends sessions)
Client satisfaction	Satisfaction with intervention methods and outcomes
Variables that Affect Inferences about the Causes of Treatment Effects	
Causal variables	Variables that affect the behavior problems or intervention goals
Functional relations	The relations between causal variables and problem behaviors
Alternative explanations for intervention inferences	For example, monitoring teacher attention when evaluating the effects of a time-out program

changes in estimated functional relations may require modification of the focus of intervention to address the most important causal variables.

Second, time-series assessment is an important component of a scholarly, "accountability" approach to clinical intervention. Time-series assessment facilitates the ability of the clinician to draw valid inferences about the effects of intervention and about the mechanisms that underlie intervention effects. Assessment within single-subject, interrupted time-series designs (e.g., Kazdin, 1998) can further strengthen the validity of inferences about intervention effects.

Third, the outcome of intervention can be enhanced by ongoing measurement. Many behavioral intervention programs involve learning experiences for the client in the natural environment. A clinically significant outcome often depends on the degree to which a client engages in these activities. For example, a client who experiences frequent episodes of severely depressed mood may self-monitor automatic negative thoughts associated with stressful situations encountered during the day. This information can serve as a measure of intermediate intervention effects and as a focus for discussion during cognitive-behavioral treatment (CBT) treatment sessions about the relation between thoughts and mood.

As indicated in Table 4-5, intervention outcomes can be ultimate, intermediate, and immediate. The *ultimate intervention outcome* with the client with depressed mood is fewer (and/or less intense, shorter) depressive episodes and more positive mood states. The degree to which this ultimate outcome is achieved covaries with the degree to which the client engages in the homework activities, such as monitoring automatic negative thoughts. These daily activities can be thought of as the "independent variables" that affect the major dependent variables—the targeted behavior problems. We can also consider these independent variables as *immediate or intermediate goals* of therapy—goals that are necessary if the ultimate goals are to be achieved (see discussion in Mash & Hunsley, 1993). They are the mechanisms through which therapeutic changes are affected and are important assessment targets.

Assessing immediate and intermediate intervention goals with a client increases the clinician's ability to quickly detect failing therapies. The expected latency to change is shorter for immediate and intermediate than for ultimate goals. Consequently, time-series measurement of immediate and intermediate goals can provide a sensitive index of intervention outcome.

Monitoring Client Adherence, Cooperation, and Satisfaction During Intervention

Client adherence, cooperation, and satisfaction with intervention are also important assessment targets. Client adherence and cooperation include behaviors that facilitate or impede the achievement of therapy goals. Lack of cooperation (sometimes called "resistance") would be indicated by frequent tardiness for sessions, frequent negative reactions to therapist's suggestions, inconsistent performance of homework assignments, reluctance to talk about particular topics or provide needed information, not returning self-monitoring records, lying in self-reports, or an argumentative style within the session.

The functions and triggers of uncooperative behaviors can vary across clients. Some uncooperative behaviors may reflect generalized styles of social interaction, such as those sometimes characteristic of a client with long-standing interpersonal difficulties (Linehan, 1993). Other uncooperative behaviors may indicate that the client anticipates that successful intervention will result in an unacceptable cost, such as, a loss of control over a spouse, a loss of attention from peers, return to an unpleasant work setting. Some clients may also be reluctant to discuss anxiety-provoking topics, such as sexual dysfunctions (La Greca, 1990) or marital violence (O'Leary, 1987).

Some uncooperative behaviors may be warranted in that they reflect reasonable reactions to poorly designed or poorly explained assessment and intervention strategies. The procedures or focus recommended by the clinician may not seem relevant or appropriate to the client (i.e., it may not have *social validity*). This issue intersects with the "informed consent" and client-focused nature of the behavioral assessment paradigm. Whenever possible, the focus and strategies of assessment are selected through informed and respectful consultations between the clinician and client.

Regardless of function, a lack of cooperation can impede intervention outcome and should be carefully monitored. Because uncooperation impedes the attainment of immediate and intermediate intervention goals, they must often be addressed before ultimate intervention goals can be attained.

Client satisfaction with the assessment-intervention process can affect the degree to which the client cooperates with assessment and intervention. Consequently, two goals of assessment are to evaluate and maintain client satisfaction with the assessment process (see for example, Parent's Consumer Satisfaction Questionnaire; Forehand & McMahon, 1981). Information obtained during assessment on important functional relations has little value if the client stops attending treatment sessions or with a client who is hospitalized and decides not to cooperate further (see Box 4-3).

Most behavior therapists assume that the interaction between the client and clinician greatly affects the client's satisfaction and cooperation. The mandate for the assessor to specify and quantify problem behaviors and causal variables and to estimate functional relations can sometimes diminish the positive ambience of the client-assessor relationship. The assessor can stress the information goals of assessment at the expense of other assessment goals.

It is important to remember that the clinician can integrate rapport-building strategies into the assessment and treatment process. The results of many studies conducted in the 1950s through the 1970s (e.g., Matarazzo & Wiens, 1972) suggest that positive paralinguistic behaviors, accurate empathy, nonpossessive warmth, positive regard, and genuineness can enhance the assessor-client relationship (see discussions in Haynes, 1978; Kohlenberg & Tsai, 1991; McConaghy, 1998; Turkat, 1986).

Additional Assessment Goals

There are several other goals of assessment, indicated in Table 4-1. These include psychiatric diagnosis, the provision of informed consent to clients, and the assessment of additional client variables.

Psychiatric Diagnosis

The psychological assessment-diagnosis relationship has been discussed in many chapters and articles (e.g., Clark, Watson, & Reynolds, 1995; Eifert, Evans, & McKendrick, 1990; Widiger, 1997). Many issues have been addressed: the dimensional vs. categorical basis of diagnosis, the internal consistency of symptom groupings, causal inferences associated with some taxonomies and taxonomy categories, the heterogeneity among persons with the same diagnosis, the communicative functions of psychiatric taxonomies, the clinical utility of psychiatric diagnoses, and the methods through which diagnostic categories and criteria are determined. Clinicians from a behavioral assessment paradigm have often commented on problems associated with the topographic rather than functional approach to assessment.

Box 4-3
Informant Satisfaction

Many assessment strategies require the cooperation of informants such as psychiatric staff members, teachers, parents, and nurses. Informants can provide helpful information during interviews and often assist in providing observation data on the client that would otherwise be unavailable to the assessor.

The validity of assessment inferences often depends on their cooperation. Consequently, all assessment participants should be treated in a respectful, professional, supportive manner. They should be kept informed of the goals and outcome of assessment, and their efforts should be formally and informally acknowledged.

Despite problems associated with psychiatric diagnostic systems, behavioral clinicians are often required to provide a psychiatric label for a client. Given this mandate, it is obligatory for the clinician to use the most valid assessment strategies available to gather the information necessary to make that judgment. Diagnosis is a meta-judgment that reflects the clinician's specific judgments about the rate, duration, cyclicity, and intensity of specific behavior problems; covariation among multiple problems; functional impairment associated with the behavior problems; the recent and historical time-course of problems; and the presence of behaviors indicative of competing diagnostic categories (e.g., for differential diagnosis). In sum, a diagnosis is a complex clinical judgment whose validity, within the constraints imposed by the taxonomic system, depends on the validity of the information obtained. Diagnostic judgments can be made more validly through the use of multiple sources of information from validated assessment instruments.

Client Informed Consent

Informed consent is another important goal of behavioral assessment. Whenever feasible, the client should be informed about, and agree to, all assessment strategies and goals and the rationale underlying them. Clients should be treated as important, knowledgeable, active participants in the assessment process.

Informed consent for assessment methods should also be obtained from responsible individuals such as parents, teachers, guardians, hospital administrators, and psychiatric team leaders, whenever the competence of a client to give informed consent is questionable. Responsible individuals should be informed of the goals, methods, and results of assessment (see Box 4-3).

The Assessment of Additional Client Variables

The goals of behavioral assessment often include the measurement of other attributes of the client and of the client's social and physical environment. These additional client variables can operate as important causal variables for a client's behavior problems and important moderators of intervention outcome. As such, they can be important components of the functional analyses.

Some important client variables are: (a) the client's knowledge, (b) the client's social environment (e.g., patterns of family interaction, social support from friends or family members), (c) important life events, and (d) the client's cognitive abilities.

Table 4-6

Areas of Client Knowledge that May Affect the Design of Intervention Strategies*

---

1. The characteristics and factors associated with the client's *behavior problem* (e.g., the time-course of blood-alcohol levels following drinking and health risks associated with excessive alcohol use).
2. *Causal variables* for the behavior problem (e.g., triggers, mediators, intervening variables, maintaining factors for excessive alcohol use).
3. *Sequelae* for, and correlates of, the behavior problem (e.g., neurological problems associated with chronic excessive alcohol use).
4. *Methods of assessment* (e.g., breathalyzer, timeline followback interview procedures).
5. *Intervention methods* for the behavior problem (behavioral and nonbehavioral; methods, cost-effectivness, benefits, side effects of various alcoholism treatment programs).
6. *Intervention goals* (necessary conditions for obtaining goals; immediate/intermediate/ultimate goals in the treatment of excessive alcohol use).

---

*These areas are also relevant for other persons (e.g., parents, spouses, staff, teachers) who would be involved with a client's intervention.

Client Knowledge

The client's knowledge about his or her behavior problems, associated medical disorders, anticipated intervention goals, causal variables, and intervention procedures can guide intervention foci and affect intervention outcome. Some important areas of client knowledge are outlined in Table 4-6.

For example, Creer and Bender (1993) noted that when working with asthmatic children it is important to assess the knowledge of children and their parents about the risk factors for the child's asthma episodes (e.g., pollen, temperature changes, mold, exercise), the time-course of the disorder, and the effects of medication.[1] Knowledge by the client of risk factors for asthma episodes is particularly important because it can facilitate the family's efforts to arrange the environment and activities in a way to reduce the incidence of the child's asthma episodes.

Similarly, assessment of client knowledge can be an important goal in family therapy with schizophrenic patients. The family's knowledge about schizophrenia and about principles of positive family communication, the importance of close adherence to a medication regime, and the deleterious effects of negative life events may affect the chance of relapse after the client returns home after hospitalization (see discussion of schizophrenia in Bellack & Mueser, 1990).

Client knowledge would be a particularly powerful mediator of intervention success in cases where the client has a basic behavioral repertoire of self-regulation skills (Watson & Tharp, 1997). When a basic behavioral repertoire exists, increasing the client's knowledge about the behavior problem may allow the client to implement existing self-regulation strategies and may lead to clinically meaningful behavior change (Cantor, 1990).

Frequently, knowledge can be measured most efficiently through self-report methods. Most specialized books on the behavioral intervention of behavior disorders contain references or examples of questionnaire measures of client knowledge. However, knowledge of behavioral skills is modestly correlated with the implementation of those skills. For example, the assessor should not presume that a parent's, teacher's, and staff member's knowledge of principles of positive reinforcement translates into the frequent use of those principles.

---

[1]Creer and Bender (1993) provided a clinically useful table that describes four questionnaires designed to measure the knowledge of children (and their parents) about asthma; four other questionnaires in the table measure the asthma knowledge of adults. The table describes items (the questionnaires range from 12 items to 100 items), content areas, and item groupings.

This redirects us to an important tenet of the behavioral assessment paradigm—phenomena of interest should be directly observed whenever possible. A questionnaire measure of knowledge of parenting skills can be very useful. However, "knowledge of parenting skills" is a different construct than "parenting behavior," and a measure of knowledge cannot substitute for the direct observation of behavior.

The Client's Social Environment

Elements of the client's social environment can serve as causal and treatment moderator variables. Social interactions often serve as important antecedent and consequent variables for clients' behavior problems and for goal attainment. The relationship between a client and his or her social environment can also be bidirectionals. Some behavior problems, such as agoraphobic, depressive, and delusional behaviors can have adverse effects on a client's social interactions. For example, chronic pain and depressive episodes can place a strain on a client's normal sources of social support (Hatch, 1993).[2]

"Social support" has been proposed as a moderator of the relation between life stressors and many behavior problems and as a direct causal factor for intervention adherence, effects, and recidivism. For example, some research suggests that a supportive family environment can attenuate the effects of life stressors on a schizophrenic client (Liberman, Kopelowicz, & Young, 1994). Conversely, a family environment characterized by frequent aversive exchanges may increase the chance of relapse among schizophrenic clients (e.g., Rehm, LePage, & Bailey, 1994).

"Social support" is a higher-order composite variable with many elements that do not necessarily strongly covary. The social support construct is used in many different ways and may include emotional support (e.g., sympathetic understanding about a problem), negative emotional expression (e.g., anger), informational support (e.g., telling a friend about side effects associated with chemotherapy), positive and negative dyadic exchanges, and tangible support (e.g., money). Further complicating our understanding of the effects of social support, the specific mechanisms through which social support affects behavior have been topics of debate.

Because "social support" is a highly abstract construct, it is important to focus on its specific components and mechanisms of effects. This is particularly true when one type of social support is necessary for successful implementation of specific intervention strategies. With increased specification, clinically useful social support variables are most likely to be identified (e.g., identifying the types of positive verbal/emotional exchanges that are most helpful following the death of a family member can suggest ways to help a client to reduce persistent debilitating grief following a loss).

Important Life Events

Important life events, particularly traumatic life events, have been implicated as nonspecific causal factors for many behavior disorders (e.g., Miller, 1996). Often, traumatic events, such as childhood sexual abuse and war-related trauma, have sequelae that function as important causal variables for behavior problems. For example, traumatic events are sometimes associated with feelings of guilt, of beliefs of personal vulnerability, or conditioned

---

[2]Complaints often operate on a DRL schedule (differential reinforcement of low-rate behaviors): Initial complaints are followed by responses of concern and sympathy from others, but such supportive comments diminish as complaints continue or increases in rate.

emotional responses to trauma-related stimuli, which can function as causal variables for mood and anxiety problems.

The most important focus of behavioral assessment with reference to traumatic events is the contemporaneous sequelae of the event. It is important to obtain detailed information on events that may help explain current behavior problems. However, it is more important to obtain detailed information on contemporaneous thoughts, behavior, and physiological responses related to those life events. These responses are the modifiable elements in a causal chain beginning with an original traumatic event and ending with a client's current behavior problems.

Summary

In this chapter we stressed the interdependence among assessment goals, the specific clinical judgments that are to be made, and the principles and strategies of assessment. Each assessment occasion provides information to guide particular clinical judgments. The goals of assessment vary across assessment occasions, depending on the client's problems, the assessment setting, and the judgments that must be made. The principles and methods of the behavioral assessment paradigm are differentially applicable for different goals.

Initial goals of behavioral assessment are the selection of assessment instruments and strategies. The assessor must select the most appropriate assessment methods, the time-course of measurement, the most important targets of assessment, and who should participate in the assessment. The assessor also must decide if consultation and referral from other sources would facilitate the goals of assessment.

The primary goal of most preintervention behavioral assessment is the development of the clinical case formulation. The clinical case formulation is composed of many lower-order judgments including the identification of problem behaviors, causal variables, and functional relations.

Intervention program design is strongly affected by the clinical case formulation. Information on the client's goals and strengths, variables that may moderate treatment effects, client knowledge, medical complications, and characteristics of the social environment also affect intervention program design.

Important goals of behavioral assessment also involve the measurement of intervention process and outcome. These include the evaluation of intervention compliance, client-therapist interaction, and other moderators of intervention outcome. Intervention evaluation also involves the assessment of immediate, intermediate and ultimate outcomes. Additional goals of clinical assessment include diagnosis, informed consent, and the assessment of additional client variables that may explain behavior problems and moderate intervention effects.

Suggested Readings

Books on the Goals of Nonbehavioral Assessment Paradigms

Butcher, J. N. (Ed.). (1995). *Clinical personality assessment: Practical approaches* (pp. 278–301). New York: Oxford University Press.

Goldstein, A., & Hersen, M. (Eds.). (1997). *Handbook of psychological assessment* (3rd ed.). Boston/New York: Pergamon.

Maruish, M. E. (Ed.). *The use of psychological testing for treatment planning and outcome assessment* (pp. 581–602). Hillsdale, NJ: Lawrence Erlbaum Associates.

Articles on the Goals of Behavioral Assessment

Barrios, B. A. (1988). On the changing nature of behavioral assessment. In A. S. Bellack & M. Hersen (Eds.), *Behavioral assessment: A practical handbook* (pp. 3–41). New York: Pergamon.

Mash, E. J., & Terdal, L. G. (1988). Behavioral assessment of child and family disturbance. In E. J. Mash & L. G. Terdal (Eds.), *Behavioral assessment of childhood disorders* (pp. 3–65). New York: Guilford.

Ollendick, T. H., & Hersen, M. (1993). Child and adolescent behavioral assessment. In T. H. Ollendick & M. Hersen (Eds.), *Handbook of child and adolescent assessment* (pp. 3–14). Boston: Allyn & Bacon.

II

Conceptual and Methodological Foundations of Behavioral Assessment

5

Scholarly, Hypothesis-Testing, and Time-Series Assessment Strategies

Introduction

In Chapter 3 we discussed strategies for increasing the validity of clinical judgments. Many of these strategies can be considered as exemplars of a scholarly approach to clinical assessment and judgment, such as the use of validated assessment instruments to aid clinical judgments. In this chapter we examine in more detail several interrelated methodological aspects of the behavioral assessment paradigm: (1) a scholarly, empirically based approach to psychological assessment, (2) a hypothesis-testing approach to psychological assessment, and (3) the use of time-series measurement strategies in clinical assessment.

A scholarly approach to assessment strategies and clinical judgments has many elements (Hayes, Follette, Dawes, & Grady, 1995; Spengler, Strohmer, Dixon, & Shivy, 1995). It involves the use of validated assessment instruments, multiple sources of information, a skeptical view of clinical judgments, time-series measurement strategies, the importance of obtaining quantitative information, and the integration of quantitative and qualitative information. Time-series assessment emerges out of the scholarly approach because behavior is dynamic, requiring multiple measurements across time.

An emphasis on a scholarly approach to assessment is also characteristic of other psychological assessment paradigms. However, a scholarly approach is manifested in different ways across paradigms, depending on the conceptual tenets of the paradigm. For example, the use of internally consistent aggregate scores of personality traits is more characteristic of personality assessment, and the use of carefully designed time-series assessment of dynamic variables is more characteristic of behavioral assessment.

Elements of a scholarly approach to psychological assessment are featured in all chapters in this book. In this chapter we emphasize several goals, principles, and strategies of a scholarly approach to psychological assessment:

1. Clinical judgments are more likely to be valid if assessment instruments have been validated in domains relevant to the client.
2. The assessment process can be guided by the empirical literature relevant to all aspects of the client's behavior problems, causal variables, and applicable interventions.
3. Clinical judgments should be approached skeptically, as hypotheses to be tested.
4. Time-series assessment strategies can help identify causal and noncausal functional relations and can help monitor intervention process and outcome.
5. A scholarly approach to psychological assessment should be promoted during interactions with other professionals, especially during clinical case conferences.
6. Clinical judgments are more likely to be valid when based on multiple sources of information.
7. The assessment process often involves the integration of conflicting information based on estimates of the relative validity of the information.
8. Assessment strategies should include behavioral observation and controlled experimentation whenever feasible.
9. A scholarly orientation toward assessment can include both qualitative and quantitative assessment strategies.
10. The future time-course of behavior can be predicted more accurately, changes in important variables can be identified more quickly, and functional relations identified more accurately if both the phase and state dimensions of variables are measured.

A Scholarly, Empirical, Hypothesis-Testing Approach to Assessment

Epistemology is an important characteristics of a psychological assessment paradigm[1] because it influences preferred strategies for understanding a client's behavior problems, for understanding the causes of those problems, the strategies for deriving clinical judgments, and the best methods of estimating intervention effects. As we noted in Chapter 1, epistemology also affects the degree to which an assessment paradigm evolves to reflect new findings about human behavior and its determinants. A central epistemological element of behavioral assessment is an emphasis on a scholarly, empirically based approach to assessment. Elements of this approach are outlined in Table 5-1.

Psychological assessment should be a scientifically based enterprise. A scholarly approach to assessment emphasizes that clinical judgments should be based, as much as possible, on valid data from clinical assessment and empirical research. The following sections discuss in greater detail several elements of a scholarly approach to psychological assessment.

The Design of an Assessment Strategy

Use Validated Instruments and Methods

The selection of an assessment strategy should be empirically informed. The assessment instruments selected for use should be those shown in previous research to provide valid measures in conditions similar to those of the target assessment occasion. There are several elements of this mandate:

- *Avoid assessment instruments that have not been adequately evaluated and validated.* It is impossible to know the degree to which measures from inadequately evaluated instruments represent the targeted construct. Consequently, judgments based on these measures must be viewed skeptically.
- Consider the *conditional nature of validation* when interpreting validity data. Has the instrument been validated on dimensions of individual difference relevant to your client?
- Know the *sources of error* that affect obtained measures, such as memory and bias effects of self-report questionnaires, observer drift, and autocorrelation of self-monitored data.

As we will discuss in Chapter 6, idiographic assessment strategies involve instruments that are individually tailored for a particular client. Consequently, validity data may not be available for these instruments. However, the method of assessment (e.g., self-monitored thought records) may have been subjected to prior evaluation, and idiographic methods are still subject to psychometric evaluation and other mandates for a scholarly approach.

[1]Epistemology is a branch of philosophy that addresses the theory and methods of acquiring knowledge, the methods and criteria used to decide when something is "known," and sources of errors in acquiring knowledge (Blackburn, 1994). Epistemological approaches can include empiricism, positivism, and skepticism. In psychological assessment paradigms, epistemology refers to the methods of collecting information presumed to best facilitate the understanding of human behavior. Recommended methods of acquiring knowledge about a client are considered "methodological" (as opposed to "conceptual") tenets of the paradigm.

Table 5-1

A Scholarly, Empirically Based Approach to Psychological Assessment

---

The Design of an Assessment Strategy

Use instruments and methods validated and relevant for the client, assessment setting, and goals of assessment.

Use multiple sources of information.

Include observation and experimentation as assessment strategies.

Use systematic approach to assessment and clinical decision making.

Assessor Training and Knowledge

Know the empirical literature relevant to a client's behavior problem, possible causal variables and mechanisms, intervention goals, and sources of individual differences (e.g., gender, age, ethnicity factors).

Know the empirical literature on the validity, sources of measurement and inferential error, and appropriate applications of the assessment instruments.

Know the empirically validated intervention strategies relevant to the client's behavior problems and goals and the assessment strategies best suited to the measurement of their outcome.

Be well trained in psychometric methods and principles, research methods, and statistics.

A Hypothesis-Testing Perspective of Clinical Judgments

Adopt a skeptical attitude about your hypotheses and judgments*

Gather data from multiple sources that could disconfirm your hypotheses about the client's behavior problems or hypothesized causal relations.

Be constructively skeptical about other clinicians' hypotheses, judgments, and inferences.

Measure outcomes of your judgments (e.g., intervention effects based on your clinical case formulation).

Retain a scholarly orientation but be receptive to new findings and ideas (i.e., do not immediately reject new ideas, assessment instruments and methods, research findings, theories, and interventions).

Assessment Strategies During and Following Intervention

Use ongoing, time-series measurement strategies.

Collect and integrate quantitative data on all aspects of the assessment/intervention process.

Measure approximations to specified immediate, intermediate, and ultimate intervention goals.

Professional Interaction

Promote a scholarly approach to psychological assessment and clinical judgments during case conferences, in clinical case reports, and in other professional interactions.

---

*Presume that in the psychological assessment process you are progressing from indubitable ignorance to "thoughtful uncertainty" (Esar, 1968), or that assessment is an "unending adventure at the edge of uncertainty" (Jacob Bronowski, as quoted in Brussell, 1988).

Base Clinical Judgments on Multiple Sources of Information

As we suggested in Chapter 3, the impact on clinical judgments of measurement error associated with an assessment instrument can often be reduced with multiple sources of information (Dumas & Serketich, 1994; Nay, 1979; Sobell, Toneatto, & Sobell, 1994). Multi-source assessment most often refers to the process of obtaining data from multiple informants (e.g., parents, teachers, spouses). However, multisource assessment has a broader meaning and can involve data from:

- *Multiple methods of assessment* (e.g., self-monitoring, psychophysiological assessment, and interviews);
- *Multiple assessment instruments* (e.g., using more than one observer or questionnaire to measure a particular variable);
- *Multiple informants* (e.g., client, parents, teachers, peers, spouse, and staff members);
- *Multiple occasions* (e.g., time-series measurement; may also involve different times of the day and different days, depending on what inferences are to be drawn);
- *Multiple contexts and settings* (e.g., different physical and social environments, client states, social contexts, times of the day).

We consider the first four multisource assessment strategies in this section. Assessment across multiple occasions (i.e., time-series assessment) is considered in a later section.

Multisource assessment addresses several measurement problems. First, different sources of information often capture unique facets of a targeted construct. For example, different informants can contribute information on unique facets of a child's depression (Frame, Robinson, & Cuddy, 1992). Self-report measures from the child can provide information on the child's depressive mood and thoughts. These facets may or may not have behavioral concomitants that are observable to others. Interviews with the child's parents and teachers can provide information about the behavioral and somatic facets of the child's depression (Kamphaus & Frick, 1996) and may identify developmental aspects, cross-situational differences in behaviors, and functional relations. Similarly, observations of interactions of the child with other persons in a structured clinic setting can provide information about the child's social behaviors that may not have been obtained through interviews or questionnaires.

As we noted in Chapter 4, different assessment instruments that use the same method and target the same construct (monomethod assessment) can also tap unique facets of the targeted construct. For example, there are several self-report questionnaires and structured interviews that measure "depression" (e.g., BDI, CES-D) (Hamilton & Shapiro, 1990; Persons & Fresco, 1998; Rehm, LePage, & Bailey, 1994). These different self-report instruments differentially weight the somatic, cognitive, and behavioral facets of depression. Consequently, the meaning of a depression "score" (i.e., the judgments that can be derived from the score) varies depending on the instrument from which it is derived.

The effect of the differences in focus between instruments occurs across all assessment methods. For example, different observation coding systems for marital interactions target unique classes of behaviors (Floyd, Haynes, & Kelly, 1997; Halford & Markman, 1997; O'Leary, 1987); different questionnaires on social anxiety and phobia provide scale scores of unique facets (e.g., Brown et al., 1997); methods of ambulatory monitoring of cardiovascular responses differ in their use of time- and event-sampling procedures, aggregation methods, and daily diary procedures (Fahrenberg & Myrtek, 1996).

Because assessment instruments and methods often differ in the degree to which they tap the various facets of a variable, a targeted variable can sometimes be estimated more comprehensively by using multiple assessment instruments and aggregating the obtained measures.

Second, each source of assessment information is associated with unique sources of measurement error. For example, data from self-report questionnaires can sometimes reflect a tendency for clients to report events in a way that presents the client in a positive or negative light, or can reflect response patterns as a function of the sequence of questions or response format used. Sources of error may also differ across informants. For example, reports from teachers and parents about the behavior of a child may reflect the characteristics, mood, and life stressors of the informant (see discussions in Edelbrock, 1988; Lovejoy, 1991).

Third, data from different sources often reflect behavior of the client in different situations. Data obtained from different methods or informants may appear to conflict because the informants are exposed to the client in different situations. In their review of over 100 studies of parent and teacher ratings of child behavior, Achenbach, McConaughy, and Howell (1987) reported that the agreement for participants from the same setting was significantly higher than the agreement between participants from different settings. This pattern of correlations is consistent with the presumption that children behave differently across settings.

Conflicting data from different assessment sources can make important contributions to the functional analysis of a client when the sources covary with important sources of variance in behavior problems. For example, significant differences in the rate of self-injurious behaviors (SIB) by a child with developmental disabilities reported by two teachers may reflect important differences in the situations in which the child is observed or in how the teachers respond to the SIB. These reported differences in rate could reflect differences in difficulty of tasks presented to the child (e.g., a high vs. low demand classroom environment) and suggest that the child's self-injurious behaviors enable him or her to escape from those situations. In this example, information about the conditional probabilities of the SIB can contribute to the functional analysis and the design of intervention programs.

In summary, multisource assessment can strengthen the validity of clinical judgments in several ways:

- It can capture unique facets of a targeted construct;
- It can reduce the impact of idiosyncratic and systematic sources of measurement error;
- It can contribute to a functional analysis by identifying important sources of behavioral variance.

Although apparently conflicting data from different sources can reflect true differences in the targets of assessment across those sources, conflicting data can also reflect error in the assessment instruments. Consider the difficulties in making clinical judgments when parents disagree about the rates of a child's aggressive behavior and how they discipline the child, or when staff members on a psychiatric unit disagree about what triggers a patient's delusional behaviors, or when spouses disagree about the rate and severity of violence in their relationship. In these cases, the assessor must differentially weight the information from different sources to construct a clinical case formulation. Methods of integrating information are discussed in chapters and by Kamphaus and Frick (1996) and Achenbach (1997).

All strategies of integrating conflicting information focus on estimating the validity of the information obtained and weighting the information according to its estimated validity. Specific strategies for integrating conflicting information include:

- Consider whether differences among sources could reflect true differences in the targeted variables (e.g., different informants may be reporting about behavior in different situations).
- Consider systematic, reliable error inherent in each instrument. For example, different questionnaires may address unique facets of the same construct. One informant may be strongly positively biased toward the client.
- Gather additional information to validate information from informants and instruments. For example, gather information from additional informants or use additional assessment instruments.
- Examine the reliability of each source. For example, interview each informant more than once, or use different prompts to examine the temporal stability of reports over time.
- Examine the psychometric foundation of each source. For example, information from some sources (e.g., retrospective self-report from unstructured interviews) may be more suspect than that from other sources.

Multisource assessment strategies are generally preferred but are not always incrementally useful. Adding more sources of data can aid clinical judgments if (a) the additional source taps aspects of the targeted construct that are untapped by existing measures, (b) additional sources are cost-effective methods of validating existing measures, and (c) measures from a new source are valid. Consider the impact on our inferences about the aggressive behavior of a patient on a psychiatric unit if we uncritically added the reports of an unreliable staff member to the reports of a reliable staff member. Judgments based on both would be less valid than those based only on the reliable source—here a multisource strategy reduces the validity of our inferences.

Include Behavioral Observation and Experimentation in an Assessment Strategy

The behavioral assessment paradigm emphasizes the direct observation of a client's behavior (Suen & Ary, 1988; Tryon, 1999). Observation can occur in several contexts and through several methods: (a) observation by external observers in the client's natural environment, (b) observation by external observers in analogue clinic settings (e.g., observing parent-child interactions in structured situations in a clinic playroom), (c) qualitative observation of clients during assessment interviews, (d) participant observations (e.g., observations of a hospitalized patient by psychiatric staff members), (f) observation through instrumentation (e.g., tape recordings of family discussions at dinner, actimeters), and (g) self-observations (e.g., self-monitoring of panic episodes).

Observations not only can provide strong evidence about functional relations and intervention effects, they can be a rich source of data for clinical hypotheses. Observing how parents and adolescents discuss a problem topic can help the assessor identify complex chains of verbal interactions and many possible sources of their distress (see discussion in Barrios, 1993). Although there are many sources of error in behavioral observation, observation is less susceptible to many errors and biases associated with self-report interviews and questionnaires.

"Experimentation" in psychological assessment refers to the acquisition of data while carefully and systematically manipulating hypothesized contingency, instructional, or contextual factors. Examples include observing the effects on a child's self-injurious behavior associated with the systematic presentation or removal of response contingent social attention (taking care to prevent injury to the child) and measuring the psychophysiological responses of a client with PTSD symptoms to slides of trauma and nontrauma related stimuli.

Experimentation has been a hallmark of experimental and applied behavior analysis (see the *Journal Experimental Analysis of Behavior* and the *Journal of Applied Behavior Analysis*). By obtaining behavioral observation measures during careful manipulation of hypothesized causal variables and contexts, the assessor can more confidently draw inferences about functional relations.

There are many strategies for the systematic manipulation of hypothesized controlling variables. Some of these strategies include ABAB designs, multiple baseline designs, and changing criterion designs. These ***interrupted time-series designs*** (i.e., single-subject, within-subject) can help increase the confidence in inferences about hypothesized functional relations (they increase confidence in the ***internal validity*** of our inferences). (Readers may consult Barlow and Hersen, 1984; Kazdin, 1998; and Kratochwill and Levin, 1992, for excellent coverage of this topic.)

Assessor Knowledge and Communication of Empirical Literature

To select the most valid and relevant assessment methods and instruments and to integrate the obtained measures for the purposes of drawing clinical judgments, the assessor must be familiar with the empirical literature relevant to the client. The assessor should be familiar with research: (a) on the characteristics of the client's behavior problems (e.g., epidemiology, time-course, prognosis, developmental considerations, sources of individual differences, comorbidity), (b) relevant to possible causal variables and mechanisms associated with the client's behavior problems, (c) relevant to the client's goals, and (d) on assessment instruments, methods, and strategies relevant to the client's problems and goals. Additionally, as we noted in Chapter 4, the clinician should be familiar with problems associated with the client's behavior problems that are outside the assessors field (e.g., genetic/physiological defects; speech, visual, motor, hearing impairments; medication effects), and empirically validated interventions for the client's behavior problems and goals, or seek outside consultation.

Consider the importance of knowledge of the empirical literature for the assessment of a client with sleeping difficulties (see discussions in Morin & Edinger, 1997). To select the best assessment strategy, the assessor must have knowledge of the empirical literatures on the characteristics of different sleep disorders (e.g., delayed sleep onset, central and obstructive apnea), methods of measuring sleep, the sequelae of sleep problems, sleep medications, and behavioral and cognitive factors associated with sleep dysfunctions.

In many situations, however, there will not be a sufficiently developed research literature relevant to a behavior problem. Alternatively, the assessor may not be able to get to the empirical literature because of pragmatic constraints (e.g., available time). Under these conditions, the assessor should draw from theoretical and strategic guidelines provided by the behavioral assessment paradigm. Additionally, the assessor can sometimes make plausible generalizations from research in related areas (see Box 5-1).

A Cautious Hypothesis-Testing, Problem-Solving Approach to Assessment and Clinical Judgment

A *hypothesis-testing strategy* is an important element of the behavioral assessment paradigm (e.g., Kratochwill & Shapiro, 1988; Repp, Karsh, Munk, & Dahlquist, 1995). Early in the preintervention assessment process, the assessor forms hypotheses about the client. These hypotheses are often preliminary clinical judgments about the client's behavior problems and possible causal variables.

A scholarly approach to clinical assessment requires that these hypotheses be carefully formulated and tested. As we reviewed in Chapter 3, there are many sources of systematic and unsystematic error in clinical judgments and hypotheses. Consequently, the assessor should

---

Box 5-1
Multisource Assessment, Shared Method Variance
(Common Method Variance) and Clinical Judgment

The magnitude of correlation between measures obtained from different assessment instruments can provide evidence for the validity of each. However, the magnitude of correlation can also reflect the degree of similarity in the methods and content of the instruments. High correlations can reflect similar sources of measurement error (e.g., if they use the same response format or contain the same biases) and overlap in the elements between different instruments. For example, when correlation coefficients reflect the similarity of items between two questionnaires, it is called *item contamination*).

Because of shared method variance, convergent and criterion validation from assessment instruments with overlapping methods and content is less convincing than convergent validation from assessment instruments with divergent methods and content.

maintain a constructively skeptical "hypothesis testing" strategy—hypotheses are evaluated by gathering additional assessment data that could disconfirm them.

As Mash has noted (Mash & Hunsley, 1990; Mash & Terdal, 1997a) the assessment-hypothesis-case formulation process is an ongoing, iterative, development and evaluation process. As information is collected, new hypotheses are formed and prior hypotheses are refined or disconfirmed. Eventually, the incremental contribution of new assessment data diminishes. When new data confirm the assessors hypotheses and do not suggest new hypotheses, the clinician integrates these hypotheses into a behavioral case formulation, from which intervention strategies are derived. Figure 5-1 illustrates the iterative process that results in a behavioral case formulation.

It is particularly important that hypotheses be stated in a testable form and that assessment strategies are selected that allow for their disconfirmation. For example, an assessor has hypothesized that a client's panic episodes are more likely to occur in social situations that include many strangers. Disconfirmatory data could be collected by additional semistructured interviews that ask about other situations associated with an elevated conditional probability of panic episodes, and self-monitoring procedures in which panic and nonpanic responses are monitored across a variety of settings. The clinician would be less likely to refine or disconfirm hypotheses if follow-up assessment involved only personality or cognitive assessment and did not ask about other panic-inducing settings.

Often, assessors form questions before they form hypotheses (see Figure 5-1). These questions can be thought of as clinical "problems" to solve, and behavioral assessment can be

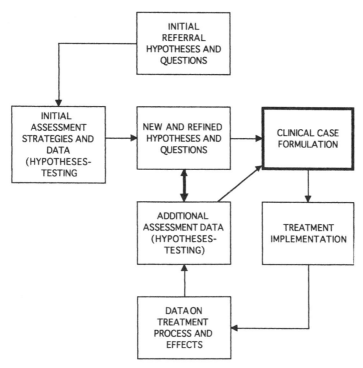

Figure 5-1. Dynamic interactions among assessment, hypotheses and judgments, clinical case conceptualization, intervention, and hypotheses testing.

thought of as a scientific, iterative approach to solving *clinical problems* (Nezu & Nezu, 1989; Nezu et al., 1997). As Nezu and Nezu stated, the assessor is initially presented with a broad problem—what is the most effective intervention for the client? A solution to the problem requires that immediate and intermediate problems be solved: (a) what are the client's main problems, (b) what life circumstances and developmental and biological factors affect those problems that might affect (i.e., facilitate, impede) intervention outcome (note that "a" and "b" are central elements of the functional analysis), and (c) what strategies should be used to gather information on "a" and "b"? As with the hypotheses-testing aspect of the assessment process, the problems addressed by the assessor often change during assessment and therapy.

A scholarly, hypothesis-testing approach strengthens the scientific foundation of the psychological assessment process and of the resultant clinical judgments. Many elements of a scholarly hypothesis-testing approach to assessment parallel the principles of maximizing the validity of clinical judgments, as outlined in Chapter 3. The assessor can facilitate a scholarly hypothesis-testing strategy by:

- Specifying hypotheses and assessment questions;
- Basing hypotheses on empirical foundations;
- Avoiding premature hypotheses;
- Maintaining a skeptical attitude toward clinical hypotheses;
- Using assessment strategies that allow for disconfirmation of hypotheses;
- Carefully considering data that disconfirm hypotheses;
- Using multisource assessment strategies to evaluate hypotheses;
- Using time-series measurement strategies.

An Emphasis on Quantification

Measurement is the process of applying numbers (or other symbols) to some attribute of a person, event, or construct. We assign numbers to help us draw inferences about the attribute (see discussion of measurement by Sarle, 1995). An important methodological tenet of the behavioral construct system is that the validity of clinical judgments can be increased if we acquire quantitative measures of variables. The numbers are amenable to summarization and statistical analysis. Quantitative data make it easier to test the validity of our hypotheses, draw inferences about how much the attribute changes over time, the degree to which the attribute was modified through therapy, how a person stands relative to other persons on that attribute, and the strength of functional and causal relation between unique attributes of a person and across persons.

We presume that if an observer in a classroom records six aggressive acts for Jeffrey and three aggressive acts for Aly, Jeffrey behaved more aggressively than Aly (for that observation period). If Lori records two panic episodes a week in the month before intervention and no panic episodes a week for the month after intervention, we presume that she has experienced a decrease in panic episodes across time. In these case, we assigned numbers (which are sums of discrete occurrences during time samples) to attributes (aggressive behavior, panic episodes) to make judgments about their relative rate, between persons and across time.

Quantitative information on constructs in psychological assessment should optimally be acquired on many *dimensions*: (a) the *rate* of behavior problems and causal factors (e.g., rate of panic episodes and aggressive acts), (b) the *magnitude* of behavior problems (e.g., intensity of headaches and social anxiety), (c) the *duration* of behavior problems (e.g., sleep-onset latency, duration of marital arguments), (d) the *time-course* of behavior problems (e.g., time-related pattern of substance use), (e) *approximation* to intervention/program goals (e.g., outcome of an aids sex-education program), (f) *conditional probabilities* (e.g., how often self-injurious behaviors follow stressful social situations), and (g) the *magnitude of covariation* (i.e., strength of functional relation) between variables.

Quantification promotes specification of clinical inferences and is particularly important in assessment interviews. Clients often report that they have sleeping troubles "many" times a week, that their children are "constantly" fighting, that their spouse "never" says something supportive. These nonspecific complaints are informative because they help the assessor understand the appraisals and beliefs of the client. However, they are insufficiently specific for many purposes of psychological assessment, such as identifying the most important behavior problems, identifying important functional relations, and judging the effects of interventions.

Limitations of Quantitative Measures

In previous sections we noted several constraints on measures obtained in psychological assessment. To reiterate some of these limitations and to introduce new ones:

- Measures are only estimates of an attribute and should not be reified. All measures underrepresent the attribute and/or include irrelevant variance.
- An attribute can be measured in different ways, resulting in different estimates of the attribute.
- No single measure captures all aspects of an attribute.
- Measurement can change the attribute being measured, or related events.
- Not all important constructs lend themselves to quantification (e.g., social skills deficits of patients; paralinguistic factors in marital problem solving).
- Although quantitative data can lead to important hypotheses, qualitative information can also be rich sources of hypotheses. Excessive dependence on quantification can impede clinical judgment and clinical case formulation.

Time-Series Measurement and Space-Phase Functions

Introduction to a Time-Series Measurement Strategy in Psychological Assessment

A *time-series measurement* strategy is an important component of a scholarly approach to psychological assessment.[2] A time-series measurement strategy is one in which variables are measured frequently, usually at regular intervals, across time (Hersen & Bellack, 1998; Kazdin, 1998; Kratochwill & Levin, 1992; see Box 5-2). Examples of time-series measurement strategies in a clinical assessment context include daily self-monitoring by a client of headaches to measure the effects of behavioral interventions; daily monitoring of thoughts during stressful social situations to identify cognitive processes that may trigger depressed mood; on-the-hour monitoring by a staff member of hitting and pinching by a child with developmental disabilities to identify triggers or reinforcers for the aggressive behavior; and completion of a question-naire on specific areas of marital distress by a couple in marital therapy before every weekly treatment session to monitor intervention effects and identify current areas of distress.

[2]Portions of this section were drawn from Haynes, Blaine, and Meyer (1995).

Box 5-2
Time Course of Variables

All variables can be described on time-related dimensions, such as rate, duration, latency, and cyclicity and also dimensions that can vary across time, such as form and magnitude. The *time-course*, or *time series plot*, of a variable refers to the representation of a dimension across time. The time-courses of variables are frequently illustrated in behavior analysis (see *Journal of Applied Behavior Analysis*; *Journal of Experimental Analysis of Behavior*), psychophysiology (Cacioppo & Tassinary, 1990), and developmental psychology (Baltes, Reese & Nesselroade, 1988). Extended time-series measurements support the maxim that behavior and functional relations can be *dynamic*, or *nonstationary*. The dimensions of behavior (e.g., magnitude, rate) and functionally related events (e.g., life stressors, parental contingencies) often change across time (see reviews in Haynes, 1992 and Haynes, Blaine, & Meyer, 1995).

Table 5-2 lists several assets of time-series measurement. Perhaps of most importance, time-series measurement is congruent with the dynamic nature of behavior, behavior problems, intervention goals, causal variables, and causal relations. Many studies have shown that these phenomena can change across time.

Phase-Space Functions and Time-Series Measurement

As discussed in Haynes (1995), a phase-space function is a plot of variable value across time. The value of a variable at a single measurement point is its *state*. The direction and rate of change of the variable are its *phase*. The state of a variable in the context of its phase is its *phase state*. Phase-space functions are elements of chaos theory (e.g., Baker & Gollub, 1990; Çambel, 1993; Heiby, 1995b; Peitgen, Jürgens, & Saupe, 1992) and have implications for a scholarly, quantitative approach to psychological assessment.

Table 5-2
The Rationale for Time-Series Measurement in Clinical Assessment

---

Behavior Is Dynamic
   The form and dimensions (e.g., rate, duration) of behavior problems can change
Intervention Goals Can Change Over Time
Causal Variables and Relations Are Dynamic
   The strength and other characteristics of causal relations can change
   New causal variables can become operational
   Variables can disappear or cease to have causal effects
   The degree of "change" of a variable can have causal properties
   The occurrence or strength of moderator variables can change
Interventions Can Be Evaluated and Modified
   Failing interventions can be identified quickly
   Time-series measurement provides more and faster feedback to assessor/therapist
   Time-series measurement is consistent with an emphasis on professional accountability (it can be used to document intervention outcome)
It Is Congruent With an Idiographic Focus of Behavioral Assessment
   Variables specific to a client can be measured across time

---

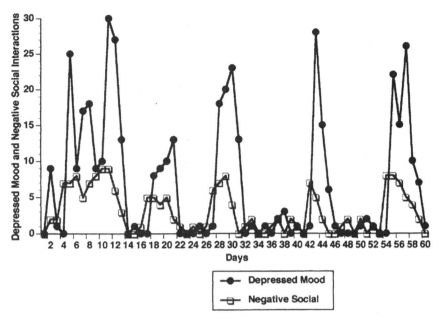

Figure 5-2. A time-course plot of magnitude of daily self-monitored mood (40-pt. scale; higher numbers = more depressed mood and negative social interactions 10-pt. scale; higher numbers = more negative social interactions) for a client with rheumatoid arthritis. (Drawn from data collected for a masters thesis by Ilisa Peralta.)

Phase-space functions are important in psychological assessment in several ways. First, clinicians are often interested in patterns of change across time in client behavior problems, such as panic episodes, mood, and blood pressure. Phase-space functions of behavior problems can help predict future episodes of behavior problems and may contribute to functional analyses. Consider the plot of an arthritis client's self-monitored mood in Figure 5-2. The time-course plot indicates that there are bursts of depressed mood, with varying durations. This plot suggests that it may be helpful to discuss with the client possible triggers of these bursts, to gather information about functional relations.

Second, assessors are often interested in changes across time in hypothesized causal variables, such as negative reinforcement, automatic thoughts, positive and negative social interactions, and exercise. Figure 5-2 also presents data on self-monitored aversive social interactions, which were hypothesized to function as a causal variable for depressed mood for this client.[3]

Finally, we are interested in the relations between the phase-space functions of behavior problems and causal variables across time. This would be illustrated by time-lagged cross-correlations between negative automatic thoughts and subsequent mood, or the time-lagged cross-correlations between aversive social interactions and depressed mood for the client with

---

[3]This multivariate time-series study, conducted by Ilisa Peralta, examined the relations among pain, depressed mood, and social interactions in clients with rheumatoid arthritis. Using time-lagged multivariate regression analysis, it was found that for three out of six clients, the relation between pain and depression in arthritis patients could be significantly explained by aversive social exchanges associated with the depressed mood. The chain included: increased pain → increased aversive social exchange → increased depressed mood.

arthritis, as illustrated in Figure 5.2. Time-lagged correlations between two variables (e.g., the correlation between sleep quality at night and pain magnitude on the subsequent day) provide information about the possible causal relations between these two variables.[4] Time-lagged cross-correlations from time-series measurement data (sometimes called *concomitant time-series analysis*) can also suggest possible causal relations because the effect of temporal precedence can be considered.

In typical psychological assessment practice a variable is measured only once. For example, a new client at an outpatient mental health center may be administered a battery of mood, anxiety, or perceived child behavior problems questionnaires, along with an intake interview on one or two assessment sessions. From this data, a diagnosis is assigned and initial intervention strategies may be determined. Formal assessment typically stops at this point.

This single-point measurement strategy only captures important phenomena in its state. However, at that measurement moment, variables exist in particular phases in their phase-space. They may be increasing, decreasing, or stable, and they may be changing quickly or slowly. A single measurement cannot inform the assessor about important phase-space contexts.

The state and phase of a variable are both important for clinical inferences and they are both likely to vary across time. The main implication of this discussion for strategies of psychological assessment is that it is important to capture the dynamic attributes of variables, and this can only be accomplished with time-series measurement strategies.

Figure 5-3 illustrates how time-series measurement and space-phase functions can affect clinical judgments (Floyd, Haynes, & Kelly, 1997). The figure presents stylized time-courses of a variable for four persons. Values of the variable are presented before and after a specific measurement point. Note that if the variable were "officially" measured only at the "measurement point," the values of the variable for all four persons would be identical (they would have identical "states"). Clearly, these single measurements are occurring within the context of unique phases for each person. To reiterate the earlier point, measures at single points in time may yield data that fail to provide important information about the dynamic time-course or phase of a variable.

Any quantifiable variable could be represented on the vertical axis of Figure 5-3: frequency of delusional thoughts, rate of interruptions during a marital argument, blood pressure, hours of exercise per week, intensity of aggressive behaviors, mood severity ratings, and the frequency of negative social interactions. If the vertical axis represented self-monitored "depressed mood" (e.g., on a 10-point daily rating scale), all four persons would have been equal on that variable at the measurement point. However, depressed mood is rapidly decreasing for Person A, rapidly increasing for Person B, stable for Person C, and highly variable (in a transitional phase) for Person D; thus the persons are in very different phases of their phase-space, although their states on the measured variable are equal. Similarly, if the vertical axis represented a hypothesized causal variable, such as the rate of aversive social interactions, all persons would have been experiencing an equal rate of aversive social interactions at the measurement point (an equal state) but would differ significantly in the phase of their phase-space for that variable.

These observations lead to an important maxim: *Different persons can be equal in the state of a variable dimension and different in the phase of that variable dimension* (Haynes et

---

[4]Cross-lagged correlations in time-series designs involve correlations between variable A at sampling point 1 (At_1) with variable B at the previous sampling point (B_{t-1}). Causal inferences from time-lagged cross-correlations should be derived cautiously. Although temporal precedence between the variables is considered, the magnitude of the correlation coefficient is sensitive to the length of the measurement interval and common effects of a third variable.

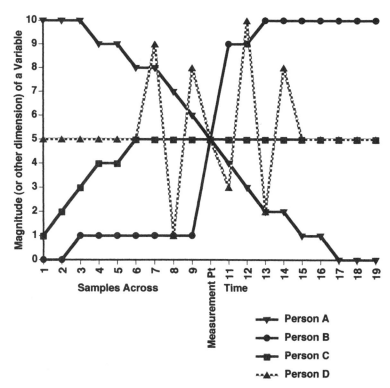

Figure 5-3. Phase-space functions for a variable that is captured at one instant in time for four persons. The ordinate could represent dimensions such as magnitude, severity, duration, and other dimensions. Variables could include most variables measured in psychological assessment: specific motor behaviors or thoughts, psychophysiological responses, mood, environmental events. (Adapted from Haynes et al., 1993.)

al., 1993). Thus, in time-series measurements for an individual, equal state values at different measurement points (e.g., measurement points 6 and 10 for Person D, in Figure 5-3) do not mean that the phases are equivalent. Additionally, in multivariate assessment, different variables can have equal state values (e.g., when using standardized scores) but be in different phases. In sum, important dynamic attributes of variables may be lost if measures are obtained at only one point in time. In turn, the lack of information about the dynamic attributes of behavior and environmental events may diminish the validity of our clinical judgments (see Box 5-3).

Estimating Functional Relations

Time-series measurement strategies can help identify ***causal and noncausal functional relations***. To illustrate, we will presume that there is a strong causal relation between negative social interaction and depressed mood (e.g., the client with rheumatoid arthritis illustrated in Figure 5-2). If we measure negative social interactions and depressed mood, concurrently, for many persons only once, we are evaluating only state measures. However, persons with identical scores may be in different phases of negative social interactions. For example, persons

---

Box 5-3
Transitional States

Time-series assessment strategies can help detect transitional states on important variables with clients (Haynes, 1992). Transitional states are conditions of a variable between two equilibrium states (illustrated by Person D in Figure 5-3, in measurement points 6–15). Transitional states are often characterized by increased variability and trend (slope) in the values of a variable dimension. Examples would be the onset, and then cessation, of extreme and rapid fluctuations in mood, blood pressure, or activity level.

Transitional states of behavior problems are important for several reasons. First, they can show important changes in causal variables and help the clinician identify causal relations. For example, significant changes in a person's social environment (e.g., changing residence, death of a family member) may be associated with increased variability and trend in mood and sleeping patterns. Transitional states are sometimes noted in initial response to pharmacological and psychological interventions.

Estimates of causal relations obtained during these transitional phases may be unreliable. Furthermore, clinicians are usually interested in the stabilized effects of a causal variable. Transient periods of varying levels of distress often follow traumatic experiences and are considered normal. Intervention is not usually warranted unless the distress continues (more than one month for DSM-IV diagnosed PTSD).

Because the underlying causal mechanisms may be in a state of flux, there may be greater susceptibility to the influence of moderating variables (e.g., behavioral intervention strategies) during the transition state than during the equilibrium state.

---

who have been experiencing an increasing rate of negative social interactions are likely to report higher depressed moods than persons who have been experiencing a decreasing rate of aversive social interactions but identical measures at the measurement point. As a result, the obtained correlation between social interaction and depressed mood would be diminished.

The covariance estimates, noted above, would be attenuated because the degree of shared variance between positive social interaction and depressed mood is reduced unless measures of both the phases and the states of the variables are included in the prediction formula. Given a causal relation between two variables, attenuation of shared variance estimates would occur regardless of whether the correlations were derived from concurrent or time-lagged measurements, from within-subject or between-subject designs, or from single or multiple time samples.

The impact of causal variables can also be affected by the phase state of the behavior problem (see discussion in Çambel, 1993). Heiby (1994b) discussed "sensitivity to initial conditions" as an example of this phenomenon. Persons may be in different phase states of depressed mood when a series of negative social interactions occurs. The effect of these aversive interactions might differ as a partial function of whether depressed mood was increasing or decreasing (e.g., aversive interactions with coworkers may have a greater impact when it occurs concurrently with increasing marital difficulties).

Phase-Space Functions and Behavioral Assessment Strategies

Phase-space concepts suggest that we can more accurately predict the future time-course of behaviors, identify changes in important variables more quickly, and identify functional relations more accurately if we measure the phase of variables in addition to their states. A valid and sensitive assessment of dynamic aspects of variables mandates the use of time-series measurement methodologies. Strategies for collecting time-series data in a clinical assessment context are outlined in Table 5-3.

Despite their utility, time-series measurement methods are rarely implemented in psychological assessment, except for research and studies in applied behavior analysis (see *Journal of Applied Behavior Analysis*). For example, none of the empirical articles published in *Psychological Assessment* from 1992 through 1998 measured the phase state of a variable.

Time-sampling parameters affect the degree to which time-series measurement captures important functional relations and the time-course of variables. The sampling rate must be sufficient to capture important aspects of a variable's time-course to place any obtained measure in the context of its phase. In time-series measurement, the rate of sampling should vary directly with the rate of change of the sampled variable (see Suen & Ary, 1989, for a more detailed discussion of time sampling).

Insufficiently frequent time samples will make it difficult to place an obtained state measure within its phase. Consequently, the sampling rate affects the clinical utility of the phase estimates and the degree to which time-series measurement enhances predictive efficacy. Most "longitudinal" assessment strategies (see review in Collins & Horn, 1991; Gottman, 1996) involve sampling rates determined by convenience or tradition (e.g., yearly measurement) and involve a sampling rate insufficient to capture important phasic characteristics of the measured variables.

Table 5-3
Strategies for Obtaining Time-Serics Measures in Clinical Assessment

1. Administration of brief behavior questionnaire before every assessment/intervention session
   A. on behavior problems.
   B. on hypothesized causal variables (e.g., on positive and social interactions, environmental stressors, response contingencies).
   C. on intervention variables (e.g., on relaxation practice, positive communication exercises, medication use).
   D. on approximations to immediate, intermediate, ultimate intervention goals.
2. Daily self-monitoring (using paper and pencil forms, handheld computers, phone calls to office answering machines)
   A. of the occurrence or other dimensions of behavior problems.
   B. of causal variables.
   C. of intervention variables.
   D. of immediate and intermediate intervention goals.
3. Automated ambulatory monitoring
   A. such as ambulatory monitoring of psychophysiological responses of patients with cardiovascular disorders.
4. Critical event sampling
   A. measuring variables contingent on the occurrence of a significant event (such as measuring thoughts during a distressing social exchange, measuring positive verbal strategies during a marital argument, measuring responses to a child's oppositional statements.
5. Other instrument-aided measurement
   A. such as actimeter/pedometer measures of movement with clients who have sleep or pain disorders.
6. Informant ratings
   A. such as frequent ratings by staff members of a patient's behaviors, or by teachers of a child's behavior in the classroom.
7. Computer-assisted measurement
   A. such as computer-assisted measures of goal attainment before every treatment session, or computer-aided self-monitoring.

Ethical, time, and institutional constraints in clinical assessment settings often limit the applicability and parameters of time-sampling strategies. Sampling parameters are often dictated by considerations other than the hypothesized rate of change of the measured variables. The sampling rate, number of samples obtained, and the duration of the sampling period are often constrained by the need to quickly make clinical decisions (e.g., diagnosis, hospitalization, the initiation of intervention), by financial considerations, and by lack of client adherence. For example, daily samples are sometimes taken of many clinically important variables, such as headache, mood, panic episodes, seizures, or negative life events. A client might record at the end of each day the number of panic episodes that occurred that day, or fill out a daily questionnaire on depressed mood. However, daily sampling is often based more on the convenience for the client or assessor than on the expected time-courses of these variables. If daily sampling does not provide a sensitive measure of a variable's phase state (e.g., if there is important nonlinear change in the variable between sampling points), the estimated strength of functional relations involving that variable will be attenuated. Additionally, it is often difficult to estimate the best sampling rate for a variable.

Cautions About an Exclusive Emphasis on Empiricism and Quantification in Behavioral Assessment

The previous sections emphasized the importance of a quantitative, empirically based orientation to psychological assessment. However, there are dangers to an excessive reliance on empirically based methods. Earlier in this chapter we reminded readers of several sources of error in measures obtained in psychological assessment. Furthermore, a scholarly orientation toward assessment can include qualitative, nonquantitative assessment strategies.

An overzealous adoption of methodological empiricism can be counterproductive—it can hamper the evolution of an assessment paradigm. Excessively molecular measures and excessive quantification can trivialize the assessment process. These strategies, when used without sufficient consideration, can render valid data with little social or practical importance and with insufficient ecological validity Unwarranted emphasis on quantification of minutia demeans the behavioral assessment paradigm and reduces the clinical utility of the assessment process. As we have stressed several times, a functional approach to assessment suggests that the methods and resultant data should be appropriate for the goals of the assessment. The type of data to be collected should be determined by its potential contribution to clinical judgments. Data should be collected on only those variables that are important to clinical judgments, at a level of specificity that is clinically useful, and only for as long as they are helpful.

An exclusively quantitative approach to assessment can also limit the validity and utility of clinical judgments, the creativity of psychological inquiry, and the evolution of an assessment paradigm. We must retain a humble stance regarding the behavioral assessment paradigm: It is a useful and cybernetic epistemological framework but nascent in its understanding of the course and causes of behavior disorders.

The evolution of all assessment paradigms is best served by an openness to new concepts and relations. Although a scientific approach is the best method of evaluating hypotheses, and while data sets can be a rich source of hypotheses, many hypotheses can be generated from qualitative observations of and thoughtful reflection about clients. By supplementing quantitative with qualitative analyses and some imagination, behavioral assessors can facilitate creative hypothesis generation.

Now, a caveat about our caveat. Although hypotheses can be generated and clinical judgments can be strengthened with qualitative methods, the importance of a quantitative, scientifically based approach to psychological assessment cannot be understated. Psychological construct systems must ultimately be based on the results of scientific, quantitatively based inquiry. Many construct systems (e.g., Gestalt, transactional, psychoanalytic) have changed little across the decades because their constructs and methods are not conducive to empirical scrutiny and refinement. They are characterized by well-defended assumptions about the nature of behavior and causality, rather than by methods of inquiry that encourage examination and refinement of these assumptions. In contrast, the evolution of the behavioral assessment paradigm, the enhanced power, and the clinical utility of behavioral assessment methods are results of a methodological emphasis, rather than an emphasis on a predetermined set of concepts.

Summary and Suggestion for Modeling a Scholarly Approach to Psychological Assessment

Several methodological tenets of the behavioral assessment paradigm were examined in this chapter. An important epistemological element of behavioral assessment is a scholarly approach to assessment. This involves the use of validated instruments and methods. Several elements of this maxim were reviewed: (a) validated instruments should be used whenever possible, (b) validity indices are conditional and can vary across assessment goals, assessment contexts, and populations, (c) assessment strategies should be used that reduce measurement error, and potential sources of measurement error should be considered when drawing clinical inferences from the assessment data, (d) data acquired from assessment should be useful for the goals of assessment, and (e) the validity of inferences can often be strengthened by using multiple sources of information.

Multisource assessment can involve data from multiple methods of assessment, multiple assessment instruments, multiple informants, and multiple occasions. There are several limitations of psychological assessment addressed by multisource assessment: (a) different sources of data often capture unique facets of a targeted construct, (b) different assessment instruments that use the same method and target the same construct (monomethod assessment) can also measure unique facets of the targeted construct, (c) a targeted construct may more validly be measured by using multiple assessment instruments and, sometimes, by aggregating the obtained measures, (d) each source of assessment data is associated with idiosyncratic sources of measurement error, (e) sources of assessment data may differ according to the situations in which they were collected, and (f) data from different assessment sources contribute to the behavioral case formulation of a client because they identify important sources of variance in behavior problems.

The assessor should be familiar with the empirical literature relevant to the client's behavior problems and associated causal variables. Additionally, the assessor should be familiar with the literature about assessment instruments and empirically validated interventions for the client's behavior problems and goals.

A hypothesis-testing strategy is an important characteristic of the behavioral assessment paradigm. The assessor initially forms preliminary hypotheses about the components of the behavioral case formulation that are then evaluated using assessment data. This hypothesis-testing process is an ongoing, iterative process, and it is important that assessment strategies be selected that allow for hypotheses to be disconfirmed. Often, clinical assessors form questions that can be thought of as clinical "problems" to solve, and behavioral assessment can be thought of as a scientifically based, iterative approach to solving clinical problems.

Problem-solving and hypothesis-testing are facilitated by clear specification of hypotheses and assessment questions. These hypotheses should be based on a firm empirical foundation. The evaluation of hypotheses should be based on a careful analysis of confirmatory and disconfirmatory data, multisource measurement of dependent and independent variables, the use of minimally inferential constructs and multimethod assessment instruments of known psychometric properties, and the use of time-series measurement.

Measurement is the process of applying numbers to some attribute of a person or an event so that we can draw inferences about the attribute. An important methodological mandate of the behavioral construct system is to acquire quantitative measures of important variables.

There are, however, many limitations to a strict adherence to quantitative methods: (a) measures are only estimates of an attribute, (b) all attributes can be measured in different ways and no single measure captures all aspects of an attribute, (c) different measures of the same attribute can differ in their relation to the attribute, (d) measures always reflect phenomena superfluous to the attribute being measured, (e) the measurement process often changes the attribute being measured, and (f) not all important constructs lend themselves to quantification.

A time-series measurement strategy is one in which variables are measured frequently, usually at regular intervals, across time. It is recommended because constructs measured in clinical assessment are dynamic. In phase-space functions the value of a variable at a single measurement point is its state. The state of a variable in the context of its direction and rate of change of the variable (its phase) is its phase state. The state and phase of a variable are likely to vary across time.

It is important to capture the dynamic attributes of variables, and this can only be accomplished with time-series measurement strategies. Different persons can be equal in the state of a variable dimension and different in the phase of that variable dimension. In time-series measurements for an individual, equal state values across time for a given variable does not mean that those state values are in equal phases. Further, different variables may have equal state values but be in different phases of their respective phase-spaces. Important dynamic attributes of variables may be lost if static measurement strategies are used.

An overzealous adoption of methodological empiricism can hamper the evolution of an assessment paradigm by trivializing the assessment process. An exclusively quantitative approach to assessment can also reduce the validity and utility of clinical judgments. Although a scientific approach is the best method of evaluating hypotheses, and while data sets can be a rich source of hypotheses, many hypotheses can be generated from qualitative observations of clients.

Suggested Readings

Hypothesis-Testing, Scholarly Approaches to Psychological Assessment

Goldstein, W. M., & Hogarth, R. M. (Eds.). (1997). *Research on judgement and decision making: Currents, connections, and controversies*. New York: Cambridge University Press.

Hayes, S. C., Follette, V. M., Dawes, R. M., & Grady, K. E. (Eds.). (1995). *Scientific standards of psychological practice: Issues and recommendations*. Reno, NV: Context Press.

Repp, A. C., Karsh, K. G., Munk, D., & Dahlquist, C. M. (1995). Hypothesis-based interventions: A theory of clinical decision making. In W. O'Donohue & L. Krasner (Eds.), *Theories of behavior therapy* (pp. 585–608). Washington, DC: American Psychological Association.

Turk, D. C., & Salovey, P. (Eds.). (1988). *Reasoning, inference, and judgment in clinical psychology* (pp. 124–152). New York: Free Press.

Evaluation in Clinical Practice. Special section in *Clinical Psychology, Science and Practice*, 1996, *3*, pp. 144–181.

Idiographic Approaches to Psychological Assessment

Cone, J. D. (1986). Idiographic, nomothetic and related perspectives in behavioral assessment. In R. O. Nelson & S. C. Hayes (Eds.), *Conceptual foundations of behavioral assessment* (pp. 111–128). New York: Guilford.

Phase-Space Functions

Çambel, A. B. (1993). *Applied chaos theory: A paradigm for complexity*. Boston: Academic Press.

Cvitanovic, P. (Ed.). (1984). *Universality of chaos*. Bristol: Adam Hilger.

Time-Series Measurement

Hersen, M., & Bellack, A. S. (Eds.). (1997). *Behavioral assessment: A practical handbook* (4th ed.). Boston: Allyn & Bacon.

Kazdin, A. (1998). *Research design in clinical psychology* (3rd ed.). New York: Allyn & Bacon.

Kratochwill, T. R., & Levin, J. R. (1992). *Single-case research design and analysis: New directions for psychology and education*. Hillsdale, NJ: Lawrence Erlbaum Associates.

Suen, H. K., & Ary, D. (1989). *Analyzing quantitative observation data*. Hillsdale, NJ: Lawrence Erlbaum Associates.

6

Idiographic and Nomothetic Assessment

Introduction

Idiographic and nomothetic research and assessment strategies differ in several ways. They differ in the degree to which their methods are standardized across clients, in the degree to which their strategies focus on groups versus individuals, the degree to which inferences about one person depend on comparisons with persons, and in the generalizability of inferences across persons. Nomothetic research strategies focus on identifying covariations between variables using data from groups of persons. They are used to develop models of behavior problems that are generalizable to the "average" person.

Idiographic research strategies emphasize the measurement and analysis of variables for a single person. Covariation estimates are used to develop models that may be valid only for that person. Inferences from idiographic research may be, but are not necessarily, generalizable across persons (see Box 6-1).

Consider nomothetic research strategies that examine covariates of panic episodes by comparing persons who do or who do not experience panic episodes (e.g., Rapee & Barlow, 1993). Between-group comparisons could be made on measures of self-reported social anxiety and psychophysiological reactivity. It would be presumed that significant between-group differences on the measured variables generalize to groups of persons who experience panic episodes.

In contrast, an idiographic research strategy would examine the relations among panic episodes, self-reported social anxiety, and psychophysiological reactivity for a single client. Data on these variables might be collected on a daily basis for many days. It would not be presumed that the observed functional relations would be generalizable to other persons with panic episodes.

Idiographic and nomothetic assessment strategies also differ in the degree to which assessment strategies and the inferences from the assessment data are generalizable across persons. Nomothetic assessment strategies are similar across persons. Furthermore, judgments based on nomothetic measures often depend on comparisons with measures from other persons (e.g., as in the use of T-scores, means, and standard deviations).

In contrast, idiographic assessment strategies involve assessment instruments that are often individually tailored for a particular client. Because of the individualized nature of the

---

Box 6-1
Idiographic vs. Ideographic

The term "ideographic" is sometimes used erroneously for "idiographic" (e.g., Campbell, 1996; Corsini, 1987). However, the root "ideo" refers to "idea" such that "ideograph" is a pictorial representation of an idea or object. This term was originally associated in early Freudian psychology with the idiosyncratic images and meanings of patients' dreams. The root "idio" refers to "personal" or "distinct." "Idiothetic" (e.g., Tallent, 1992) has also been used, but this term does not appear in Webster's *Universal Unabridged Dictionary*. "Nomothetic" is an adjective, derived from the Greek term *Nomothete* (law giver), which means "giving, enacting or based on laws" (Webster's *New Unbridged Universal Dictionary*, 1983).

An early distinction between idiographic and nomothetic approaches to knowledge was made by Wilhelm Windelband (1848–1915) (Blackburn, 1994). Idiographic strategies in psychology were advanced by Gordon Allport (1937) who advocated the intensive study of the individual.

assessment instrument, it is more difficult to compare obtained measures across clients, to integrate measures from many clients, and to draw inferences that are generalizable across clients.

An assessment strategy can be individualized in two ways. First, an array of nomothetic assessment instruments can be selected on the basis of the characteristics of each client. For example, clients seeking services at an outpatient mental health center could be given different combinations of assessment instruments, such as a Wechsler Adult Intelligence Scale (WAIS), MMPI, and neuropsychological tests, based on the clients' behavior problems. Second, individual assessment instruments can be constructed for a client on the basis of the client's unique behavior problems, hypothesized causal variables, and variables that are hypothesized to moderate treatment outcome for the client. This chapter focuses on idiographic assessment instruments rather than on idiographic arrays of nomothetic instruments.

The first section of the chapter presents the rationale underlying nomothetic assessment. The next section describes the rationale underlying idiographic assessment and the role of idiographic assessment in clinical judgment. Later sections of the chapter examine Goal Attainment Scaling, advantages and disadvantages of idiographic assessment, and psychometric considerations. Methods of idiographic assessment are then discussed, followed by a discussion of the integration of idiographic and nomothetic assessment strategies.

We emphasize several points about nomothetic and idiographic assessment:

1. Idiographic assessment strategies are congruent with a functional approach to psychological assessment and can aid clinical judgments.
2. Idiographic assessment strategies are often unstandardized and, consequently, inferences from idiographic assessment are not always generalizable across clients.
3. Psychometric principles, particularly content and criterion-related validity and sensitivity to change, are applicable to idiographic measures.
4. Goal Attainment Scaling is a flexible idiographic method of measuring treatment outcome and can be congruent with a behavioral assessment paradigm.
5. The advantages of idiographic assessment strategies are conditional: The assets and liabilities of idiographic assessment vary across clients; the variables that are targeted in assessment, the goals of assessment, how the instrument is administered, and the specific focus and content of the assessment instrument.
6. The best assessment strategy will often involve a combination of idiographic and nomothetic instruments.
7. The validity of idiographic measures can be strengthened by careful specification of the assessment goals, the elements and dimensions measured, and by using multiple informants and methods of assessment.
8. Standardized methods can be used to develop idiographic assessment instruments.

Nomothetic Assessment

There are several characteristics of nomothetic assessment instruments. First, nomothetic assessment involves methods standardized across persons. For example, when intelligence and projective tests are administered, clients are presented with the same stimuli, in the same manner, in similar settings, using the same prompts, and involving the same response formats.

Second, nomothetic assessment instruments provide measures of the same variables on the same dimensions for all respondents. For example, the constructs measured and scales used for their measurement on the MMPI are the same for every client.[1]

Third, clinical judgments based on nomothetic assessment instruments are influenced by comparisons of the client with other persons. These comparisons can take the form of deviations from established norms, scale scores, rankings, and the degree of fit within diagnostic categories.

Consider the use of standardized questionnaires to measure the effects of behavior therapy on persons with panic disorder (e.g., Beck & Zebb, 1994; Craske, 1993). Standardized anxiety questionnaires can be used for all persons experiencing panic episodes. Furthermore, total scores and scale scores from these questionnaires can be compared to norms for each instrument. We can judge the status of a client on panic-related variables relative to other clients with panic episodes and those without panic episodes. We can classify a client as "moderate" or "severe" based on comparisons with other persons with panic episodes.

This example touches on a point to which we will return—the conditional utility of nomothetic and idiographic assessment strategies. Although idiographic assessment strategies are very congruent with the behavioral assessment paradigm, nomothetic strategies can also aid clinical judgments (Meier, 1994).

In both nomothetic and idiographic assessment strategies the assessment instruments are selected for use with a client on the basis of prior research involving persons with similar behavior disorders. For a panic disorder case, an assessor might decide to use the Anxiety Disorders Interview Schedule (ADIS-IV) (see McGlynn & Rose [1998] for a review of this and other anxiety assessment instruments) because it has been found valid and sensitive in prior studies. However, in idiographic assessment, research is more likely to guide the selection of the method of assessment rather than the specific elements of the instrument. That is, a clinician may decide that the use of self-monitoring strategies is well supported and then design a self-monitoring instrument that fits the needs of a particular client.

In summary, nomothetic assessment instruments: (a) involve methods that are standardized across persons, (b) provide measures of identical variables on identical dimensions across persons, (c) depend on aggregated measures obtained from other persons to derive judgments, and (d) are selected for use with a particular client from prior research with persons with similar behavior.

Idiographic Assessment

Definition and Characteristics

Idiographic assessment strategies[2] involve methods, instruments, measures, and contexts designed specifically for an individual client. Differences between idiographic and nomothetic assessment strategies are summarized in Table 6-1.

[1]The MMPI illustrates a point discussed later in this chapter, that the nomothetic and idiographic strategies are often compatible and that assessment instruments can have idiographic and nomothetic features and uses. While T-scores on clinical scales of the MMPI are usually obtained for all clients, assessors often select from a wide array of content scales and conduct individual item analysis for different clients (Butcher, 1995).
[2]It is useful to remember the difference between assessment instruments and strategies. An assessment instrument is a specific procedure for deriving measures on the behavior of a person (e.g., a specific self-report depression questionnaire). An assessment strategy is the general plan for deriving measures. An assessment strategy can involve a set of assessment instruments, instructions to client, time-sampling decisions, and an assessment setting.

Table 6-1
Comparison of Idiographic and Nomothetic Approaches to Clinical Assessment

Aspect of Clinical Assessment	Nomothetic Approach	Idiographic Approach
Assessment method (e.g., self-monitoring, analogue observation)	Standardized across clients	Standardized or individually selected for each client
Elements of assessment instrument (e.g., specific stimuli, codes, and situations in assessment instrument)	Standardized across clients	Individually selected for each client
Relevance and representativeness of instrument elements	May contain irrelevant elements and may not capture important variables for a client	All elements are relevant to client and more likely to capture important variables
Level of specificity of measured variable (e.g., higher-level trait variable vs. molecular behavior)	Can vary in level of specificity	Can vary in level of specificity
Obtained measures	Identical across clients	Can be identical or can vary across clients
Selection of assessment instruments (assessment strategy)	Based primarily on data from assessment of other persons	Based primarily on data from client
Basis for clinical judgments from obtained measures	Based on comparison of the same measures obtained from other clients	Based on criteria specific to the client, sometimes in conjunction with measures from other clients
Data aggregation across clients	Can aggregate data from same instrument across clients	Can aggregate across clients for different measures of the same construct if a standardized format is used
Generalizability of inferences	Inferences from measures are generalizable across persons	Inferences from measures are not necessarily generalizable across persons
Applicability of psychometric principles	All forms of reliability and validity can be applicable	All forms of reliability and validity can be applicable but especially content validity, criterion-related validity and sensitivity to change

The advantages of idiographic assessment strategies have been emphasized by many behavioral assessment scholars (e.g., Cone, 1986; Linehan, 1993; Mash & Hunsley, 1990; Nelson, 1983; Silva, 1993; Wolpe, 1986). This emphasis derives, in part, from the emphasis on single-subject, idiographic research strategies emphasized in applied and experimental behavioral analysis (e.g., Kazdin, 1978; Sidman, 1960). These research strategies have been used for many decades to estimate functional relations that operate for single organisms within carefully control situations (Kazdin, 1998; Kratochwill & Levin, 1992).

There are four main characteristics of idiographic assessment instruments and measures:

- The assessment strategy and elements of the assessment instrument (e.g., observation time samples, items on a questionnaire, scenarios in role-play assessment) are individually designed for each client.
- The measures obtained are individually selected for each client.
- Clinical judgments from obtained measures are based on individually determined criteria rather than on data from other persons.

- There are restrictions on the way in which data from idiographic assessment instruments can be aggregated across persons.

There are several other characteristics of idiographic assessment. First, idiographic assessment is congruent with a functional approach to psychological assessment. That is, the assessment strategies in an idiographic approach are strongly influenced by the goals and characteristics of the client and of the assessment occasion. For example, the variables measured on a visual analogue scale for a client with anxiety or mood problems could differ across clients, depending on the specific problems or hypothesized causal variables for each client.

Second, idiographic assessment strategies are useful across a variety of assessment goals. They can be used to measure all phenomena targeted in psychological assessment, regardless of the level of specificity of the variables. Variables measured in idiographic assessment may include high-level trait-based measures as well as highly specific behaviors and events. Furthermore, idiographic assessment can include a variety of dimensions. Idiographic measures can include many assessment methods and response modes. Individualized assessment instruments can involve interviews, behavioral observation, psychophysiological and self-report instruments.

Third, idiographic assessment instruments can have nomothetic characteristics. The elements of an assessment instrument and of an assessment strategy can differ in the degree to which they are idiographic or nomothetic. Consider the prototypic idiographic self-monitoring form shown in Figure 6-1, designed to be filled out by a client before bedtime. Some elements of this self-monitoring assessment strategy are nomothetic, in that they would apply to all persons using the instrument: (a) The time-sampling strategy (measures obtained daily, before bedtime), (b) the response format (five-point scales), and (c) the data collection method ($3'' \times 5''$ card or handheld computer). This method of assessment is also nomothetic in that it can be used with all persons with sleep-related behavior problems and can be based on prior research. A standardized construction increases the applicability of an idiographic assessment instrument across clients and the generalizability of inferences from obtained measures.

Finally, because data are often collected on different variables for different clients, the generalizability across clients of inferences from idiographic assessment strategies is limited. Generalizability is restricted because, for example, not all clients using the instrument in Figure 6-1 would monitor their level of pain. However, as we discussed above, idiographic assessment strategies can contribute to generalizable inferences if conceptually related phenomena are aggregated. Clement (1996) illustrated how idiographic assessment measures (Goal Attainment Scaling) can be used to draw inferences about groups of clients.

Bases for Clinical Judgments

Nomothetic and idiographic assessment strategies sometimes differ in the bases for clinical judgments. Three overlapping bases for clinical judgments are:

- *Norm-based judgments.* Clinical judgments are based on comparing measures obtained from the client with norms for those particular measures (e.g., MMPI, Beck Depression Inventory [BDI]).
- *Client-based judgments.* Clinical judgments are based on criteria determined for the client that may or may not reflect norms (e.g., individualized treatment goals).
- *Criterion-based judgments.* Clinical judgments are based on criteria that may or may not reflect norms (e.g., statistical criteria for determining the clinical significance of treatment effects).

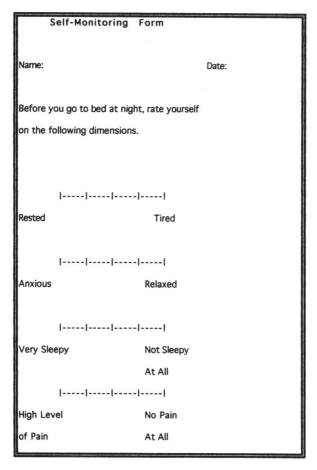

Figure 6-1. A self-monitoring form (e.g., on a 3″ × 5″ card) that has both nomothetic (e.g., consistent scaling, time-sampling) and idiographic (dimension labels) elements.

Nomothetic strategies more often use norm-based judgments, and idiographic strategies more often use client- and criterion-based judgments, although all bases can be used by each strategy.

Applications to Clinical Assessment

Idiographic assessment instruments can be used to gather data about all elements of the functional analysis and to measure treatment process and outcome. Idiographic assessment instruments can be used to identify and rank-order a client's behavior problems and to estimate the type and strength of relations between behavior problems. They can also be used to identify causal variables, moderator variables, mediating variables, causal chains, and to estimate the type and strength of relations among these variables and between them and the client's behavior problems. Idiographic assessment instruments can be used to monitor the behavior problems of a client in response to specific stimuli, situations, or interventions. The diverse applications of idiographic assessment strategies are outlined in Table 6-2.

Muran and Segal (1992) described an idiographic assessment instrument, "self-scenarios," based on models of self-schemas and emotional processing that can be used to evaluate the

Table 6-2
Examples of Idiographic Applications in Behavioral Assessment

Reference	Population	Measures	Assessment Method	Description
Blanchard et al. (1994)	Car accident victims	Heart rate, BP, EMG, electrodermal	Laboratory psychophysiological assessment	Audiotaped descriptions of each victim's accident
Chadwick et al. (1994)	Outpatient psychiatric	Delusional beliefs	Self-monitoring	Measured conviction, preoccupation, and anxiety to five statements about delusions
Hillbrand & Waite (1994)	Sex offenders	Sexual thoughts	Self-monitoring	Recorded activity and thoughts when paged
Kern (1991)	University students	Assertion skills	Role play	Subjects tested in assertion situations from own experience
Muran & Segal (1992)	Anxious and depressed outpatient adult	Extended vignettes of highly distressing events	Self-report questionnaire	Vignettes measured on five dimensions (frequency alternatives …)
Pitman et al. (1990)	Clients with PTSD or anxiety disorder	Heart rate, EMG, electrodermal	Laboratory psychophysiological	Individual vignettes of trauma experiences presented in lab
Shalev et al. (1993)	Patient with PTSD	HR, electrodermal	Laboratory psychophysiological	Individually constructed audiotape of trauma event

effects of cognitive-behavioral treatment. This assessment instrument involved the construction of vignettes designed to measure a client's responses to distressing events. The vignettes were individually constructed for each client on the basis of interviews. The client is presented with the vignettes during assessment sessions and rated his or her responses along several dimensions.

Examples of self-scenarios in the case study described in Muran and Segal included: (1) "When I am in social situations, I feel extremely nervous and high-strung, almost manic. I desperately try to get everyone to like me. I am always questioning whether people like me. It's awful if they don't. It is so important for them to like me in order to feel worthwhile." (2) "When people mislead or mistreat me, I often become enraged, and I lose my temper. I usually think, 'No one has a right to treat me that way! They're bastards!' If I let them treat me like this, then I am really worthless." The self-scenarios involved a stimulus situation, affective responses, motoric responses, and cognitive responses.

The client rated each scenario on several dimensions: (a) frequency of occurrence, (b) degree of preoccupation with the scenario, (c) the degree to which the scenario can be imagined, (d) how easily an alternative scenario can be imagined, (e) confidence in enacting the alternative, (e) the degree to which the scenario is relevant to the client, and (f) chronicity. In this case, the client rated five individually constructed scenarios on these dimensions, six times, across the course of therapy.

Pitman and associates (1990) developed individualized scripts describing the trauma or anxiety experiences (e.g., a stressful combat experience, and precombat, positive, and neutral experiences) of clients diagnosed with either combat-related PTSD or an anxiety disorder. Each client described his or her experience in writing and then identified the psychophysiologic reactions that accompanied the experience. The assessor reviewed and clarified the client's descriptions and then composed a 30-second script that described each experience, incorporating the client's psychophysiologic reactions. The experiences were then presented to the client, via an audiotape, in a laboratory setting while multiple psychophysiologic and subjective measures were obtained. The authors found significant differences in the responses of PTSD clients and anxious clients to the idiographic scripts—most PTSD patients were highly reactive to scenes of their past combat experiences.

McGlynn and Rose (1998) discussed individually tailored strategies for the assessment of clients with anxiety and fear disorders. Clients were exposed (through verbal descriptions by the assessor, videotape/audiotape presentations, from written and verbal descriptions by the client) to idiosyncratic and specifically described feared stimuli. Behavioral, cognitive, and emotional responses of clients were measured during these presentations.

These idiographic "exposure" assessment methods can also involve behavior avoidance tests (BAT). In a BAT, the client is requested to approach feared stimuli (e.g., to approach a window on high floor, to walk out of house, speak before a small audience) either in a controlled clinic or natural environment situations. Clients may also be asked to role-play anxiety-arousing or difficult social situations, such as meeting a new person or disagreeing with a friend. Measures are usually obtained of subjective distress, thoughts, and degree of approach to the feared stimuli.

Kern (1991) discussed the relative costs and benefits of standardized and individualized role-play assessments. Kern described a "standardized idiographic" strategy for measuring social anxiety and social skills. The client provided details of recent distressing social experiences. Examples were solicited within six categories of experiences (e.g., "You want someone to do something which he or she had previously promised to do or was supposed to do, but never did"). The client specified the other interactant's words, voice tone, and nonverbal behavior. The assessor then acted as the other person during subsequent role plays, which were videotaped for later scoring. Role plays involved two to six interchanges between the testee and the tester and were repeated if either party's behavior in the role play did not accurately represent the naturalistic interaction. The client's responses in the role plays were scored, with the help of ratings guidelines, into six response classes ranging from assertion to submission and aggression.

These examples illustrate various strategies of idiographic assessment. All involve a standardized approach to the development of individually tailored assessment instruments. Although the specific elements of the assessment instruments used by each author (e.g., the trauma scenarios, the feared objects approached) were personalized for each client, standardized methods were used to determine these elements. Furthermore, the higher-level construct each instrument was intended to measure (e.g., "multimodal responses to a traumatic event") was identical across clients.

There are many other examples of idiographic assessment in the literature. For example, systematic desensitization involves a standardized approach to idiographic assessment—clients report their magnitude of subjective distress to individually tailored hierarchies of feared stimuli, developed from interviews. In this example, the higher-order construct targeted by the instrument is the same, but there are differences across clients in the specific anxiety-provoking scenes and situations contained in the hierarchy. Halford, Sanders, and Behrens (1994) discussed idiographic approaches to the analogue assessment of the communication strengths and deficits of distressed marital couples. Torgrud and Holborn (1992) discussed the validity of role-play assessment of social skills and suggested that their external validity could be increased by using individually constructed scenarios that included the salient stimuli and contexts from each client's recent problematic interactions.

Goal Attainment Scaling

Goal Attainment Scaling (GAS) is a frequently used idiographic approach to the measurement of treatment outcome (Kiresuk, Smith, & Cardillo, 1994). Despite deficiencies in its usual manner of application, GAS is a flexible and standardized approach to idiographic assessment that can be used in a manner congruent with a behavioral assessment paradigm.

GAS was originally developed in 1968 with support from the National Institute of Mental Health and has been applied in many educational, mental health, and business contexts and within many psychological assessment paradigms. GAS is often implemented at a level of specificity and using response formats that are incompatible with the behavioral assessment paradigm. For example, as part of a treatment outcome measure, a client might rate him- or herself on "degree of self-esteem."

GAS was developed to address several deficiencies associated with the assessment of treatment outcome with nomothetic instruments. Most nomothetic instruments (e.g., personality inventories, trait-based questionnaires) for measuring treatment outcome are broadly focused, include elements and scales that are irrelevant for a client, and emphasize unidirectional measures of behavior pathology rather than positive treatment goals.

Item-irrelevance is an unavoidable characteristic of most nomothetic measures and can lead to clinical judgment errors. For example, at pretreatment assessment a client will score highly only on some scale items or on some scales of a questionnaire with multiple scales. Similarly, only some behaviors in a behavioral observation system for coding problematic family interactions will be relevant for a particular client. While data from multiple scales and multiple items can be useful for guiding subsequent pretreatment assessment strategies and for constructing a functional analysis, they are sometimes less relevant and less sensitive measures of treatment outcome. Because aggregated scale scores often include items that are irrelevant for a client, their specificity and sensitivity can be compromised. Judgments about treatment effects based on nomothetic aggregated scale scores are insufficiently specific and can be attenuated by floor effects associated with stability of the irrelevant items (or, the irrelevant items can contribute error to the judgments).

Consider a questionnaire that contains nine items that cover the domains of depressive behaviors (e.g., sad mood, eating and sleeping problems, anhedonia, fatigue, impairment in concentration, thoughts of death or suicide, and feelings of worthlessness). If a total score from the questionnaire is used to measure treatment outcome for a client who is experiencing problems in only three of the domains, scores on six domains would not be expected to change as a function of treatment and their inclusion would dampen the sensitivity to change of the questionnaire for this client.

Goal Attainment Scaling is designed to measure the individual motor behaviors, thoughts, emotions, and events that are the most salient targets of intervention for an individual client. The items in GAS are those that are most relevant and representative of the problems and treatment goals for each client. Consequently, obtained measures should be more sensitive than most nomothetic assessment instruments to treatment effects.

Goal Attainment Scaling assessment strategies involve several steps (Smith, 1994): (1) behaviors that should change with effective therapy are identified, (2) specific goals are determined for the identified target behaviors, (3) a title is selected for each goal, (4) behavioral indicators are selected as measures of goal attainment, (5) the expected outcome from treatment is specified, (6) goal and outcome indicators are reviewed and refined, and (7) outcomes and indicators above and below expected outcomes are identified.

As illustrated in Table 6-3, goal attainment is typically measured on a five-point scale, with "0" representing the expected level of outcome after treatment. Sources of error in GAS are those applicable to all assessment instruments and those particular to idiographic assessment strategies. Error can also be introduced in GAS through imprecise definitions of criteria and faulty designations of goals. Usually, the designation of degree of goal attainment is a subjective judgment. These judgments are most likely to be valid if based on multiple informants and multiple situations.

Table 6-3
Illustration of Goal Attainment Scaling

Cardillo and Choate (1994) illustrated the use of GAS with a 72-year-old man who was undergoing inpatient treatment for a right-hemisphere stroke. One goal for discharge established for this client was increased socialization, measured on the following level of attainment scale (see p. 22 of Cardillo and Choate for illustration).

Level of Attainment	Description of Level	Indicator
−2	Much less than expected	No social conversations; spends free time in room
−1	Somewhat less than expected	Leaves room occasionally; no social conversations
0	Expected outcome	Converses socially outside of room when approached
+1	Somewhat more than expected	In addition to "0" initiates conversations
+2	Much more than expected	In addition to "+1" participates in group activities inside or outside facility

Advantages and Disadvantages

Advantages and disadvantages of idiographic assessment were introduced in Table 6-1 and are summarized in Table 6-4. As with all assessment methods, the advantages and disadvantages of idiographic assessment are conditional—they vary across clients, the variables targeted in assessment, the goals of assessment and the inferences that are to be derived, the assessment method, how the instrument is administered, and the specific focus and content of the assessment instrument. Thus, advantages outlined in Table 6-4 are potential and conditional—they will pertain to some but not to other idiographic instruments, on some but not other assessment occasions.

Two of the most important advantages of idiographic assessment are *sensitivity to change* and a *flexibility in level of specificity*. "Sensitivity to change" is the degree to which a measure reflects true changes in the targeted construct. Idiographic measures can be very sensitive to change because their variance is not dampened by irrelevant sources. Idiographic measures are

Table 6-4
Advantages and Disadvantages of Idiographic Assessment Instruments

Aspect of Assessment	Explanation
	Advantages
Relevance for client	All elements of the assessment instrument (e.g., questionnaire items, scenarios) are relevant for each client.
Level of specificity	Flexible. Data can be collected at a level of specificity that is best suited for each client.
Sensitivity to change	Can be highly sensitive to change across time in measured variables.
Face validity	Methods and elements can seem relevant and appropriate to clients.
Generalizability; external validity	Variable, but can be high because elements of the assessment instrument are close representations of behaviors and events in the natural environment.
Congruence with behavioral assessment paradigm	Congruent with assumptions regarding multiple causality and multimodal nature of behavior disorders, emphasis on functional relations and constructional approaches, and a scholarly approach to clinical assessment.
Comparison across clients	Allows comparisons of clients with different goals if the elements of the assessment instruments (scales, time-frame, method of measurement) are the same.
Constructional orientation to assessment	Allows for a focus on the achievement of positive treatment goals, in addition to the measurement of the parameters of the behavior problems.
Treatment utility	Can be used to measure changes in treatment targets and can help identify failing therapies.
Amenability to different assessment targets	Can be used with a wide array of client problems, goals, and causal variables.
Promotion of empirically based assessment and treatment	Can be use with controlled single-case designs in clinical settings.
	Disadvantages
Errors in assessment instrument and methods	Because of nonstandardized nature of assessment, the assessor may make errors in the construction of the instrument and in its implementation.
Normative comparisons	Difficult unless standardized methods are used to construct the idiographic instrument.
Cost-efficiency	Assessment may require construction of new instrument for each client.
Utility for program evaluation (aggregation across clients)	Can be difficult to use for program evaluation unless the instrument is constructed to allow for aggregation of data.

also congruent with the emphasis in the behavioral assessment paradigm on time-series assessment.

Although one advantage of idiographic assessment instruments is that they can target variables at different levels of specificity (and different response modes), the level of specificity of obtained measures affects their sensitivity to change. Higher-order, more aggregated variables, such as self-esteem, are composed of multiple elements and indicators, only some of which are relevant for a particular client. Consequently, only some elements of the aggregate would be expected to change over time or to change as a function of treatment for a particular client.

Idiographic assessment is congruent with the behavioral assessment paradigm in other ways. First, it is congruent with a multivariate model of behavior problems and their causes. Second, as we noted earlier in this chapter, idiographic assessment is congruent with the emphasis in applied and experimental behavior analysis on the intensive study of the individual. In the functional analysis, we are most interested in estimating functional relations relevant to important behavior problems for a client, and these judgments often do not depend on normative comparisons or data from standardized instruments. Third, idiographic assessment is congruent with the emphasis on a constructional approach to assessment and treatment. It can be used to measure approximation toward positive treatment goals, behaviors targeted for strengthening, and positive alternatives to problem behaviors.

The strengths of idiographic assessment are also a source of limitation. First, the increased relevance of obtained measures for individual clients is accompanied by a decreased utility for drawing inferences regarding other clients with the same behavior problems. Second, errors can be introduced anytime a new instrument is constructed. Specifically, a clinician may select the wrong variables for a client, use the wrong response scale, define the measured variables poorly, and construct erroneous instructions. Data may also be obtained from informants who are unqualified, unknowledgeable, or biased.

Usually, the advantages of idiographic assessment are hypothesized rather than empirically demonstrated. As we note in the following section, idiographic assessment instruments have seldom been subjected to psychometric evaluation.

Psychometric Considerations

Many psychometric principles are relevant to idiographic assessment generally and GAS specifically (see discussions by Cardillo & Smith, 1994; Smith & Cardillo, 1994). *Content validity* is an important evaluative dimension of clinical assessment instruments, particularly idiographic assessment instruments. Given that the goal of idiographic assessment is to measure behaviors and events that are relevant for each client, the content validity of an idiographic assessment instrument is the degree to which the behaviors and events measured by the instrument are those most relevant to the client.

Referring to the examples in Table 6-2, content validity is the degree to which: (a) the audiotaped descriptions of auto accidents used in the study by Blanchard et al. (1994) captured the salient features of traumatic experiences of each client; (b) the role-play scenarios used in the study by Kern (1991) included the most problematic assertion situations encountered by each client; and (c) the vignettes of distressing experiences used in the study by Muran and Segal (1992) incorporated the most distressing social situations encountered by each client.

In GAS, content validity is the degree to which the goals, levels, and indicators are relevant to, and representative of, the behavior problems and goals of each client. There are four important considerations in constructing content valid goal attainment scales:

- All of the client's major goals should be represented.
- All goals included in the GAS should be relevant to the client (no minor or inapplicable goals should be included).
- Levels of attainment should be relevant to the client (they should be appropriate for the client's initial level and for the expected outcomes of treatment).
- Indicators of goal attainment should be relevant to the client (they should be observable and measurable).

Referring to the example of GAS in Table 6-3, content validity is the degree to which: (a) "conversation outside the patient's room" is a relevant treatment goal for this patient, (b) the degree to which this goal captures all important goals for this client, (c) the degree to which social conversation outside the room is an appropriate indicator of goal attainment, given the characteristics of this client, the expected course of recovery, and expected treatment effects.

Convergent and criterion-related validity also affect confidence in judgments based on data from idiographic assessment instruments. Given that measures from every assessment instrument reflect true variance in the targeted construct, systematic variance not associated with the targeted construct, and random measurement error, it is important to estimate and strengthen the degree to which measures from an idiographic assessment instrument reflect variance in the targeted constructs.

The strategies to strengthen the validity of clinical judgments outlined in Chapter 3 are also applicable to judgments based on idiographic assessment instruments. Judgments from idiographic measures are more likely to be valid if they are based on multiple methods of assessment, multiple informants, multiple measurement occasions, clearly defined and minimally inferential criteria and variables, and multimodal assessment.

We must remember the conditional nature of psychometric evaluations. General statements about the validity of idiographic assessment strategies are unwarranted. Inferences about the validity of idiographic measures depend on the confluence of assessment method, target of assessment, response format, and client characteristics, among other variables. Thus, GAS may be a valid or invalid method of assessment, depending on the goals, indicators, client, and setting of the assessment occasion.

Given these constraints, many studies (see Table 6-2) have supported the convergent, discriminative, and criterion-related validity of idiographic assessment instruments. For example, Blanchard et al. (1994) found that heart rate responses to idiosyncratic audiotaped descriptions of the victim's own auto accidents was a sensitive indicator of PTSD.

The uniqueness of idiographic assessment instruments makes it difficult to draw general inferences about the validity of the method. The extant data only suggest that properly constructed idiographic assessment instruments can show a high degree of content, convergent, and discriminative validity.

Reliability is also an important consideration in idiographic assessment. For example Lambert (1994) reviewed several studies on GAS and noted that low reliability has been a problem. That is, different goals and criteria are often identified for the same patient by different persons. However, as Lambert noted, reliability of GAS and all idiographic assessment instruments can be increased with a carefully standardized approach to their construction.

Lambert (1994) noted other threats to the reliability and validity of GAS: (a) goals set for a client may reflect the therapist's biases, (b) excessively difficult or easy goals may be included (a threat to the content validity of the instrument), which would affect inferences about treatment outcome, and (c) measures of goal attainment on GAS may not correlate highly with other treatment outcome measures.

Methods of Idiographic Assessment: Integrating Idiographic and Nomothetic Strategies

Integrating Idiographic and Nomothetic Measures

Given the relative advantages of idiographic and nomothetic strategies, the best assessment strategy will sometimes involve a combination of both (Nelson-Gray, 1996). Clinical judgments are often aided by data from standardized, nomothetic instruments and data from instruments that are unique for a client. Thus, idiographic and nomothetic assessment strategies are complementary rather than exclusionary (Meier, 1994).

Nomothetic instruments can be particularly useful for broad-spectrum assessment in the early phases. Behavior problem checklists and structured interviews can often help identify variables of special relevance for a client, which can be the focus of subsequent idiographic assessment. In the evaluation of treatment outcome, idiographic instruments can sometimes be used to monitor functional relations and treatment effects on variables identified with nomothetic instruments. This nomothetic-idiographic sequence is congruent with the "funnel" approach to assessment often recommended by assessment scholars (Hawkins, 1986; Mash & Hunsley, 1990). Assessment instruments with an increasingly greater specificity are used sequentially as client behavior problems, goals, and causal variables are identified.

Norm-based judgments can be particularly useful in the assessment of children (Ollendick & Hersen, 1993b). Normative comparisons can help track a child's relative developmental level over time in language, motor skills, cognitive abilities, self-help skills, interpersonal relationships, and height and weight. Significant changes relative to developmental level across time (e.g., a child at an average level of weight who begins to quickly fall into lower percentile categories as he or she ages) suggest the need for more intensive assessment (Batshaw, 1997; Wicks-Nelson & Israel, 1997) of potential causal factors.

Finally, nomothetic assessment instruments can be used idiographically. An example would be an item analysis of a client's MMPI or Beck Depression Inventory. In this example, clinical judgments, such as treatment effects, would be based on the client's responses to specific items, rather than on comparisons of the client's scores with norms.

Principles of Idiographic Assessment

Several principles guide idiographic assessment strategies. These methodological principles emphasize the use of carefully standardized, psychometrically sound strategies for developing idiographic instruments.

- Ensure that the method of idiographic assessment is congruent with the goal of the assessment.
- Select assessment targets on the basis of standardized and validated assessment methods: Whenever possible, use standardized interviews and questionnaires to select variables to be measured in idiographic assessment.
- Content validity is a particularly important consideration: Select targets that are rele-

vant and representative of the problems and goals of the client. In analogue observation and role-play assessment, this includes the relevance and representativeness of the situations encountered by the client in his or her natural environment (see discussion by Torgrud & Holborn, 1992).

- All elements of idiographic assessment instruments should be specified and standardized (e.g., for role plays, this includes the behavior of confederates and instructions to clients; for GAS and self-monitoring this includes the response dimensions and format).
- When treatment outcome measurement is the goal of idiographic assessment, select multiple targets that should be sensitive to positive and negative treatment effects.
- When feasible, include multiple response modes, dimensions, methods, situations, and informants.
- Attend to the principle of informed consent. Clients should understand and agree with the methods and selected variables.
- Instruments should be administered in carefully designed time-series format when possible.
- When possible, instruments should measure functional relations, not simply target behaviors and events.
- The contexts of measurement should be carefully defined.
- When assessment occurs in the natural environment, methods of data collection should be established to maximize reliability and cooperation by the client.
- When feasible, measures should be collected frequently and reviewed with the client.

The use of standardized methods to construct idiographic assessment instruments is particularly important (Cone, 1988). The degree of standardization of idiographic assessment instruments affects the degree of confidence that obtained measures reflect the targeted constructs and the degree to which data from different client can be compared. For example, Torgrud and Holborn (1992) emphasized the need for standardized functional analytic interviews to develop idiographic role plays to allow for comparisons of data across client and clinicians.

Goal Attainment Scaling is "informally standardized" (e.g., Kiresuk, Smith, & Cardillo, 1994), in that general outlines for constructing individual Goal Attainment Scales have been offered. These methods are best described as "semistructured" and the relative validity and utility of the recommended procedures have not been evaluated. Without standardization, obtained measures are more likely to reflect systematic or unsystematic errors by the assessor.

Summary

Idiographic and nomothetic assessment strategies differ in the degree to which the inferences depend on normative comparisons and the degree to which inferences are generalizable across persons. Nomothetic assessment instruments are more likely to be identical, and inferences are more likely to be generalizable across persons. The unique construction of some idiographic assessment instruments can reduce the generalizability across clients of inferences based on obtained measures.

Nomothetic assessment involves: (a) methods standardized across persons, (b) clinical judgments that are often based on comparisons with measures on the same instrument obtained from other persons, and (c) instruments selected from prior research with persons with similar behavior disorders.

The boundaries between nomothetic and idiographic assessment strategies are ambiguous at times. However, there are three primary characteristics of idiographic assessment instruments: (a) the assessment strategy and elements of the instrument are unique for each client, (b) clinical judgments from obtained measures are based on individually determined criteria, and (c) there can be restrictions on the degree to which measures can be aggregated across persons. Idiographic assessment is congruent with a functional approach to psychological assessment and can be used with most clients and variables targeted in psychological assessment.

Idiographic measures can contribute all elements of the functional analysis and can be used to monitor treatment process and outcome. Idiographic assessment can help identify a client's behavior problems, estimate the type and strength of relations between behavior problems, identify causal variables and causal relations among variables, monitor the behavior problems of a client and the responses of a client to specific stimuli, situations, or interventions.

Goal Attainment Scaling is a flexible idiographic approach to the measurement of treatment outcome that can be implemented in a manner congruent with a behavioral assessment paradigm. It is designed to measure the behaviors and events that are most salient for an individual client and most sensitive to treatment effects. Two important advantages of idiographic assessment instruments are their sensitivity to change and flexible level of specificity. They can be sensitive to change because variance in obtained measures is less affected by irrelevant variance.

Idiographic assessment strategies are congruent with the behavioral assessment paradigm in many ways: (a) with the complex causal and behavior disorder models, (b) with the emphasis on the intensive study of the individual, (c) and with the emphasis on a constructional approach to assessment and treatment. However, gains in the relevance of obtained measures for each client are associated with a decreased ability to draw normative comparisons.

Content validity is a particularly important evaluative dimension for idiographic assessment instruments. The content validity of an idiographic assessment instrument is the degree to which the elements of the instrument are relevant to the client and the degree to which measures represent the array of the client's behavior problems. In GAS, it is important that all of the client's major goals be represented, and all goals, indicators, and levels of attainment should be relevant to the client.

Convergent and criterion-related validity of idiographic measures also affect confidence in judgments based on them. It is important to estimate the degree to which idiographic measures reflect variance in the targeted construct and to strengthen the validity of judgments from idiographic measures. Acknowledging the conditional nature of psychometric evaluation, many studies have supported the validity of measures obtained from idiographic assessment instruments.

Several guidelines for idiographic assessment were offered: (a) match the method to the goals of assessment, (b) select assessment targets on the basis of validated assessment methods, (c) use standardized methods to construct idiographic instruments, (d) attend to the content validity of the instrument, (e) control all aspects of idiographic assessment instruments, (f) when treatment outcome measurement is the goal, select a variety of targets that should be sensitive to treatment effects, (g) collect data on multiple response modes, multiple dimensions, multiple methods, in multiple situations, and from multiple informants, (h) ensure that the client understands and agrees with methods and variables, (i) collect time-series data, (j) measure functional relations when possible, (k) carefully define the contexts of measurement, (l) during assessment in the natural environment, establish methods of data collection to maximize reliability and cooperation, and (m) review assessment data with the client.

Suggested Readings

Goal Attainment Scaling

Kiresuk, T. J., Smith, A., & Cardillo, J. E. (Eds.). (1994). *Goal attainment scaling: Applications, theory, and measurement*. Hillsdale, NJ: Lawrence Erlbaum Associates.

Idiographic Strategies in Psychology Research

Pervin, L. A. (1984). Idiographic approaches to personality. In N. S. Endler & J. M. Hunt (Eds.), *Personality and the behavior disorders* (pp. 261–282). New York: John Wiley & Sons.

Idiographic Assessment

Cone, J. D. (1986). Idiographic, nomothetic and related perspectives in behavioral assessment. In R. O. Nelson & S. C. Hayes (Eds.), *Conceptual foundations of behavioral assessment* (pp. 111–128). New York: Guilford.
Nelson-Gray, R. O. (1996). Treatment outcome measures: Nomothetic or idiographic? *Clinical Psychology, Science and Practice*, *3*, 164–167.
Silva, F. (1993). *Psychometric foundations and behavioral assessment*. Newbury Park, CA: Sage (chapter 3).

7

Specificity of Variables

Introduction

This chapter examines the level of specificity of variables in psychological assessment. "Specificity" refers to the number of facets and dimensions subsumed by a variable. For example, the assessment of marital aggression can include specific variables such as "rate of verbal criticisms," less specific variables such as "rate of negative verbal interactions" (verbal criticisms is one of several facets), or even less specific variables "degree of communication problems" (negative verbal interactions is one of several facets).

Specificity affects the utility and validity of clinical judgments. Specific variables facilitate the identification of behavior problems, functional relations, and treatment effects but can be less reliable. Less specific variables are sometimes more reliable but can pose problems for deriving more specific judgments about clients.

The behavioral assessment paradigm is characterized by an emphasis on specific variables such as discrete observable behaviors, discreet thoughts, response contingencies, and physiological responses. The measurement of specific variables is often the optimal approach to addressing the goals of behavioral assessment, such as the development of a behavioral case formulation and judging the effects of intervention.

"Unit of analysis" is a related concept and refers to measurement units that contribute to clinical judgments. For example, we may measure heart rate by measuring beat-by-beat intervals (IBI). However, our inference about treatment effects may be based on the unit of analysis of "average IBI during a five-minute stress exposure period." Similarly, we may measure discrete self-injurious behaviors, during 15-second time samples, by a child with developmental disabilities, but our unit of analysis is more likely to be "rate of SIBs," composed of an aggregate of many unique behaviors across time.

This chapter examines the rationale, clinical utility, assets and liabilities, and sources of errors of variables with different degrees of specificity. We emphasize several points about specificity and units of analysis.

1. Specificity refers to the number of sources of variance in a variable or measure.
2. Variables can differ in the number of facets they subsume, in the degree to which their dimensions are specified, and in the degree to which they reflect or aggregate situational and temporal sources of variance.
3. Clinical judgments can differ in their degrees of specificity.
4. There are fewer alternative explanations for variance in specific compared to non-specific variables.
5. The specificity of a variable is relative, and an assessment method can include variables and measures with different levels of specificity.
6. The most useful specificity depends on the goals of the assessment occasion.
7. Psychological assessment instruments often provide data that are not sufficiently specific for the goals of behavioral assessment.
8. A unit of analysis refers to the part of a phenomenon that serves as the target of measurement and inference.
9. The identification of functional response classes can help identify positive alternatives to problem behaviors.
10. Specific variables promote the use of observational methods and the use of time-series measurement strategies.
11. Specific variables promote the measurement of functional relations.
12. Specific variables reduce the number of alternative explanations for obtained measures and strengthen clinical judgments.
13. Specific variables aid judgments about the process and outcome of interventions.

Specificity in Psychological Assessment

Types of Specificity

Four components of the psychological assessment process can vary in specificity. First, *variables targeted* in psychological assessment and the *measures obtained* from psychological assessment instruments can differ in the diversity and number of facets they subsume. Some variables, such as "quality of life" Lehman (1996) are very nonspecific because they include many facets. The quality of life variable (and quality of life measures) can subsume physical health, financial status, spirituality, safety, and satisfaction with relationships.

In turn, "marital satisfaction" is often considered one facet of quality of life. It is more specific than quality of life because it has a narrower domain and it does not include other facets of the more molar quality of life variable. However, marital satisfaction also has multiple facets, one of which could be "communication satisfaction." "Satisfaction with problem solving communication" is at a still higher degree of specificity, but could be decomposed into multiple facets such as "interruptions" and "agreements" (see Box 7-1).

Figure 7-1 illustrates six levels of specificity of behavior problems for one client who was assessed for depressive symptoms. The least specific variable (depressive disorder) is composed of several component variables (e.g., somatic, cognitive behaviors), each of which is composed of several lower-level variables. As we discuss later, the specificity of variables can be increased indefinitely, and the assessor must determine the degree of specificity that is most consistent with the goals of assessment.

Second, variables can differ in the degree to which *dimensions and modes* are specified. The variable "panic episodes" is specific relative to the variable "panic disorder" (APA, 1994). However, it is nonspecific in terms of dimensions. Panic episodes could be measured on different response modes (thoughts, physiological states, overt behavior) and on different dimensions, such as "frequency," "duration," and "magnitude." A description of panic episodes on one dimension and mode would increase its specificity because it narrows the domain of possible inferences.

Third, variables can differ in the degree to which *situational and temporal conditions* are specified. For example, "trauma-related feelings of guilt" is more specific than "feelings of guilt"; "negative thoughts in response to an aversive social situation" is more specific than "negative thoughts"; "alcohol use in the last seven days" is more specific than "recent alcohol use."

Fourth, *clinical judgments* can differ in their specificity. The three components of

---

Box 7-1
A Variables, Measures, and Specificity

A *variable* is an attribute that can change and a *measure* is a number that represents that variable (see Glossary). Variables and measures can differ in specificity, and comments made about variables in this chapter also apply to measures.

A variable can be measured in different ways, and measures of a variable can differ in their specificity. "Anxiety" is a nonspecific variable (because it has multiple facets) that can be measured with nonspecific methods, such as projective, tests moderately specific methods, such as a self-report questionnaire, or specific methods such as behavior avoidance tests. Thus, *specificity* of a measure refers to the range of facets or dimensions of a variable tapped by a particular assessment instrument.

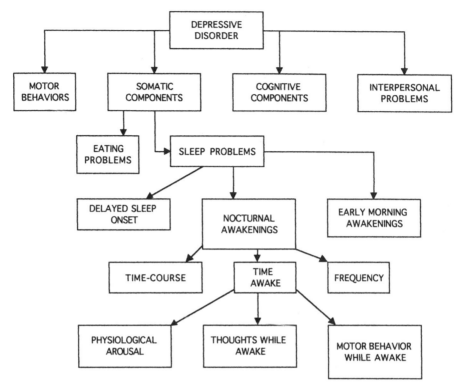

Figure 7-1. Six levels of specificity reflecting the facets and dimensions of a higher order variable. The highest level variable (depressive disorder) is composed of several lower level variables (i.e., facets; e.g., somatic, cognitive components). Each of these facets is composed of several lower level variables (e.g., eating and sleeping for somatic components), each of which is composed of several lower level variables, and so forth.

specificity discussed above affect the specificity of clinical judgments. Judgments about behavior within a specific period or situation, or about particular facets of a variable, are more specific than unconditional judgments. For example, judgments about the conditions likely to lead to a child having panic episodes at school are more specific than judgments about whether a child is prone to panic episodes due to "personality" characteristics.

Characteristics of Specific and Nonspecific Assessment

These examples illustrate several attributes associated with the specificity of variables and judgments.

- *Specificity* refers to the number of sources of variance in a measure. More specific variables reflect fewer sources of variance. If we examine Figure 7-1, we note that the number of sources of variance for a construct is shown by the number of variable boxes subsumed by it. There are fewer sources of variance as specificity increases. A measure of "depressive disorder" reflects variance in four major facets (e.g., motor behavior, somatic components), each of which reflects variance in many more facets, and so forth.

However, a measure of one facet, such as "somatic components of depression," omits variance from three of these four major facets.[1]

- Because there are fewer sources of variance, there are fewer alternative explanations for variance in more specific compared to less specific variables. Consequently, confidence in inferences can be increased by the use of more specific variables. For example, there are many ways that a client could obtain a high score on a self-report depression questionnaire but fewer ways that a client could obtain a high score on one subscale on that questionnaire. Similarly, we cannot be sure about the basis for a person's score on a quality of life instrument—did a low score indicate current financial or marital troubles? Thus, the range of permissible judgments decreases as specificity increases.

- As these examples illustrate, specificity is inversely related to the degree of aggregation. An aggregated variable reflects multiple facets, joined additively or multiplicatively. Measures of nonspecific variables, such as "magnitude of depression," are composites of all of the facets of the variable. The problem associated with aggregation is also that associated with the use of nonspecific variables—aggregation can mask important sources of variance. A measure of "assertiveness" can mask important differences in assertive behavior across situations and important differences among the various facets and modes of assertiveness. Importantly, these specific data are most useful to planning and evaluating a behavioral intervention strategy.

- As we noted with Figure 7-1, the specificity of a variable is relative. Because variables can always be further decomposed and aggregated, the specificity of a variable can be judged only in relation to other variables and to the goals of assessment. "Self-injurious behavior" can be decomposed into head-banging, face-slapping, which could be further specified as to particular head location and hand. But, at some point, further specificity does not facilitate, and can impede, clinical judgments.

- Specificity does not necessarily covary with the method of assessment. Although variables targeted in behavioral observation are often more specific than those targeted in self-report questionnaires, this is not always the case. We could obtain a nonspecific observation measure and specific self-report measures of social skills (e.g., observed rate of "positive social behaviors" and self-reported rate of "initiating conversations with strangers") (see Box 7-2).

A Functional Approach to Determining the Best Specificity

There are assets and liabilities to both specific and nonspecific variables, and it is often difficult to select the best degree of specificity for an assessment occasion. For example, First et al. (1992) discussed the assets and liabilities of specific and nonspecific diagnostic categories and criteria in DSM (see also discussion of psychiatric diagnosis in *Behavioral Assessment*, *1*[10], 1988). First and colleagues noted that nonspecific constructs (e.g., diagnostic categories such as "PTSD") can help organize related ideas into useful categories. A molar-level diagnostic category, or functional response class, can describe a set of covarying behaviors and can facilitate communication among scholars and clinicians. However, nonspecific variables are also more susceptible to idiosyncratic interpretation by clinicians, may be associated with lower agreement among raters, and can erroneously imply a higher-than-warranted magnitude

---

[1]The inference about the association between specificity and the sources of variance presumes that the facets have no functional relation (are not highly correlated). However, even for correlated facets, the range of sources of variance and the number of alternative explanations for obtained scores are reduced as the specificity of variables increases.

Box 7-2
Different Terms for "Specificity"

Different terms have been used to refer to "specificity." The terms "global," "molar level," "higher-level" or "macrolevel" are often used to refer to less specific variables. Similarly, "micro level" or "lower-level" are often used to refer to more specific variables. "Level of abstraction," "level of reduction," and "level of inference" are sometimes used synonymously with "specificity" (e.g., First et al., 1992). "Precision" is sometimes used to mean "specificity," but refers to the degree to which a measure approximates the "true" value of a variable (see Glossary).

---

of covariance among facets (e.g., consider the difference in specific behavior problems of patients with similar diagnostic labels).

From a functional approach to assessment, the most useful specificity depends on the goals of the assessment occasion (Barrett, Johnston, & Pennypacker, 1986; Lees & Neufeld, 1994). To select the best specificity, the assessor must ask, "What judgments are to be made and what specificity will best contribute to those judgments?"

In Figure 7-1, if the main assessment goal is prescreening with a large community sample (e.g., "Should this individual be referred for additional assessment for depressive symptoms?"), a one- to three-item, nonspecific depression screening inventory could be sufficiently specific. Such a screening instrument might include a few nonspecific questions, such as, "I have been feeling depressed lately—Y, N." Queries about specific thoughts, social interactions, sleeping habits, time frames, or magnitude of depressive symptoms would be unnecessary and possibly irrelevant for a judgment about further screening.

In contrast, if the goal of assessment is to evaluate the effects of an intervention program on cognitive and behavioral aspects of depression (e.g., "What are the effects of a cognitive-behavioral intervention program on the facets of depression?"), measures of the specific facets would be necessary. A global depression score would be insufficiently specific to make judgments about specific treatment effects.

The client discussed in Haynes, Leisen, and Blaine (1997) illustrates the differential utility of specific and nonspecific variables. This client reported significant sleep difficulties. One possible source of variance for this client's sleep difficulties was worry after she went to bed. A global measure of "anxiety" might initially focus the assessment but, if used by itself, would be insufficiently specific to guide treatment decisions. A high score on an anxiety questionnaire would not have informed the assessor about an important functional relation—that presleep worry was an important trigger for delayed sleep-onset. Furthermore, a nonspecific measure would not suggest that attention-focusing or relaxation strategies at bedtime might aid sleep maintenance.

Nonspecific variables hamper clinical judgments primarily when used in isolation. Hypotheses derived from the measurement of global variables should be followed by more specific assessment. Often, psychological assessment instruments provide data that are not sufficiently specific for most behavioral assessment goals. An "intellectual/cognitive functioning" score for a client with neurological impairments, and an "introversion/extraversion" score for a client with severe social anxiety are insufficiently specific to aid most treatment-related clinical judgments and the design or evaluation of intervention programs.

Variance in nonspecific variables between persons and across time and settings can have multiple explanations. Additionally, alternative explanations of variance and covariance are more difficult to evaluate with nonspecific variables. Consequently, the use of nonspecific variables can also inhibit the development of basic and applied behavioral sciences.

Degree of Specificity, Units of Analysis, and the Function of Behavior

Degree of specificity is related to **units of analysis** in psychological assessment (see Box 7-3). A unit of analysis refers to the part of a phenomenon that serves as the target of measurement (Johnston & Pennypacker, 1993). For example, in behavioral observation of a child who is engaging in self-injurious behaviors, should we count occasions in which a child bites himself, bangs his head, and pinches himself as occurrences of the aggregate variable "self-injurious behavior"? If we do, the unit of analysis would be a less specific and more aggregated composite of three behaviors. Alternatively, should we count and analyze the three behavioral measures individually? If we do, the unit of analysis would be more specific, less aggregated.

Johnston and Pennypacker recommended a functional approach to selecting the best unit of analysis. That is, the most useful units of analysis will depend on the functional relations that are of most interest. Behaviors with common functions, similar responses to environmental stimuli, and high magnitudes of covariation can be treated as elements of a **response class**. In the example above, if biting, head-banging, and pinching strongly covaried and had similar effects on their environment, the best unit of analysis might be the composite "self-injurious behavior." Alternatively, if the child bit himself more often in some situations and banged his head more often in others, the most useful units of analysis would be the individual behaviors. Similarly, head-banging and pinching should be analyzed separately if one functioned to escape an aversive situation and the other functioned to garner physical contact from others.

Box 7-3
The "Unit"

The **unit of analysis** in psychological assessment derives from mathematics. "Unit" can refer to a standard of measurement used as the basis for counting (James & James, 1992); examples include an hour, foot, and pound. Any *dimension*, such as length, can be measured with multiple units.

In physics, units are divided into two classes: *fundamental*, or base, and *derived*. Derived units are always expressed as multiples of the fundamental unit. The fundamental units of physics have been established by international agreement in 1960 to ensure consistent use across researchers. Fundamental units include the meter (as a measure of length), second (as a measure of time), and mole (as a measure of substance) (Lerner & Trigg, 1991). The most frequently used fundamental unit in behavioral observation is "rate of response occurrence." Measures such as conditional probabilities, rate, and change over time can be considered as derived units because they are based on this fundamental unit.

In psychological assessment, there is frequent disagreement about the phenomena to be measured, the dimensions on which the phenomena should be measured, and the base units that should be applied to the dimensions. Inconsistency in dimensions and units is particularly evident in the measurement of situations and contexts, which are important components in functional analyses (McFall & McDonel, 1986). "Derived" units are similar to the concept of "aggregated" measures. However, aggregation can also involve types of units (e.g., a time unit and a frequency unit).

Response Topography and Response Class

Response topography refers to the form or characteristics of a behavior. It is often a qualitative characteristic and often involves a description of behavior occurring in space (e.g., a specific definition of what motion constitutes a "hit").

A ***response class*** is a set of responses that have common sources of influence. A ***functional response class*** (i.e., a functional response group) is a set of responses that differ in form/topography and other characteristics but are under the control of the same contingencies.

As Donahoe and Palmer (1994) noted, functional response classes are formed through environmental selection. The environment, such as contingencies provided by a parent for a child's oppositional behaviors, provides similar reinforcement to a set of different responses. This set is "functional" because the responses are similar in their effect on the environment rather than in their form.

Functional response classes are important in behavioral assessment in several ways. Sometimes, more adaptive responses can be substituted for maladaptive responses in the same functional response class. For example, simple communication skills may sometimes be taught to children as substitutes for severe behaviors used to gain attention from adults or to escape from aversive situations.

Because behaviors in a functional response class often covary (although sometimes they are mutually incompatible), estimates of difficult-to-measure responses can sometimes be derived from measures of easier-to-observe behaviors in the same response class. For example, measures of noncompliance and verbal aggression may help estimate stealing and lying, if these behaviors are part of the same functional response class for an adolescent. A behavior can be a member of multiple response classes because it can have multiple functions. (See discussion in Johnston & Pennypacker, 1993).

The identification of functional response classes is an important assessment goal for two reasons. First, behavioral interventions are often designed to modify sources of variance for sets of behavior problems. For example, if social contingencies help maintain self-injurious behaviors, a behavioral intervention strategy would attempt to change the contingencies for the self-injurious behaviors.[2] This behavioral management strategy would be effective for all behaviors maintained by social contingencies but would be less effective for behaviors affected by different response contingencies.

Second, the identification of functional response classes can help identify positive alternatives to problem behaviors. For example, Durand (1990) discussed a functional communication training intervention for clients with severe behavior problems. He noted that many severe behaviors, such as self-injury in children with developmental disabilities, affect persons in the child's environment. He suggested that severe behaviors sometimes serve as a way to communicate with others. Considering severe behaviors as elements of a communication functional response class, it may be possible to substitute more adaptive communication behaviors for the maladaptive ones. For this and other types of maladaptive behaviors, the assessor asks, "What is the function of the behavior and can we help the person learn more adaptive behaviors that have the same function?"

[2]For the efficiency of discussion we simplify the descriptions of behavioral interventions. For example, behavioral assessment and intervention with a child exhibiting self-injurious behaviors would be multifaceted and long term. It could involve medical and nutritional interventions; strengthening family support systems (e.g., support groups with other parents, respite); an assessment of the child's strengths; programs to help the family achieve positive educational, communication, and social goals for the child; and a focus on family systems, such as other siblings and the marital relationship.

We implicitly endorse the idea of a functional response class when we teach clients how to relax or exercise, instead of eating or injuring themselves, when they feel anxious. Shiffman (1993) implemented a functional response class strategy when he recommended that the intervention for smoking should depend on the "motives" for smoking. For example, he recommended that a client who smokes to relax should be given relaxation training.[3]

It is important to note that functional response classes are often *idiographic*, that is, the same behavior may have different functions across persons and, consequently, functional response classes may be composed of different behaviors for different clients.

Degrees of Specificity and Inferential Errors

As we emphasized earlier, nonspecific measures can lead to clinical judgment errors because there are more sources of variance for obtained data. Data collected by O'Leary, Vivian, and Malone (1992) illustrate this point. Their research suggests that if the focus of assessment is to know if a person is being hit, kicked, or shoved by their spouse, specific terms must be used during the assessment interview. If the assessor asks if the client is being "physically abused," the response may reflect the degree to which the client believes these violent acts were: (a) due to external circumstances (e.g., drinking or job stress), (b) "caused by" other marital problems (e.g., communication), (c) triggered by something the client did or said, (d) benign in intent (the spouse did not mean to hurt the client), (e) just a temporary event, and (f) followed by an apology.

Azar (1994) made a similar point regarding assessment in organizational psychology. She discussed the assessment of the reasoning processes of job applicants. If the goal is to measure the *way* persons think about problems, measurement of thinking "outcome" (i.e., was a specific problem solved) may not be sufficiently specific because it does not necessarily reflect the reasoning process. She illustrated this issue with students learning how to fix electrical circuits in the U.S. air force. A computer model simulated a malfunctioning electrical circuit and the trainee was asked to repair it. Beyond measuring successful repair of the circuit, the computer tracked the pattern of moves to determine whether the student understood proper diagnostic techniques. Outcome ("successful circuit repair") was a nonspecific variable and only partially reflected the variable of most interest to the assessors—the degree to which circuit diagnostic procedures were followed.

In a similar manner, specific measures help the assessor to select the best targets in an intervention program. For example, a single questionnaire item on global marital satisfaction may help identify individuals and couples for whom additional marital assessment might be appropriate. However, this measure would be insufficiently specific to help focus those intervention efforts. More specific measures of marital distress and interaction, such as the Areas of Change Questionnaire (clients rate each of 34 specific behaviors on how much they want their partner to change) (Margolin, Talovic, & Weinstein, 1983) and the Spouse Observation Checklist (each partner monitors the occurrence of common pleasing and displeasing

---

[3]Both Durand and Shiffman used questionnaires to help identify functional relations for a client's behavior problems. Shiffman (1993) used the "Reasons for Smoking Scale," which includes items on motives, antecedents, consequences, patterns of smoking, and on the effects of not smoking (he also uses the "Occasions for Smoking Scale" and "Motives for Smoking Scale" in the functional analysis of smoking). Durand (1990) used the 16-item "Motivational Assessment Scale" (MAS) to help identify the contextual determinants of self-injurious and other severe behaviors exhibited by persons with developmental disabilities. The MAS can help determine if a severe behavior is maintained by tangible rewards, attention, or escape from aversive situations.

marital behaviors by their spouse) (Weiss & Perry, 1983) are more helpful in identifying specific problems and strengths in a marital relationship.

There are many other cases in which nonspecific measures can lead to errors in clinical inferences. Patterson and Forgatch (1995) noted that global parent ratings of change among adolescents in family intervention programs may reflect how the parents feel about themselves and the child, rather than changes in the behavior of the child. The authors cited four studies in which global maternal ratings of problem children were more highly correlated with the mothers' self-ratings of depression than with the observed behavior of their children.

Specificity in Behavioral Assessment

The behavioral assessment paradigm acknowledges the utility of nonspecific variables but emphasizes the advantages of greater specificity (e.g., Barrett, Johnston, & Pennypacker, 1986; Goldfried & Kent, 1972; Haynes, 1978; McFall & McDonel, 1986). The emphasis on specificity in behavioral assessment is partly based on dissatisfaction with the nonspecific variables associated with traditional psychological assessment. Molar variables do not optimally aid clinical case formulation and the design of intervention programs.

Specific variables help clinical judgment in psychological assessment in several ways:

- Specific variables *promote the use of observation assessment methods.* For example, if "trouble initiating conversations" is identified as a potential problem with a patient in an inpatient psychiatric unit (as opposed to less specific variables such as "introversion" or "social inhibition" or "low self-esteem"), the assessor is more likely to use analogue observation of conversation scenarios to observe the patient's conversational skills than if the targeted variable is "social anxiety."
- Specific variables are more likely to *promote an examination of the contexts, situations, response contingencies, and antecedent events* associated with behavior problems. An assessor is more likely to evaluate the situations and responses associated with "trouble initiating conversations" than with "low self-esteem."
- Specific variables are *more amenable to time-series measurement.* Because of their sensitivity to change, they facilitate the analysis of the time-course of variables as well as the identification of variables that may be associated with changes across time.
- Specific variables *reduce the number of alternative explanations* for obtained measures. Consequently, they reduce the chance of differences across assessors in judgments based on the same measures. For example, there are many ways to interpret a nonspecific variable such as "low self-esteem," but fewer ways to interpret the more specific facet of that variable, such as "expectations of rejection when meeting new people." With fewer alternative explanations, the biases of the assessor are less likely to affect judgments based on data.
- Specific variables *are more useful for constructing functional analyses of clients.*
- Specific variables *are more useful for the design of behavioral intervention programs.* Behavioral intervention programs are often designed to modify specific behaviors and the causal variables that maintain problematic behaviors.
- Specific variables *are sensitive to change and more useful for evaluating the process and outcome of interventions.* When molar variables are used to evaluate intervention process or outcome, one cannot be sure which facets of the variable are responsible for observed changes. Additionally, clinicians and researchers are often interested in

specific, rather than global, effects of the intervention (Mohr, 1995). Therefore, with nonspecific variables, it is more difficult to identify the specific effects of interventions and the specific variables that affect intervention outcome.

Approaching the Best Degrees of Specificity in Behavioral Assessment

Behavioral assessors are sometimes presented with nonspecific assessment requests from other professionals. Requests for assessment seldom take the form of "please provide functional analysis of the client's frequent thoughts of persecution." Requests for assessment can take the form of a "referral for psychological/psychiatric evaluation," "please provide psycho-educational evaluation," "obtain psychological testing and intervention recommendations," "need family assessment," or "refer for behavioral assessment." Given that the best assessment strategy depends on the goals of assessment, nonspecific referral questions do not provide sufficient guidance about the goals of assessment.

From a functional approach to assessment, the assessor must specify with the referring professional the exact goals of assessment before deciding on an assessment strategy. The referral agent becomes the client, and the assessor uses behavioral interviewing skills to specify the referral question.

The most useful strategies for specifying assessment questions with other professionals involve a constructive, educational, and collegial approach, emphasizing open-ended questions, followed by appropriate prompts for more specific information: What use will be made of the information? What questions will be addressed with the assessment information? What are the particular concerns, issues, and goals of the client to be addressed in the assessment?

The principles and skills applicable when interviewing other professionals about a referred client are identical to those applicable when interviewing the adult client about his or her behavior problems: (a) the professional should be informed about the purpose of the interview, (b) open-ended, nonleading questions should be used when possible, (c) reflections and summaries are judiciously used, (d) a major goal is specification of issues and concerns, (e) more specific questions and prompts should be used when necessary, and (f) a positive interpersonal ambience and reinforcement of the professional are important.

The interview continues until the assessor understands the specific clinical judgments that are to be based on the assessment data. If the questions asked and the judgments to be made are relevant, the assessor can then design an assessment strategy that provides the needed information. One effect of such an approach is that other professionals are shaped into framing more specific assessment questions in the future.

Behavioral assessors are sometimes presented with excessively specific, restricted, or irrelevant assessment questions. This occurs most often when referring professionals are not knowledgeable about the importance of systems-level, multimodal assessment and the need to identify functional relations. Often, these professionals are interested in estimating the "status" of a client. An example would be the referral of a four-year-old child diagnosed with Asperger disorder for "assessment of intellectual level." While such information might be useful for monitoring changes in cognitive abilities over time, it neglects the important communicative, cognitive, and interpersonal deficits associated with this diagnostic classification and the importance of situational factors and social response contingencies. Given time and financial considerations, and the problems with obtaining reliable estimates of intellectual abilities with a four-year-old boy with communication problems, an intellectual evaluation may not be the most clinically useful and cost-effective focus for assessment efforts.

Sometimes, clients and referring professionals do not, or cannot, specify problems, goals, and causal variables. This occurs most often in early phases of assessment. Parents can have concerns about their child's "irresponsibility," a newly married client can express concerns because of vague feelings of "lack of mutual support" with a spouse, a teacher can refer a child for evaluation because of "low self-esteem," an adult can seek help because of "lack of meaning or purpose in my life." These are molar constructs with many facets and the relevance and importance of these facets can differ across clients with the same complaint. It is difficult for the assessor to identify functional relations, develop a behavioral case formulation, and to recommend intervention strategies when problems and goals are expressed at this degrees of specificity. In cases such as these, the task of the assessor is to get additional data through behavioral interviews and other assessment methods to further specify problems, goals, and functionally related variables.

Summary

Components of the psychological assessment process can differ in their degrees of specificity. Variables can differ in the diversity and number of facets they subsume and in the degree to which their dimensions or parameters are specified. Variables can differ in the degree to which relevant situational and temporal conditions for the target variable are specified. Additionally, clinical judgments can differ in their degrees of specificity.

There are several characteristics of specific and nonspecific variables and judgments: The specificity of variables reflects sources of variance, the specificity of a variable is inversely related to the degree of aggregation, specificity estimates are always relative, and specificity does not necessarily covary with the method of assessment.

The best specificity for psychological assessment depends on the goals of the assessment and the clinical judgments that are to be made. Often, measures obtained in psychological assessment are insufficiently specific for most goals of clinical assessment, and the use of such measures can preclude the development of a behavioral case formulation and the design of behavioral treatments.

A functional approach to assessment guides selection of the best units of analysis. That is, the best units of analysis depend on the goals of assessment and on which functional relations are of interest. Behaviors with common functions, similar responses to environmental stimuli, and high magnitudes of covariation can be treated as elements of a response class. A functional response class is also a useful concept in the identification of positive alternatives to undesirable behaviors.

The behavioral assessment paradigm emphasizes the use of specific variables. Several advantages to using specific variables were noted: (1) specific variables promote the use of observation assessment methods, (2) specific variables are more likely to promote an examination of the contexts, situations, response contingencies, and antecedent events associated with behavior problems, (3) specific variables are more amenable to time-series assessment, (4) specific variables reduce the number of alternative explanations for obtained data, (5) specific variables are more useful for constructing functional analyses of clients, (6) specific variables are more useful for the design of behavioral intervention programs, and (7) specific variables are more useful for evaluating the process and outcome of interventions.

When presented with nonspecific assessment questions a preliminary objective is to specify the exact goals of assessment, using a constructive, educational, and collegial approach, that emphasizes open-ended questions, followed by appropriate prompts for more specific information. The same strategies are used to respond to irrelevant assessment questions or excessively specific assessment questions.

Suggested Readings

Degrees of Specificity

Barrett, B. H., Johnston, J. M., & Pennypacker, H. S. (1986). Behavior: Its units, dimensions, and measurement. In R. O. Nelson & S. C. Hayes (Eds.), *Conceptual foundations of behavioral assessment* (pp. 156–200). New York: Guilford.

McFall, R. M., & McDonel, E. (1986). The continuing search for units of analysis in psychology: Beyond persons, situations and their interactions. In R. O. Nelson & S. C. Hayes (Eds.), *Conceptual foundations of behavioral assessment* (pp. 201–241). New York: Guilford.

8

Assumptions About the Nature
of Behavior Problems

Introduction

We have noted that assumptions about the nature of behavior problems affect three aspects of psychological assessment: the focus of assessment, the strategies of assessment, and the behavioral case formulation. For example, if a client's problems are considered internal, stable personality traits (e.g., "overdependence"), as is characteristic of many psychodynamically based paradigms, then assessment will focus on the detection of these traits, and assessment strategies will most likely involve projective methods and personality inventories. Finally, the ultimate case formulation will reflect the presumed importance of these causal variables.

This chapter examines assumptions about the nature of behavior problems within a behavioral assessment paradigm. We emphasize in this chapter several assumptions about behavior problems and the effect of these assumptions on behavioral assessment strategies:

1. Clients can have multiple behavior problems that can be functionally interrelated.
2. Behavior problems can have multiple modes, facets, and dimensions, which may not strongly covary.
3. Behavior problems are conditional and dynamic; they can vary across situations and time.
4. Clients classified as having the same behavior disorder can have different behavior problems.
5. Assessment strategies, the behavioral case formulation, and treatment decisions are facilitated when behavior problems are well specified.
6. Assessment strategies, the behavioral case formulation, and treatment decisions can sometimes be facilitated by a focus on client goals.
7. There are individual differences among clients in the importance of behavior problem dimensions.
8. Assessment strategies should be appropriate for the most important dimensions of a client's behavior problems.
9. Assessment strategies should be appropriate for the conditional and dynamic nature of behavior problems.

The Complex Nature of Client Behavior Problems

Clients often present with a complex array of behavior problems. They often have multiple behavior problems, each problem can involve multiple response modes, and each response mode can be measured on multiple dimensions. In this section we examine the complex nature of client behavior problems and implications for assessment strategies.

Clients Often Have Multiple Behavior Problems

Many persons have multiple behavior problems. In a study involving 20,000 interviews in several communities, Regier et al. (1990) found that 53% of persons who had received a lifetime diagnosis of alcohol abuse or dependence also met the criteria for at least one other DSM disorder. Beck and Zebb (1994) reported that 65 to 88% of patients with panic disorder and 51 to 91% of patients with panic disorder and agoraphobia had coexisting disorders. Beck and Zebb presented a table of 11 studies on comorbidity with panic disorders, the most frequent comorbid disorders being other anxiety and mood disorders. Silverman and Kurtines (1996) noted that many children with anxiety disorders can meet criteria for four to six diagnoses.

Persons and Bertagnolli (1994) reported that persons with personality disorders usually have multiple problems: They often have multiple axis I and axis II disorders. Hatch (1993) noted that persons with chronic pain, such as chronic headache, often experience sleep disturbances, occupational difficulties, disruption in social relationships, medication overuse, financial difficulties, and depression. Blanchard (1993) found that 42% of a sample of patients with irritable bowel syndrome also had panic, obsessive-compulsive, social phobia, or PTSD disorders, 28% had generalized anxiety, and 6% had mood disorders.

As suggested above, most studies on comorbidity address the cooccurrence of psychiatric diagnostic categories. Many more clients have multiple but more specific behavior problems that do not meet criteria for formal psychiatric diagnosis. Clients may experience important sleeping difficulties, loneliness, prolonged sadness, excessive anger, marital conflict, concentration difficulties, parent-child conflicts, occupational difficulties, and worry.[1]

Why Clients Often Have Multiple Behavior Problems

The likelihood that a client will evidence multiple behavior problems depends on the paradigmatic assumptions of the assessor, how problems are defined, the assessment strategies of the assessor, and characteristics and causes of the behavior problems. To illustrate how definitions affect apparent comorbidity, behavior disorders such as social phobia, panic disorders, agoraphobia, and PTSD (DSM-IV; APA, 1994) include various permutations of the same symptoms, such as subjective anxiety, physiological arousal, avoidance behaviors, and worry. Consequently, a person who meets criteria for one of these disorders has an increased likelihood of meeting criteria for another because of symptom overlap among the categories.

Similar symptom overlap has been noted among other classes of behavior disorders, such as the personality disorders (Persons & Bertagnolli, 1994), childhood anxiety disorders (Last, Strauss, & Francis, 1987), and severe childhood behavior disorders (Mash & Terdal, 1997a). In essence, many behavior problems are not uniquely associated with a particular diagnostic category.

The probability that multiple behavior problems will be identified by a clinician also depends on which assessment strategies are used. Sometimes, clinicians focus their assessment strategies on a particular client problem and fail to survey for additional problems. This is particularly likely when initial problems are highly salient to the clinician or client, such as suicidal behaviors, major depressive episodes, debilitating panic episodes, or severe anorexia. Such a premature focus decreases the chance that the clinician will detect other important problems that may have important functional relations to the initially identified problem.

An assessment strategy that begins with a broadly focused interview and questionnaire survey of possible behavior problems is more likely to detect multiple problems than an assessment strategy that quickly focuses on a problem identified early in the assessment process. Semistructured interviews that ask about a variety of problems and broadly focused behavior problem checklists can help in identifying multiple behavior problems (Sederer, Dickey, and Eisen [1997] reviewed some broadly focused behavior problem inventories and interviews). A strategy that proceeds from broadly focused to more narrowly and specifically focused assessment is sometimes called a **multiple gating** or **funnel** approach to assessment (Mash & Hunsley, 1990; Sisson & Taylor, 1993).

Multiple behavior problems can also result from various permutations of functional relations among causal variables and behavior problems. Figure 8-1 illustrates several types of

---

[1]Persons and Bertagnolli (1994) noted that multiple behavior problems can hinder assessment. For example, some behaviors associated with personality disorders can interfere with the clinician's ability to identify behavior problems: A client with "narcissistic" behaviors may be hesitant to acknowledge some important problems.

causal relations that can account for covariance among clients' multiple behavior problems. As path diagram B illustrates, multiple behavior problems can occur when a behavior problem functions as causal variables for other problems. That is, behavior problems may be functionally related or form a functional response class. Sometimes, one problem may serve as a causal variable for other behavior problems (Alessi, 1988) or, as we have noted, serve as a "keystone" behavior problem. For example, a client who is experiencing marital distress may experience a reduction in positive social interactions and an increase in conflict in his or her daily life. Given these effects of marital distress, depressed mood might be a consequence for some persons. Depressed mood and its associated behavioral concomitants could, in turn, further impair the quality of marital interactions (see discussions of marital distress and depression in Beach, Sandeen, & O'Leary, 1990).[2] Similarly, depressive symptoms might be a consequence for some parents whose children have severe childhood behavior problems, for persons who are experiencing severe family conflicts, or for persons who are exposed to chronic pain.

As Figure 8-1 shows, behavior problems can occur together when they share a common cause—when they are maintained by the same environmental consequences (path diagram A) or are triggered by the same antecedent stimulus or mechanism (path diagram C). For example, severe behavior problems of a child (e.g., self-biting, head-banging, physical aggression toward others, and screaming) may all be maintained by negative reinforcement, escape from aversive situations, or positive attention (see discussions in Durand, 1990; Newsom & Hovanitz, 1997; *Journal of Applied Behavioral Analysis, 27,* 1994). In this example, multiple behavior problems may be characterized as a functional response class because they covary and are maintained by similar contingencies.

Some clients are exposed to multiple, concurrently occurring, and sometimes functionally related causal variables. Although each causal variable may affect different behavior problems (Figure 8-1, path diagram D), a functional relation between the causal variables can result in the cooccurrence of the behavior problems. For example, a parent with a sick child may also be experiencing work-related stressors, personal health problems, marital conflict, and decrements in social support (note the potential functional relation among some of these causal variables). A possible outcome for a person facing these multiple life events would be multiple behavior problems such as sleep loss, eating disorders, depressive symptoms, and anxiety.

The Relative Importance of Behavior Problems for a Client

Judgments about the relative importance of, and relations among, behavior problems are important elements of the functional analysis. Importance estimates can be considered as "weights" assigned to each behavior problem. These judgments help the clinician estimate the potential benefits to the client (the relative *magnitude of effect*) of focusing treatment on each causal variable. Furthermore, the focus on estimating the relative importance of a client's behavior problems reflects critical differences among clients and is another element of the idiographic nature of behavioral assessment.

It can be difficult to estimate the relative importance of a client's behavior problems and goals. "Importance" of a behavior problem is a higher-order clinical judgment based on

---

[2]The relationship between marital distress and depression for a client would be expected to be moderated by several variables, such as an individual's degree of social support from family and friends, beliefs about the causes and likely outcome of the marital distress, and skills in coping with interpersonal conflict. Marital assessment strategies are discussed in Floyd, Haynes, and Kelly (1997) and O'Leary (1987) and treatment of marital distress is discussed in Halford and Markman (1997).

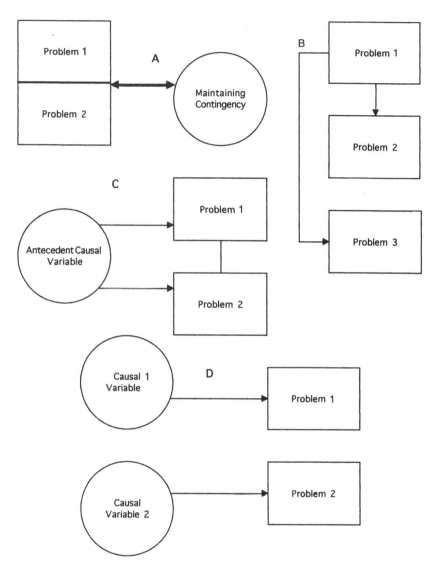

Figure 8-1. Four types of functional relations that can result in multiple behavior problems for a client. A = Two behavior problems operate as a functional response class because they are maintained by the same reinforcement contingencies (e.g., two different disruptive behaviors in the classroom are maintained by peer reinforcement). B = One behavior problem serves as a causal variable for two others (i.e., is a "keystone" problem) (e.g., chronic pain is a cause of sleep disorder and marital distress). C = Two behavior problems result from the same causal variable (e.g., excessive alcohol intake and self-injury are both triggered by interpersonal conflict; in the figure the behavior problems are correlated, but need not be so). D = Different behavior problems may be a result of multiple, uncorrelated causal variables operating concurrently (e.g., a client may be experiencing depressed mood as a result of a marital separation and nightmares as a result of a previous trauma, unrelated to marital distress).

several interrelated lower-order assessment-based judgments. Estimates of the relative importance of a client's behavior problems are derived from:

- Judgments about the *rate and magnitude of a behavior problem* (e.g., the relative importance of panic episodes or oppositional behaviors for a client is influenced by the frequency and severity of each).
- Judgments about the *probability that the behavior problem will lead to harm* (e.g., the relative importance of head-banging and domestic violence for a client increases with the likelihood that these behaviors will lead to physical injury).
- Judgments about the *degree of impact on the client's quality of life* (e.g., clients will differ on the degree to which their subjective quality of life is affected by marital distress, problems with their children, occupational stressors, and health problems).
- Similarly, the degree to which a behavior problem is associated with *functional impairment* in the client's life (e.g., the degree to which a chronic pain problem interferes with work or family functioning).
- *The degree to which a behavior problem functions as a cause of other behavior problems.*

Koerner and Linehan (1997) discussed how their dialectic treatment strategies, primarily with persons diagnosed with personality disorders, focus on problems in a descending order of their importance. The first stage of therapy focuses on suicidal/homicidal or other life-threatening behavior. Subsequently, the focus turns to therapy-interfering behavior, behavior that impairs the client's quality of life, and behaviors necessary to promote positive changes in the client's life.

Usually, importance estimates are based on multiple sources of assessment information. Probably the most frequent source is from client estimates. For example, a clinician can ask a client to rate, on a five-point scale, the importance of each of several behavior problems. Persons and Bertagnolli (1994) suggested that the clinician and client make a "problem list" and rate the importance of each entry.

Judgments about the relative importance of behavior problems (and goals) are sometimes based on estimates from informants (Alessi, 1988). However, informant reports can partially reflect the aversiveness of behavior problems to the informant, rather than to the primary client (Mash & Hunsley, 1990). Parents, teachers, or psychiatric staff may rate as more important those behavior problems that they find more troublesome. Importance judgments can also be influenced by data from naturalistic observation, analogue observation, and self-monitoring on the frequency and severity of behaviors.[3]

Behavior Problems Have Multiple Response Modes

As we have noted previously, a "response mode" refers to the form or type of behavior.[4] In contrast to functional response classes, response modes are organizational categories (a

---

[3]"Importance" is sometimes estimated by degree of deviation from the norm. However, this is a criterion associated with complex social value issues (Alessi, 1988). The main goal of the behavior therapies is to promote competent, creative, happy, adaptive persons. That may or may not involve approximation to normative behavior. Deviance is a highly contextual judgment in that some behaviors may be deviant in some cultures and environments and adaptive in others. In addition, many people who behave unusually have high quality lives and make important social contributions.

[4]Response modes are sometimes called "response systems," "response channels," and, less accurately, as "response dimensions."

schema or taxonomy) for *types* of behavior, irregardless of their function or functional relations.

Several taxonomies have been proposed for response modes. In behavioral assessment, response modes have traditionally been divided into "motor" (observable behavior), "cognitive" (thoughts, beliefs, attitudes), and "physiological" (e.g., cardiovascular) systems (Nelson & Hayes, 1986; Rachman & Hodgson, 1974). Other taxonomies for response modes have also been proposed, such as "affective," "cognitive," "sensory-motor"). One well-developed taxonomy is Arthur Staats's "language-cognitive," "sensory-motor," and "emotional-motivational" behavioral repertoires (Staats, 1986; also see Box 8-1).

Some taxonomies are specific to a particular behavior problem. McGlynn and Rose (1998) noted that the multimodal concepts of anxiety (e.g., cognitive, behavioral, psychophysiological aspects of anxiety) remain popular but evolving. For example, "anxiety" is usually associated with "emotion," which is considered by some emotion theorists to have separate cognitive and affective facets. The main point is that there are multiple response mode taxonomies and the most useful taxonomy may vary across behavior problems.

Response modes are important in behavioral assessment for five reasons:

1. Many behavior problems have multiple response modes.
2. Response modes are often discordant and asynchronous across time and persons (Gannon & Haynes, 1987).
3. There are important differences across clients in the importance of various modes of a behavior problems.
4. Response modes may differ in their functional relations (e.g., they may be under the control of different causal variables).
5. Some behavioral treatment strategies may have differential effects across response modes.

Box 8-1
Staats's Basic Behavioral Repertoire

Arthur Staats (1986, 1995), in discussing a general theory of behavior, learning, personality, and psychopathology, has presented the role of complex systems of behavior in three interrelated areas: the *basic behavior repertoires* (BBR). Repertoires are composed of sequentially learned and continually evolving skills and attributes. BBRs include language-cognitive, sensory-motor, and emotional-motivational repertoires. These complex "areas of personalty" are elicited by situations, they affect an individual's behavior across situations, and are changed through an individual's interaction with his or her environment.

The "basic behavioral repertoire" schema provides an organizational structure for understanding client behavior problems that is an alternative to traditional response mode schema (i.e., behavioral, physiological, cognitive). Basic behavioral repertoires can be viewed as mediators of client behavior problems and, therefore, as important multimodal targets of assessment. For example, deficits in a child's language repertoire may partially account for his or her use of physical aggressive behaviors to "communicate" with others. The concept of BBR broadens the assessment focus. It mandates that assessment of a physically aggressive child should focus on the child's communication skills (language-cognitive BBR) in addition to emotional-motivational repertoire of the child (e.g., reinforcers for aggressive behaviors).

"Synchrony" refers to the degree to which two events covary across time—the degree of congruence between the time-course of two events. Asynchronous, or dysynchronous, events differ in their time-courses (e.g., in periodicity, latency, or duration). Consequently, asynchronous events manifest low magnitudes of covariance across time. Consider the differential latencies of heart rate and diastolic blood pressure response to a laboratory stressor. Interbeat intervals can be affected within a second of stimulus onset, while diastolic blood pressure can take many seconds to show a measurable response.

The relations among response modes can also be discordant across persons. For example, the importance, cooccurrence, and covariation of the behavioral components of PTSD, mood disorders, autistic disorders, psychotic disorders, and others vary across persons with the same disorder (see discussions in Achenbach & McConaughy, 1997; Turner & Hersen, 1997).

Examples of Dysynchrony Among Response Modes

There are many examples of dysynchrony and discordance among response modes, across time, and persons (Meier, 1994). For example, anxiety disorders can involve behavioral avoidance or escape from anxiety-arousing situations, subjective distress, elevated physiological arousal, catastrophic thoughts, and anticipatory worry (Forsyth & Eifert, 1998; McGlynn & Rose, 1998). The importance of each response mode, and the functional relations among modes, varies across persons. Some persons experience intense subjective distress without avoiding anxiety-provoking situations while others evidence different patterns of response across modes. The magnitude of synchrony can also vary across persons. Some persons show a high, while other persons show a low, magnitude of covariance among the multiple behavior problem modes.

Asynchronous and discordant response patterns have also been noted for many other behavior problems and disorders. Examples include discordance among psychophysiological responses of persons with PTSD (Blanchard et al., 1994); between affective and overt behavioral responses of persons with social phobias and other anxiety disorders (Glass & Arnkoff, 1989); among response modes for children with anxieties and fears (Finch & McIntosh, 1990); among behavioral, physiological, and cognitive responses in substance use (Sobell, Toneatto, & Sobell, 1994), and male behavioral, cognitive, and physiological modes of erectile disorders (Carey, Lantinga, & Krauss, 1994).

Explanations for Response Mode Dysynchrony

Dysynchrony and discordance among response modes across time and persons may reflect operation of causal factors but may also reflect differences in measurement strategies. First, behavioral, cognitive, and physiological response modes may be a function of different causal relations and variables. For example, social contingencies may more strongly affect how a client talks about his or her depressed mood than the biochemical correlates of depression.

The underlying physiological mechanisms and time phases of responses may also differ. For example, physiological mechanisms that affect heart rate (e.g., vagal innervation) can result in immediate heart rate changes in response to a stimulus, while physiological mechanisms that affect blood pressure (e.g., smooth muscle contractions) do not have significant effects until seconds after a stimulus. Because of these different physiological mechanisms, heart rate and blood pressure often show time-lagged, asynchronous responses to environmental stressors.

The observed magnitude of covariance among response modes depends on how each mode is measured. When dynamic variables are measured, time-sampling parameters and data analytic strategies can affect estimates of covariance magnitude. As illustrated by the example of blood pressure and heart rate, concurrent measurement of responses that have identical but time-lagged response magnitudes can underestimate the covariance between the two responses unless the lagged characteristics of their time-course is considered.

Figure 8-2 illustrates the importance of time-sampling strategies when drawing inferences about the covariation between time-lagged dynamic phenomena. The two responses in Figure 8-2 have identical magnitudes and time-courses, except one is delayed in comparison to the other. Our estimate of the degree to which these responses are synchronous or covary will depend on how we sample and analyze data. If we correlate data collected at each sampling period, we obtain a correlation coefficient of .5. If we conduct time-lagged correlation analysis, with a lag of 2 (A_{t1}:B_{t3}; A_{t2}:B_{t4}, ...) the obtained correlation coefficient approximates 1.0. In sum, judgments regarding dynamic phenomena are affected by the time-sampling strategies used to obtain data and the methods used to analyze the obtained data.

Estimates of the magnitude of covariance between response modes are also affected by the similarity in the methods used to assess them—the degree to which they reflect ***common method variance***. For example, high correlations between two questionnaire measures of anxiety symptoms can be inflated because both use subjective self-report methods, both are paper-and-pencil questionnaires (as opposed to interview self-report), and both use similar response formats (e.g., both could have a four-point Likert scale).

Estimates of covariance between different response modes are often based on different methods of assessment. During exposure to anxiety-provoking stimuli in the laboratory, we use psychophysiological assessment to estimate autonomic responses, self-report measures of thoughts, and observation of behavior. Each method is associated with unique sources of error

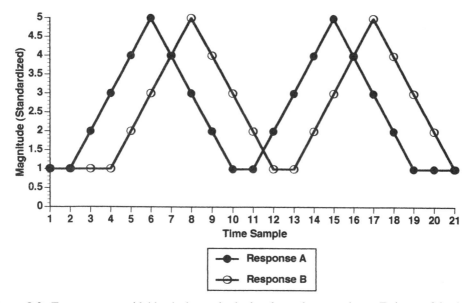

Figure 8-2. Two responses with identical magnitudes but dysynchronous phases. Estimate of the degree to which these two responses covary will depend on how data are analyzed. If correlations are calculated simultaneously at each sampling period, we obtain a correlation coefficient of (.5). If we conduct time-lagged correlation analysis, with a lag of 2 (A_{t1}:B_{t3}; A_{t2}:B_{t4}, ...) the obtained correlation coefficient is (1.0).

variance, which serve to dampen the obtained estimates of covariance among the responses. Cone (1979) called this "confounded" comparisons among response modes because the mode of response is confounded with the method of measurement, dampening estimates of covariance.

The dimensions of response modes can also be dynamic: The relative importance, magnitude, and functional relations of a response mode may change across time. Cognitive modes (e.g., intrusive imagery, attributions of self-blame) may be more characteristic of a client diagnosed with PTSD at one point in time, and avoidant strategies may be more characteristic for that client at another point in time.

The relations between the predominant response mode of a client's behavior problem and the outcome of mode-specific treatments have been the focus of extensive research and discussion (see reviews Hersen & Ammerman, 1994). Given that some treatments can have differential effects across response modes, effects that are mostly behavioral might be expected from contingency management interventions, and effects that are mostly cognitive might be expected from cognitive therapies. Thus, one goal of the functional analysis is to identify the most important response mode of a client's behavior problem so that the appropriate mode-specific treatment can be selected.

Mixed outcomes have resulted from research on the incremental benefits of matching treatments to the predominant mode of a behavior problem for a client. The issue of response mode-treatment matching has been discussed by Shiffman (1993) for smoking, by Linehan (1993) for personality disorders, by Michelson (1986) for agoraphobia, by Ost, Jerremalm, and Johansson (1981) for social phobia, for depression by Imber et al. (1990), for hypertension by Haaga et al. (1994), and for anxiety and fear by McGlynn and Rose (1998). Matching treatment to the characteristics of a client's problems has also been discussed in psychoanalytic treatments (e.g., Luborsky, 1984).

The treatment-response mode association is complicated by the fact that many response modes are functionally related, and many treatments have nonspecific effects across multiple response modes. Also it is likely to be more important for some behavior problems than for others. As discussed by Haynes, Leisen, and Blaine (1997), Kratochwill and Shapiro (1988), and many others, strategies have not been well developed for making intervention recommendations on the basis of assessment data on the multiple response modes of behavior problems.

A Functional Approach to Selecting the Best Type and Level of Response Mode Taxonomy

Multimodal assessment is an important principle of the behavioral construct system—often the assessment of multiple response modes is necessary to capture important aspects of behavior problems. However, as we noted earlier, response mode taxonomies are only constructs (Jensen & Karoly, 1992). They are methods of organizing behavior problems to guide the measurement, explanation, and modification of behavior.

As with all assessment principles the utility of measuring multiple response modes is conditional. Multiple response mode measurement complicates the clinical assessment task, and the assessor must decide if its benefits outweigh its costs. Several issues guide decisions about whether to emphasize multimodal assessment and about which response mode taxonomy is most useful. First, does the research evidence suggest that response modes are differentially important? Is there evidence that a behavior problem consists of different modes that sometimes do not covary highly. Are different response modes affected by different causal variables?

Second, if response modes do not strongly covary, are different response modes sufficiently important to warrant their measurement? If so, what modes should be measured? Would the goals of assessment be advanced if we measured verbal and cognitive aspects of a client's panic episodes, chronic pain, or oppositional behaviors? What are the benefits of gathering subjective reports from an aggressive child with severe developmental disabilities? Does psychophysiological data add to our understanding of a patient's PTSD?

The clinician's decisions about the incremental utility and focus of response mode measurement with a client are affected by data from research and by the results of initial assessment with a client (i.e., from nomothetic and idiographic data). Our earlier examples of response mode dysynchrony illustrated the extensive research on multiple response modes that can be used to guide assessment with many behavior problems. Additionally, initial assessment information can suggest whether multimodal measurement may be warranted.

These examples also illustrate that response modes can vary in their magnitude of functional relations, have different levels of specificity, and have fuzzy boundaries (see Box 8-2). The physiological, behavioral, and cognitive response modes in anxiety disorders are not orthogonal because, for example, overt behavior often occurs concurrently with, and has bidirectional causal relations with, thinking and physiological responses. Furthermore, each of these response modes can be endlessly subdivided into lower-level, more specific modes (see Chapter 7).

Decisions about which response modes to measure should be approached from a functional, assessment goal-oriented perspective. Which measurement modes will best strengthen the validity of clinical judgments about the client? Which measurement modes will facilitate the identification of important causal variables, the description of the time-course of the behaviors, and the selection of intervention strategies?

Box 8-2
Modes, Facets and Patterns of Behavior Problems

The concepts of "response modes" and "facets" sometimes overlap. A "facet" of a behavior problem refers to an internally consistent and clinically relevant aspect of a problem. For example, in cases of chronic pain, facets of the problem may involve tissue pathology, the subjective experience of pain, pain complaints, and the ingestion of pain medication (Turk & Melzack, 1992). Facets of marital distress may include problem solving and conflict resolution tactics, emotional and psychophysiological responses during conflict, and commitment to the relationship (Gottman, 1998).

Some criteria for DSM-IV disorders can be considered facets. For example, unexpected travel away from home and confusion are two facets of "Dissociative Fugue" (APA, 1994, p. 484). There can be multiple facets of a behavior problem within the same response mode. Trauma-related guilt may involve several cognitive facets, such as hindsight bias, beliefs of personal responsibility for the traumatic event, and violation of a personal value.

Facets are (preferably) unidimensional, internally consistent aspects of a behavior problem. Facets often are clinically important aspects that help define the domain of the problem and may be only moderately intercorrelated. Understanding of the facets of a behavior problem can help the assessment process focus on the most important aspects of a behavior problem.

In the initial construction of assessment instruments, it is often helpful to identify the facets of the measured construct to ensure that the assessment instrument taps the entire domain of the construct (Haynes, Richard, & Kubany, 1995; Smith & McCarthy, 1995). Elements of facets (e.g., behavior codes and items on a questionnaire designed to measure an unidimensional facet) should be highly correlated.

To summarize, the idea that behavior problems have multiple response modes, which can vary across clients and across time, have several implications for behavioral assessment strategies:

- Assessment should be *multimodal.* Assessment should focus on the multiple response modes of behavior problems and goals when data regarding one mode of a behavior problem for a client cannot be used to draw inferences regarding another mode.
- Response mode assessment may be *individualized.* The most useful and important response modes to measure can differ across clients with the same behavior problems.
- *Time-sampling strategies* should be selected to be sensitive to the different dynamic characteristics of different response modes.
- *Functional relations* should be examined separately for separate response modes.
- A *diagnosis* (e.g., a DSM-IV diagnosis; APA, 1994) is insufficient to draw inferences regarding the most important response modes for a client because high levels of covariance among behaviors subsumed by a diagnostic category cannot be assumed.
- Acknowledging these mandates, the assessor should consider the *incremental utility and validity* of measuring different response modes.

Behavior Problems Have Multiple Dimensions

Most behavior problems (and the modes and facets of behavior problems) can be described on multiple **dimensions** ("dimensions" are sometimes called "parameters"). A dimension is a fundamental or derived quantitative attribute of an event. "Frequency," "duration," "magnitude," "cyclicity," "variability," and "rate" are typical dimensions of behavior (see Glossary).[5]

The multidimensional nature of behavior problems has several aspects and implications for assessment. First, there can be differences between clients in the relative importance of different dimensions of the same behavior problem. One client may have frequent short duration headaches while another may have infrequent but long duration headaches. Clients with episodes of depressive behaviors may differ in the frequency, severity, and duration of those episodes; children may differ in the frequency, duration, and severity of night terrors (see Box 8-3).

Second, different dimensions of behavior problems often do not strongly covary. Consequently, knowledge about how often a behavior problem occurs does not necessarily help us estimate its severity or duration.

Third, and perhaps most importantly for the functional analysis, different dimensions of a behavior problem may be affected by different causal variables. Consequently, the functional analysis and the best treatment strategy for a client may vary, depending on which dimension of the behavior problem is most important.

There are many examples of a differential effect of causal variables across dimensions of a behavior disorder. Barnett and Gotlib (1988) suggested that the duration and magnitude, but not the onset, of depressive behaviors may be affected by learned helplessness beliefs. That is, the onset of depressive episodes may be triggered by life stressors, which may also trigger beliefs that then affect the magnitude and duration of the episodes. Catastrophic thoughts may affect

---

[5]As with other assessment concepts, "dimension" assumes different meanings in different contexts. The "dimensionality" of a scale, factor, or other aggregate often refers to the internal consistency or patterns of covariance among its elements. Items of a "unidimensional" scale measure a single variable or facet, as suggested by high inter-item correlations. One "dimensionalizes" a set of items or codes by examining patterns of covariance.

Box 8-3
Estimates of the Correlation Among Dimensions
of a Behavior Problem Are Affected by Sample Composition

In epidemiological samples significant correlations among dimensions of behavior problems would be expected because durations and magnitudes > 0 are possible only when frequency is > 0 (unless "0" occurrences are omitted from these analyses). However, the focus in clinical assessment and clinical research is with a subset of the general population that meets minimal criteria for "caseness." For these persons, we are interested in the degree to which estimates of one dimension of a client's behavior problem allows us to estimate other dimensions.

Significant covariation among dimensions can be a function of diagnostic inclusion criteria. Some diagnoses (e.g., anxiety disorders) include frequency, duration, and severity criteria. In clients who meet diagnostic criteria, the clinician can presume that multiple dimensions are significantly elevated. However, the relative importance of different dimensions cannot be estimated from a diagnosis because the diagnosis can result from different combinations of criteria.

---

the duration and severity of panic episodes but not their onset or rate (see discussions in Rapee & Barlow, 1993; Whittal, Goetsch, & Eifert, 1996). The responses of family members may affect the severity and duration of medical conditions, such as asthma, more than the onset of those conditions (Creer & Bender, 1993; Wicks-Nelson & Israel, 1997). The events that trigger paranoid delusions (e.g., ambiguous social stimuli) may be different from the events that affect the duration and content of the delusions (e.g., responses of others to the client's behavior when delusional) (Haynes, 1986b).

Fourth, because behavioral interventions are often designed to modify hypothesized causal variables for behavior problems, and causal variables can have differential effects across the dimensions of a behavior problem, behavioral interventions may have differential effects across dimensions of behavior problems. Referring to the previous examples of panic episodes, interventions that reduce catastrophic thoughts associated with the physiological sensations may have a stronger effect on the severity and duration than on the rate of a client's panic episodes. Thus, multidimensional assessment is often helpful for the construction of a valid behavioral case formulation and for designing the best intervention strategy for a client.

The multiple dimensions of behavior problems have several implications for assessment strategies.

- Assessment should focus on *multiple dimensions of behavior problems*.
- Multidimensional assessment should be *individualized*.
- Assessment should focus on the *functional relations* and *causal variables* of the most important dimensions of a behavior problem for a client.
- *Different assessment methods* may be necessary to identify causal factors for different dimensions of behavior problems. For example, self-monitoring headaches at preset intervals (e.g., 4×/day) may be useful to gather data for persons with frequent, short duration headaches. However, self-monitoring headaches when they occur, such as through critical incident sampling, may be more useful for persons with infrequent, but long duration migraines.
- A *psychiatric diagnosis* for a client (e.g., a DSM-IV diagnosis; APA, 1994) suggests that there may be elevated indices of all dimensions of a behavior problem but is insufficient to estimate the most important dimensions of that problem for a client.

In sum, differences between clients in the importance of behavior problem dimensions and modes further emphasize the need for specification of variables and assessment strategies matched to the characteristics of the behavior problem. Molar-level constructs (e.g., "anxiety," "depression") that aggregate across modes and dimensions are not optimally useful for drawing clinical inferences. They do not help the clinician specify important sources of variance and functional relations, and they do not help the clinician identify and evaluate treatment effects.

The Conditional and Dynamic Nature of Behavior Problems

Two additional assumptions about the nature of behavior problems strongly affect behavioral assessment strategies: Behavior problems can vary systematically across situation and time.

The Conditional Nature of Behavior Problems

A central assumption of the behavioral assessment paradigm is that behavior problems are often *conditional*. For many clients, behavior problems do not occur randomly but vary systematically, particularly as a function of variables in the client's environment but also as a function of "states" of the client. Many studies have shown that the conditional probability, form, rate, magnitude, and duration of behavior problems can vary across settings and contexts and as a function of variance in antecedent and discriminative stimuli.

The conditional nature of behavior problems varies across clients. For some clients, self-injurious behaviors are more likely to occur in demanding than in nondemanding learning situations; panic episodes are more likely to occur in the high-anxiety than in low-anxiety mood states (which themselves covary with environmental contexts); aggression against a spouse is more likely to occur in intoxicated than in nonintoxicated states; paranoid thoughts are more likely to occur in ambiguous than in highly structured social situations; oppositional behavior is more likely to occur with one parent than another; headaches are more likely to occur during stressful than during nonstressful work times. However, for other clients there is no evident covariance between these behavior problems and environmental variables or states[6] (see discussions in Gatchel & Blanchard, 1993; Glass, 1993; Ollendick & Hersen, 1993a).

There are differences in behavior problems in the degree to which they covary with environmental variables. Some behavior problems tend to have strong and reliable functional relations with environmental variables while others are more stable across situations. For example, short-term memory deficits of persons following a stroke or acquired head injury may vary across situations as a function of stressfulness and stimulus complexity of the situation. However, for most persons memory deficits can be observed in all contexts in which short-term memory plays an important role (see discussions in Cushman & Scherer, 1995). Similarly, children can exhibit reading, speech, and hearing difficulties across multiple situations. However, an assumption by the assessor that a client's behavior problems may show elevated conditional probabilities in some but not other situations can often lead the assessor to discover

[6]The failure to identify covariates of a behavior problem does not necessarily mean that the problem is "endogenous." A behavior problem may appear unconditional when the wrong dimension is measured (e.g., examining functional relations for onset rather than magnitude of a behavior problem) and when the wrong environmental covariates are measured. An a priori assumption that a behavior problem is endogenous discourages the clinician from searching for covariates that might be useful in the functional analysis and treatment of the client.

Box 8-4
Conditional Probability and Sequential Analysis

The analysis of conditional probabilities has been applied to chains of behavior in dyadic exchanges and environment-behavior chains. For example, we may be interested in sequences of verbal behaviors that lead to critical comments by spouses when they are discussing a marital problem. We can sequentially code verbal and nonverbal behavior in real time or by using short time samples. We can then calculate the conditional probabilities of a behavior, such as a critical comment, given some prior event(s) such as another critical comment or a disagreement.

Analyses of sequences and chains of events can provide information about functional relations. For example, we can calculate the conditional probability of a critical event, given combinations of prior events, response latencies, and other temporal factors. Sequential analyses usually necessitate the video or audio recordings of interactions and careful coding by trained coders. Consequently, sequential analyses are most useful in clinical research.

Discussion, examples, and methods of data analysis in sequential analysis are provided by Bakeman and Casey (1995); Fletcher, Fischer, Barkley, and Smallish (1996); Haccou and Meelis (1992); and Heller, Sobel, and Tanaka (1996).

---

clinically important sources of variance for the behavior problem (remember, indices of shared variance are important indices of possible causal relations) (see Box 8-4).

The differential conditional probabilities of behavior across situations (and states) has important implications for the functional analysis of a client because conditional probabilities can serve as markers for the operation of causal variables. There are important causal inferences, and implications for the design of intervention strategies, associated with the identification of triggers of a client's asthma episodes (Creer & Bender, 1993), the social situations that are most likely to precipitate a patient's panic episodes (Craske & Waikar, 1994) or the antecedents of a couple's marital violence (O'Leary, Vivian, & Malone, 1992). In each case, the conditional probabilities point to possible causal relations that may be addressed in an intervention program.

The cross-situation variability in the dimensions of many behavior problems strengthens our oft-repeated axiom that aggregated measures of a behavior problem are often insufficiently specific for a functional analysis. A "score" for a behavior problem from a standardized assessment instrument (e.g., a depression, anxiety, social anxiety score) provides a nomothetically based index of the probability that a person will exhibit a behavior problem or disorder, relative to others. However, a score does not help in identifying the situations in which the problem is most likely to occur. Functionally oriented assessment instruments allow the assessor to examine the conditional probabilities of behavior problems or the magnitude of shared variance between the behavior problem and multiple situational factors. Assessment methods such as functionally oriented structured interviews, self-monitoring, situation-specific questionnaires, and observation are all conducive to gathering data about the conditional nature of behavior problems.[7]

---

[7]Personality traits, although based on aggregated indices, can also be conditional. Traits are not exhibited randomly across situations: Behaviors that compose a trait are more likely to occur in some situations than in others (Kendrick & Funder, 1988; Wright & Mischel, 1987). The concept of "trait" suggests the relative degree to which a person will evidence a particular set of behaviors in a particular context (see discussion of traits and behavioral assessment in *Behavior Modification, 17*[1], 1993).

The conditional nature of behavior problems has several implications for assessment strategies. Usually, assessment should focus on the behavior problem in *multiple situations*. Assessors should gather data to determine if the dimensions and facets of behavior vary across situations. This mandate has implications for every assessment method: (a) during interviews clients and informants should be asked about differences in behavior in different situations; (b) questionnaires should adopt a functional approach and query as to situational factors associated with behavior problems; (c) self-monitoring data should be identified as to the situation in which it was collected, (d) analogue observation methods should carefully control and systematically manipulate situational factors, and (e) observation in the natural environment should occur in several situations.

The Dynamic Nature of Behavior Problems

The facets, form, and dimensions of behavior problems are often dynamic—they can change over time in the following ways:

- *Dimensions* (e.g., magnitude, occurrence, and duration).
- The *form* or characteristics of a client's behavior problem.
- The *functional relations among behavior problems*. For example, marital distress may strongly affect a client's mood sometimes but not others.
- The *elements in a behavior disorder category*: A client with PTSD may evidence strong avoidance of trauma cues during one period but not another. Thus, the *relative importance* of elements of a disorder may change over time.
- The *conditional nature* of a behavior problem. For example, aggressive behavior may be affected by particular consequences during one period but not another.

Changes in the nature of behavior problems over time can result from several sources. First, they can reflect changes in controlling variables. For example, some conditions that promote substance abuse, such as facilitation by a peer group, may change over time. Second, they can reflect natural changes associated with repeated occurrences of a behavior. For example, repeated substance abuse can affect the density of neurotransmitter receptors, which affects the individual's behavioral and cognitive responses to the substance as use continues, which can affect the frequency and magnitude of substance use.

As we discussed in earlier chapters, sensitive measurement of dynamic variables requires the frequent measurement of specific variables, using time-sampling assessment strategies, that are appropriate for the rate of change of the behavior. Collins and Horn (1991), Heatherton and Weinberger (1994), Kazdin (1998), and Kratochwill and Levin (1992) discuss strategies and issues in the time-series measurement of dynamic variables.

Summary

Assumptions about behavior problems differ across psychological assessment paradigms. These assumptions affect the selection of assessment strategies, the clinical case formulation, and treatment strategies. We emphasized the multivariate and idiographic nature of clients' behavior problems, the importance of functional relations among behavior problems, and functional relations between behavior problems and environmental events. We also examined the implications of these assumptions for strategies of behavioral assessment.

Many persons have multiple behavior problems. Multiple problems may reflect the way in which behavior problems are defined and the strategies used to assess behavior problems. Because of symptom overlap in the definition of disorders, a person who meets criteria for one disorder often has an increased likelihood of meeting criteria for another disorder. The probability that multiple behavior problems will be identified is reduced if a clinician focuses assessment too quickly on a particularly salient presenting problem. Thus, broadly focused assessment strategies are more likely to detect multiple problems.

The emphasis on the multivariate nature of client problems leads to an emphasis in the behavioral assessment paradigm on: (a) identifying multiple behavior problems, (b) estimating the form and strength of relations among the behavior problems, and (c) estimating the relative importance of the behavior problems. Importance estimates are based on: (a) judgments about the rate and magnitude of a behavior problem, (b) judgments about the probability that the behavior problem will lead to harm, (c) judgments about the degree of impact on the client's quality of life, and (d) the degree to which a behavior problem functions as a cause of other behavior problems.

Behavior problems have multiple response modes, which are organizational categories for types of behavior. Several taxonomies have been proposed for response modes, although "motor," "cognitive," and "physiological" classes are the most commonly used. The assessment of response modes are important because (a) many behavior problems have multiple response modes, (b) response modes are often discordant and asynchronous, (c) there are important differences across clients in the importance of various modes of a behavior problems, and (d) effects of a behavioral treatment strategy may differ across response modes.

Because of unique causal factors and measurement strategies, many response modes are asynchronous across time and discordant across persons. Estimates of covariance among response modes depend on how each mode is measured, the time-sampling strategies used to obtain data, and the similarity in the methods used to assess them. Additionally, the relative importance, magnitude, and functional relations of a response mode may change across time.

The measurement of multiple response modes is difficult and the assessor must decide if the benefits outweigh the costs. The assessor must consider if there is evidence that different modes should be measured, if multiple response modes are sufficiently important to warrant their measurement, and if the degree to which response modes covary is great and thus requiring separate measurement. The decision about the utility and type of response mode measurement is affected by data from published studies and by the results of initial assessment with a client.

The concept of response modes suggests that: (a) assessment should be multimodal, (b) reponse mode assessment should be individualized, (c) time-sampling strategies should be selected to be sensitive to the different dynamic characteristics of different response modes, (d) functional relations should be examined separately for separate response modes, and (e) a diagnosis is insufficient to draw inferences regarding the most important response modes for a client.

Most behavior problems have multiple dimensions, such as frequency, duration, magnitude, cyclicity, and variability. Clients can differ in the relative importance of these different dimensions of the same behavior problem. Also, different dimensions of behavior problems often display low magnitudes of covariation. Different dimensions of a behavior problem may display different functional relations with causal variables. In turn, this variation in dimensional relations has an impact on the ultimate functional analysis of a client. Because causal variables can have differential effects across the dimensions of behavior problems, behavioral interventions may have differential effects across behavior problem dimensions.

The multiple dimensions of behavior problems have several implications for assessment strategies: (a) assessment should be multidimensional, (b) multidimensional assessment should be individualized, and (c) functional relations should be examined for the most important dimensions of a behavior problem—a diagnosis is insufficient to draw inferences regarding the most important dimensions for a client.

Behavior problems can be conditional and dynamic. For many persons, behavior problems do not occur randomly but covary with variables in the person's environment and over time. The conditional nature of behavior problems varies across clients and behavior problems. The conditional nature of behavior problems has several implications for assessment strategies. Typically assessment should focus on the behavior problem in multiple situations. Assessors should gather data to determine if the dimensions and facets of behavior vary across situations. This mandate has implications for every assessment method: (a) during interviews, clients and informants should be asked about differences in behavior in different situations; (b) questionnaires should adopt a functional approach and ask about situational factors associated with behavior problems, in addition to measuring the magnitude and facets of a behavior problem; (c) self-monitoring data should identify the situation in which it was collected; (d) analogue observation methods should carefully control and systematically manipulate situational factors; (e) observation in the natural environment should occur in several situations; and (f) time-series assessment is necessary to capture important aspects of the time-course of behavior problems.

Suggested Readings

Paradigms of Psychopathology

Achenbach, T. M., & McConaughy, S. H. (1997). *Empirically based assessment of child and adolescent psychopathology practical applications* (2nd ed.). Thousand Oaks, CA: Sage.

Frame, C. L., & Matson, J. L. (Eds.). (1987). *Handbook of assessment in childhood psychopathology applied issues in differential diagnosis and treatment evaluation* (pp. 79–106). New York: Plenum.

Turner, S. M., & Hersen, M. (Eds.). (1997). *Adult psychopathology and diagnosis* (3rd ed.). New York: John Wiley & Sons.

Characteristics of Behavior Problems

Evans, I. M. (1986). Response structure and the triple-response-mode concept. In R. O. Nelson & S. C. Hayes (Eds.), *Conceptual foundations of behavioral assessment* (pp. 131–155). New York: Guilford.

Nelson, R. O., & Hayes, S. C. (1986). The nature of behavioral assessment. In R. O. Nelson & S. C. Hayes (Eds.), *Conceptual foundations of behavioral assessment* (pp. 1–41). New York: Guilford.

Comorbidity

Clarkin, J. F., & Kendall, P. C. (1992). Comorbidity and treatment planning: Summary and future directions. *Journal of Consulting and Clinical Psychology, 60,* 904–908.

Lilienfeld, S. O., Waldman, I. D., & Israel, A. C. (1994). A critical examination of the use of the term and concept of "comorbidity" in psychopathology research. *Clinical Psychology: Science and Practice, 1,* 71–83.

Persons, J. B., & Bertagnolli, A. (1994). Cognitive-behavioral treatment of multiple-problem patients: Application to personality disorders. *Clinical Psychology and Psychotherapy, 1,* 279–285.

9

Basic Concepts of Causation

Introduction

Causation has been discussed and debated for centuries. It has been a focus in philosophy, metaphysics, religion, biology, and the behavioral sciences. The earliest documented integrative thesis on causation was by Aristotle (384–322 B.C.), who critiqued the ideas of causality of philosophers who had preceded him. To Aristotle, ultimate knowledge was the knowledge of causation, the "explanation" of things. Particularly important was knowledge of the "final cause" of something—the ultimate purpose or effect of an event.[1]

Concepts of causation in the behavioral sciences have been energetically debated from a time when philosophy and psychology were integrated disciplines. These debates have centered on competing definitions of causality, the kinds of events that can serve as causes, the infinite regress of causation (one can always ask what was the cause of a cause), the subjective nature of causal inferences, the conditions necessary for inferring causality, the direction of causal relations, the best degree of specificity in causal inferences, temporal dimensions of causal relations, social and political ramifications of causal inferences, and problems in ruling out alternative explanations when inferring causal relations.

This chapter only touches on some of these issues. Principles and competing models of causality have been discussed in many books, including Feigl and Brodbeck (1953), Hume (1740), James (1893), Locke (1690), Mill (1843), Nagel (1961), and Salmon (1984). Concepts of causality in the behavioral sciences have been discussed by Asher (1976), Blalock (1964), Bunge (1963), Cook and Campbell (1979), Haynes (1992), Hyland (1981), and James, Mulaik and Brett (1982).

Assumptions about the causes of behavior problems are the elements of a psychological assessment paradigm that most strongly affect its strategies of assessment. Psychological assessment paradigms often differ in assumptions about the type of causal variables and causal relations relevant to behavior problems and the mechanisms underlying causal relations: Causal assumptions guide the methods of assessment, the variables targeted in assessment, and the functional relations that are of primary interest.

This chapter introduces concepts of causation: definitions of causal and functional relations, necessary conditions for inferring a causal relation between two variables, and limitations of causal inference.

We emphasize several aspects of causation and causal relations:

1. Necessary conditions for inferring a causal relation between two events are: covariation, temporal precedence of the causal variable, a logical mechanism for causal effects, and a reasonable exclusion of alternative explanations for the covariation.
2. Causal relations and models are subjective and hypothesized.
3. Causal relations and models have a limited domain.
4. Causal relations and models can be expressed at various levels of specificity.
5. Causal relations and models can be dynamic.
6. The dynamic qualities of causal relations may be a result of repeated exposure to, and

---

[1]In Book Alpha and Book Delta (of *Metaphysics*) Aristotle reviews previous thoughts on causality and proposes four types of causes (focusing mostly on the causes of physical substances): *material* (that of which something is made), *formal* (the plan or idea by reference to which something is made), *final* (the ultimate purpose of something), and *efficient* (the act or event that produces the result) (Magill & McGreal, 1961). Most of the causal variables proposed in the behavioral sciences would be classified by Aristotle as *efficient* causes—"external" agents presumed to be responsible for a particular event (the event to be explained would be called the "explandum-event" in philosophy) (Salmon, 1984).

duration or action of, a causal variable, changes in causal variables, new causes triggered by a behavior problem, and natural maturational changes.

7. Causal relations are nonexclusive and imperfect.
8. Causal relations often differ across clients.
9. A causal relation can be nonlinear across time or across values of the variables.
10. Causal hypotheses affect decisions about the best methods of assessment, the variables and functional relations targeted in assessment, data obtained, and the resultant functional analysis.
11. Contiguous elevation of measures of behavior problems and hypothesized causal variables or cooccurrence of a behavior problem and hypothesized causal variable is insufficient to infer a causal relation.

Differing Concepts of Causal and Functional Relations

Disagreements about the role of causation in the behavioral sciences partially derive from different definitions of causation. If one assumes that a cause is a necessary or immediate cause (see Box 9-1), few variables in the behavioral sciences would qualify as causal. This would preclude considering alcohol as one cause of automobile accidents or domestic violence.[2]

If one assumes that a "cause" must be a first cause, then one could argue that the only cause of long-term speech deficits of a client with head trauma is the head trauma, or that the only cause of adult sexual dysfunctions in a client who was sexually abused as a child is the abusive sexual experience. Similarly, if one assumes that a cause must be the immediate cause, temporally distant events (e.g., the relation between childhood trauma and adult interpersonal difficulties) would not be considered as causal.

Causal vs. Functional Relations

The role of causation has also been debated by behavioral scientists. Many behavioral scientists, particularly scholars in behavior analysis, have proposed that the essential goal of science is to "describe," rather than to "explain" behavior. They have suggested that if we can describe behavior (e.g., describe its rate of occurrence, how it covaries with other events, such as response contingencies or its conditional probabilities), then we can make reliable and useful predictions about it. Prediction implies control. Thus, these scholars have proposed that reliable prediction and the identification of functional relations are the essential goals of science, and causal constructs introduce unnecessary connotations and inferential errors.

A noncausal, descriptive approach to understanding behavior has appealing features. Foremost, it avoids problematic connotations and the subjective inferences associated with "causality." For example, from a descriptive approach, we can know that changing how a parent responds to a child's persistent tantrums will reliably change the frequency and duration of those tantrums. The concept of "causation" is unnecessary for this descriptive understanding. Furthermore, inserting "causation" concepts into this observation introduces superfluous

---

[2]Some professionals who work with battered women do not like to label alcohol as a "cause" of domestic violence, even though alcohol is often implicated in domestic violence episodes. They believe that labeling alcohol as a "cause" diminishes the responsibility of the batterer for the aggressive behavior. In causal language, they are concerned that such a label implies that alcohol is a "sufficient" cause, and that it is an "exclusive" cause. An appropriate stance is that alcohol has a causal relation with domestic violence but that many other important factors contribute to domestic violence.

Box 9-1
Types of Causes

Sufficient causes	Y occurs whenever X occurs; therefore, X is sufficient to cause Y.
Insufficient cause	That cause that, by itself, is insufficient to produce the effect, but can function as a causal variable in combination with other variables.
Necessary cause	Y never occurs without X.
Necessary and sufficient cause	Y occurs whenever X occurs, and Y never occurs without X.
First cause	That cause upon which all others depend—the earliest event in a causal chain.
Principal cause	That cause upon which the effect primarily depends.
Immediate cause	That cause that produces the effect without any intervening events.
Mediate cause	A cause that produces its effect only through another cause (Byerly, 1973).

connotations, such as considering the parent as the original cause of the tantrums or that the parent is to "blame" for the tantrums. Retaining a functional-relation, descriptive approach avoids these inferential errors and encourages a constructive approach to assessment and intervention.

Despite the philosophical and epistemological issues that have surrounded ideas of causation and the utility of a strictly functional approach to describing behavior (see Box 9-2), we promote concepts of causality in the behavioral assessment paradigm. We believe that causal concepts can guide research on behavior problems, assessment strategies, and clinical judgments. Models of causality for behavior problems help the assessor focus on variables that are most likely to be important determinants of a client's behavior problems, to select the best assessment strategies to measure and understand the complex relations among variables in clinical assessment, to predict behavior, and to estimate which interventions are most likely to be effective. Additionally, clinicians and clients often think in causal terms—the clinician often wants to know "why" a behavior problem is occurring and what events are affecting it (Goldstein & Hogarth, 1997; Turk & Salovey, 1988).

A causal focus is also mandated by the focus of behavioral interventions. Behavioral interventions are often designed to change the variables presumed to cause a behavior problem, or to introduce new causal variables to moderate another causal relation.

There are several caveats to the causal language and concepts adopted in this book. First, readers can retain a descriptive, functional approach to behavior problems and clinical assessment. The causal concepts presented herein are easily translatable into a functional language. Second, we recognize that there are no consensually accepted rules for causal inference across and within the sciences. The concepts promoted in this book are those that we believe are most useful for guiding assessment strategies and strengthening the validity of clinical judgments.

Conditions Required for Inferring a Causal Relation

A causal relation is a judgment. It is inferred on the basis of multiple indicators, and an emphasis on different indicators of causation can lead to different causal judgments. Further complicating causal judgments, there is disagreement about which indicators are most useful for inferring causal relations. Conditions for inferring that two variables are causally connected

---

Box 9-2
A Historical View of Functional, Structural, and Causal Concepts

The emphasis on functional (rather than causal and topographical) relations in behavior therapy has two interdependent origins: (a) a rejection of a structuralist approach to understanding behavior problems, and (b) an avoidance of some epistemological problems associated with the concept of causality. The early proponents of functionalism (e.g., Angell, Carr, Cattell, Dewey, Thorndike, Titchner, Woodworth), who were heavily influenced by Darwin, emphasized problems with an epistemology for behavioral science that stressed the description of structure or topography of behavior. They reasoned that effective understanding and prediction of behavior required an analysis of its "utility" and context, in addition to its form (Boring, 1957; Rachlin, 1970).

Conflicts between structuralists and functionalist have continued for almost a century and are evident in contemporaneous exchanges regarding psychiatric diagnosis (DSM-IV, American Psychiatric Association, 1994). The DSM-IV is a taxonomy of behavior disorders and adheres to a structuralist approach. Symptoms are generally clustered according to presumed topographical covariation, which is taken as evidence that some common unmeasured underlying or latent variable is operational. In contrast, a functional approach focuses on the covariation between topography and the putative controlling variables. Topographical covariation, per se, is considered meaningful only to the extent that it aids the identification of these controlling variables (see miniseries Behavioral Assessment and DSM-III-R, *Behavioral Assessment*, *10*, 1988, pp. 43–121).

Functionalism is also an accommodation to more than 2,000 years of debate concerning the nature of causality. To avoid the semantic and conceptual ambiguities associated with the concept of causality, behavioral scientists stressed functional relations in their discourses about the phenomena of their respective disciplines.

A focus on functional relations is useful because they are unencumbered with most of the necessary conditions for causal inference. As Bunge (1963) noted, in the famous functional equation $E = mC^2$ a functional relation between energy, "E," and the speed of light, "C," is described, without implying a causal relation between the two. Also, the temporal precedence and directionality are not of concern.

---

have included **covariation** (X and Y must covary), **contiguity** (X and Y must be closely associated in time or place), **temporal precedence** (X must precede Y, if X is a cause of Y), **necessity** or **constant conjunction** (X must always occur when Y occurs, if X is a cause of Y), **logical connection** (there must be a logical explanation for the causal connection), and the exclusion of **alternative explanations** for the covariation between X and Y (i.e., the covariation between X and Y is unlikely to be due to the common effects of Z).

Not all conditions that have been proposed as necessary for causal inferences are useful in psychological assessment. For example, "contiguity" and "necessity" are not useful conditions for causal inference. First, there is evidence from multiple sources that some important causes of behavior problems can occur long before the behavior problem. Second, the same behavior problem can sometimes result from different permutations of causal variables, rendering any single causal variable unnecessary (although sometimes sufficient) (e.g., Alessi, 1992).

We propose four critical conditions for inferring that two variables have a causal relation in psychological assessment.

- *The two variables must covary*—they must have a functional relation, across persons or across time for one person. Two variables have a functional relation when they have shared variance: A dimension of one variable covaries with a dimension of another variable (Blalock, 1964; Haynes, 1992; James, Mulaik, & Brett, 1982).[3]

- *The hypothesized causal variable must reliably precede the behavior problem.* With response contingency, it is the contingency that is the causal variable, rather than the response contingent event. With reciprocal causation, temporal precedence is difficult to establish because two variables are sequentially affecting each other.
- *There must be a logical mechanism for the hypothesized causal relation.* Sometimes a logical mechanism is presumed but not identified. For example, the mechanisms that underlie the behavioral effects of new psychotropic medications and new psychological interventions are often unidentified.
- *Alternative explanations for the observed covariance must be reasonably excluded.* This is perhaps the most difficult condition to address. Although the possibility of a "third variable" effect can never be completely precluded, it is important to address the possibility that the covariance between two variables with a presumed causal relation is a result of the common influence of a third variable.

The Limitations on Causal Inferences

Several other characteristics of causal relations for behavior problems guide psychological assessment strategies and the development of the functional analysis. These characteristics emphasize the limitations and conditionality of causal inferences: Causal relations are subjectively estimated and hypothesized, have a limited domain, can be expressed at different levels of specificity, and are dynamic, tentative, and nonexclusionary.

Inferences About Causal Relations Are Subjective and Hypothesized

As we discussed in Chapter 3, a model of the causal relations relevant to a client's behavior problems (i.e., the functional analysis) represents the clinician's best estimate based on available information. It is an integrative judgment based on nomothetic research and clinical assessment data relevant to the client. Causal models of clients' behavior problems are sets of hypotheses that guide assessment and intervention strategies. Causal inferences about a client also reflect errors in information acquired during assessment and in the clinician's judgments based on assessment information.[4]

Assessment data may be consistent with, but cannot prove, causal hypotheses. Whatever the predictive utility and efficacy of a causal model for a client, we cannot preclude the possibility that additional data will be inconsistent with our causal hypotheses. Consequently, the clinician should view causal relations as tentative and open to evaluation and revision.

---

[3]Covariation can be difficult to detect. When multiple causal variables affect a behavior problem, other variables can moderate or mask the functional relation between two others. Additionally, the conditions necessary for observing the functional relation may not be extant. Sometimes it is necessary to use experimental or statistical controls to observe the covariation between two variables that have a causal relation.

[4]A "causal model" of a client's behavior problems is a set of hypothesized causal relations relevant to that problem. It is an idiographic model, in that there is no presumption that the hypothesized functional relations would be valid for other clients with the same behavior problems. We are not using the term "causal model" as it is used in structural equations modeling (SEM) (Loehlin, 1998). SEMs for behavior problems are nomothetic, in that estimates of functional relations are based on data from many persons.

Causal Relations Have a Limited Domain

The "domain" of a causal relation refers to the conditions under which it is operational. Most causal relations have limited domains. The effects of praise, aerobic exercise, presleep worry, humor, traumatic life events, and sleep loss can depend on the social setting, biological state of the person, or recent experience with the causal variable. Praise may serve as a reinforcer when delivered by some persons but not others. The behavioral effects of a traumatic life event upon reexperiencing the event may depend on a history of exposure to similar events and concurrent life events (Wilson & Keane, 1997).

A domain of a causal relation may also apply to an individual client, and it may account for differences in causal relations across groups of persons. The effect of a causal variable for a client's behavior problem may be confined to a specific response mode of the client or to a specific setting or context in which the behavior occurs. It may also covary across persons with a dimension of individual differences (e.g., sex, ethnicity, age) (Butcher, Narikiyo, & Vitousek, 1993).

The fact that a causal relation operates in some but not other domains does not negate its importance. The identification of the conditionality of a causal relation is an important finding. It suggests the operation of additional causal variables. The facets of the domain may differ in important ways, such as in discriminative stimuli, the operation of moderating variables, and differential reinforcement histories.

Causal Relations Can Be Expressed at Different Levels of Specificity

Causal variables and relations can vary in their degree of specificity—the number of causal variables and relations subsumed by a causal variable and relation. As we noted in Chapter 7, "specificity" applies to four components of psychological assessment: (a) the number of elements subsumed by a causal variable, (b) the dimensions specified by a causal variable, (c) the degree to which relevant situational and temporal conditions are specified by a causal variable, and (d) the specificity of clinical judgments about causal relations.

For example, the construct "life stressors" has been included in causal models of depression, psychophysiological disorders, schizophrenia, sleep disorders, and substance abuse (e.g., Davison & Neale, 1990; Kessler, 1997; Lazarus, 1993). A "stressful life experience" may include cocaine addiction, divorce, an auto accident, medical illness, a change in residence, death of a parent, assault, or a parking ticket. A "traumatic life event" is a more specific exemplar of a "life stressor" construct but can still include multiple events such as physical assault and combat-related trauma.

The mode of impact, the duration and magnitude of impact, and the breadth of impact are likely to vary across different life stressors. Furthermore, the impact is likely to vary with other aspects of each life stressor, such as its magnitude, predictability, history of prior exposure to similar stressors, and concurrent stressors (Wilson & Keane, 1997). The main point is that nonspecific causal variables inhibit the development of specific inferences about causal relations that are necessary in behavioral assessment.

As another example, in a causal model for a child's high-rate, aversive, manding behaviors, we could include "social-environmental factors" as a molar-level (i.e., nonspecific) causal variable (in addition to other elements of the model such as "nutritional" or "biological" causal factors). At a more specific level, "social-environmental factors" could subsume "parent-delivered response contingencies" (besides other elements such as sibling provocations and a chaotic home environment). At a still more specific level, "parent-delivered response contingencies" could subsume "parental intermittent positive reinforcement for manding behaviors," which can subsume the lower-level "response-contingent positive verbal attention" (in addition to tangible rewards, hugs).

In this latter example, all levels of specificity of the causal variables and relations can be valid: Each satisfies the criteria of covariation between the causal variable and the behavior problem, temporal precedence of the causal variable, a logical connection between them, and, to a lesser degree, exclusion of an alternative explanation for the covariation.

As we noted in Chapter 7, a major drawback to the use of nonspecific variables is that assumptions of high magnitudes of covariation among their components are often unwarranted. Components of higher-level causal constructs may strongly covary for some persons and not others, in some situations but not others, and at some times but not others.

We have advocated a functional approach to selecting the best degree of specificity. The degree of specificity of a causal relation influences the best assessment strategy, affects the resultant functional analysis, and affects treatment decisions. For example, for community-based assessment and prevention efforts with AIDS, "safe-sex practices" may be a useful degree of specificity for causal variables. However, to decide how to intervene with a sexually active individual at-risk for HIV infection, more specific causal factors such as particular sex practices, beliefs about risk and personal vulnerability, and assertive skills in intimate situations may be more useful causal variables.

Causal Relations Are Dynamic

The causal variables and causal relations associated with a behavior problem can change across time. A causal relation may be operational and clinically relevant at some times and not others, the magnitude of effect of a causal variable can change, and the same behavior problem may be influenced by different causal variables at different times. Changes across time are sometimes observed in the reinforcers for aggressive behavior, the particular airborne allergens that trigger a client's asthma episodes, the reinforcement value of particular stimuli (e.g., particular toys, approval from a particular person) for a child, the effects of nicotine and caffeine on a person's cardiovascular response to stressors, the effects on aggressive and delusional behaviors of a particular medication dose level, and the impact of particular life stressors on a client's depressed mood (see discussions in Gatchel & Blanchard, 1993; Sutker & Adams, 1993).

The dynamic qualities evident in the prior examples suggest causal relations may be affected by several factors:

- *Repeated exposure* to a causal variable. Such effects are observed with extinction, habituation, and sensitization processes.
- *Duration of action of a causal variable.* For example, the effects of causal variables, such as, positive reinforcement, blood alcohol levels, and exercise, show U-shaped or inverted U-shaped relations with behavior problems (with the magnitude or probability of the behavior on the vertical axis, and the duration or frequency of the causal variable on the horizontal axis).
- *Changes in moderating or mediating variables.* Causal effects can be interactive in that the effect of one variable depends on the values of another. For example, the probability that a life stressor will lead to increased alcohol use by a client can be affected by changes in "alcohol expectancies" (Goldman, Brown, Christiansen, & Smith, 1991).

- *Natural and sometimes unpredictable changes in the occurrence of causal variables* (Bandura, 1982). New causal variables can occur (e.g., a supervisor is hired who uses coercive methods of behavior control) and earlier ones can disappear (e.g., a coercive supervisor is transferred).
- Changes in *contextual and situational factors*. For example, a disruptive child can change classrooms and be exposed to different response contingencies, learning demands, or social stimuli.
- *New causes triggered by a behavior problem.* For example, smoking that was initially influenced by peer pressure can come under the influence of the addictive properties of nicotine as it continues.
- *Natural maturational or developmental changes.* For example, the effects of alcohol, medications, social interactions, and physical activity can change as a person ages.

Causal Relations Are Not Exclusionary

The multivariate, multidimensional, conditional, and unstable nature of causal relations suggest that causal models of behavior problems are nonexclusionary. That is, a hypothesized causal model for a client's behavior problem does not preclude the possibility of other, equally valid, causal models for that client's behavior problem. Alternative causal models for a client's behavior problem can involve different classes of variables and degrees of specificity. Consequently, alternative causal models can include compatible variables and relations.

Different models can account for a significant proportion of variance in a client's behavior problem. For example, a cognitive causal model that accounts for a significant proportion of variance in post-trauma symptoms of a client does not preclude the possibility that an environmental-learning and neurophysiological causal model could also account for a significant proportion of variance in those problems and be equally useful for a clinical case formulation.

Alternative causal models for behavior problems are often viewed, unnecessarily, as competing and incompatible. A presumption of model incompatibility leads to literature reviews that artificially contrast, and research programs that artificially compare, noncompetitive models. This presumption also leads to disagreements at clinical staff meetings when different causal models for clients are presented as competitive rather than as complementary.

Although causal models can be complementary, it is important to note that not all causal models of a behavior problem are equally valid and useful. The behavioral assessment paradigm emphasizes variables and functional relations that are most likely to have important and clinically useful causal functions of behavior disorders. Other paradigms rely on causal models that have received little empirical support, are dysfunctionally molar and inferential, are poorly elaborated and specified, include difficult-to-measure variables, and are not amenable to scientific evaluation. Consequently, these models have little clinical utility and verifiability. Such causal models often fail to evolve because they are not amenable to scientific methods of testing and refinement.

Causal Variables and Paths Differ across Persons

Causal relations relevant to a particular behavior problem often differ across clients. Individual differences in causal relations for self-injurious behavior by persons with developmental disabilities were illustrated by Iwata and others (see the special issue on functional analysis and self-injurious behaviors; *Journal of Applied Behavior Analysis, 27*[1], 1994). Iwata and his colleagues systematically varied social and nonsocial antecedents and consequent stimuli while observing their effect on the self-injurious behaviors of 156 developmentally disabled clients. The authors concluded that self-injurious behavior for each client was maintained by one or more of four classes of response contingencies: (a) positive social reinforcement, (b) negative social reinforcement (e.g., escape from close contact with someone), (c) escape from aversive tasks or demands, and (d) "automatic" or self-reinforcement associated with the behavior.

Differences across persons in the array of causal variables for a behavior problem may result from differences in learning history, current contexts and stimuli, the operation of moderating variables, and biological predispositions. For example, Hohlstein, Smith, and Atlas (1995) and Smith (1994) noted that there are important individual differences in the expected effects of eating and alcohol intake. The expected effects of these behaviors (e.g., tension reduction, social facilitation, positive reinforcement) function as causal variables and may reflect a client's idiosyncratic learning history mediated by biological predispositions. Learned expectancies may interact with different levels of biological vulnerability across clients to affect the probability that each will develop alcohol or eating problems.

Causal Relations Can Be Nonlinear

Many causal functions are nonlinear (Haynes, 1992; Kazdin & Kagan, 1994). A causal relation can be nonlinear across time or across values of the variables, can have nonlinear time-courses when their dimensions (e.g., magnitude) change across time, and can be nonlinear across values of the variables in that the magnitude of the causal relation can vary across the values of either or both variables. For example, the effect of weight loss on blood pressure may not be linear (e.g., Rosen, Brondolo, & Kostis, 1993): Blood pressure reductions may not occur until a minimal weight loss has been obtained, and blood pressure reductions may asymptote after moderate weight loss.

One type of nonlinear causal relation is *sensitive dependence* on initial conditions (Heiby, 1995b). One aspect of this type of nonlinear function is that the effects of a causal variable can vary depending on small differences in the initial values of the dependent variable. For example, the effect of the loss of a close friend or chronic work stress on a client's depressive behaviors can be significantly affected by the person's magnitude of depressive behaviors when the loss or work stressor occurs. Similarly, the effects of a pharmacological or behavioral intervention may be influenced by the "state" and "phase" of the client on the affected variable when intervention begins—the magnitude of the behavior problem and whether it is increasing or decreasing when intervention occurs.

As Peitgen, Jürgens, and Saupe (1992) noted, sensitivity to initial conditions also implies that small differences between persons on initial values of a variable can, by iteration, increase to large differences over time. This iterative magnification is consistent with the research on the importance of early learning. The effects of any early learning experiences can be iterated throughout life (Bornstein, 1987).

Several other nonlinear functions have been outlined in Haynes (1992). Some of these include:

- *Sensitive periods* (i.e., critical periods) in causal relations occur when the magnitude of effect of a causal variable varies as a function of a person's age or developmental stage.
- *Causal discontinuity* occurs when covariation between variables occurs under some but not other conditions.
- *Functional plateaus* are a form of causal discontinuity in which a variable has no causal relation to another variable while its values remain within a particular range, but

significant causal relations are observed if its values fall below or rise above that range (e.g., daily stressors may have no effects on behavior if they remain within a "normal" range of frequency or magnitude).

- *Critical (threshold) levels* are a form of causal discontinuity in which a causal effect occurs only if the value of the causal variable exceeds a particular magnitude (or other dimension). There may be critical levels for the effects of a punishing stimulus, drugs and medications, weight loss or gain, traumatic life events, stressful family interactions, viral infection, sleep loss, and aerobic exercise.
- *Parabolic (hyperbolic) functions* occur when the magnitude and direction of effect changes as the magnitude of the causal variable increases (e.g., small quantities of ethyl alcohol often have mood-elevating effects while larger quantities often have mood-depressing effects.)
- *Log-linear functions* occur when the effect of a causal variable is best represented by a log function. Log-linear functions have been invoked in causal models of vomiting in bulimia (Schlundt, Johnson, & Jarrel, 1986) and alcohol use as a function of genetic and environmental factors (Cloninger, Bohman & Sigvardsson, 1981).

Summary

We reviewed basic concepts of causation and causal inference. We addressed concepts of causation and causal models because they affect clinical assessment and treatment strategies. Causal hypotheses dictate the best methods of assessment and the variables and functional relations targeted in assessment. Consequently, they also affect data obtained and the resultant functional analysis.

Many conditions for inferring a causal relation have been proposed. We offered a set of conditions that are most useful for inferring causation relevant to client behavior problems. However, many scholars have rejected concepts of causation and focused on description of behavior, especially through the identification of functional relations. By acknowledging the assets of an approach to the behavioral sciences that promote functional as opposed to causal relations, we promote concepts of causality in the behavioral assessment paradigm because we believe that it is helpful—causal models of behavior problems can aid research on behavior problems, guide assessment strategies, and strengthen the validity of clinical judgments.

Four necessary conditions for inferring a causal relation were suggested: (1) covariation, (2) temporal precedence, (3) logical connection, and (4) the exclusion of alternative explanations for the covariation.

There are other characteristics of causal relations for behavior problems that affect strategies of assessment and guide the development of the functional analysis. Causal relations are subjectively estimated and hypothesized. Causal models should not be presumed to be "real," they always remain heuristics for the assessor. Further, causal models can change over time, have a limited domain of validity, can be expressed at different levels of specificity, are idiographic, and do not preclude other valid models.

Suggested Readings

Concepts of Causation

Aristotle. (1947 translation). *Metaphysics*. Cambridge, MA: Harvard University Press.
Asher, H. B. (1976). *Causal modeling*. Beverly Hills, CA: Sage.

Blalock, H. M. (1971). *Causal models in the social sciences*. Chicago: Aldine Atherton.

Bunge, M. (1959). *Causality: The place of the causal principle in modern science*. Cambridge, MA: Harvard University Press.

Haynes, S. N. (1992). *Models of causality in psychopathology: Toward synthetic, dynamic and nonlinear models of causality in psychopathology*. New York: MacMillan.

James, L. R., Mulaik, S. A., & Brett, J. M. (1982). *Causal analysis; Assumptions, models and data*. Beverly Hills, CA: Sage.

Popper, K. R. (1959). *The logic of scientific discovery*. (Die Logik der Forschung). New York: Basic Books, 1959 (originally published in 1935).

Salmon, W. C. (1984). *Scientific explanation and the causal structure of the world*. Princeton, NJ: Princeton University Press.

Functionalism

Block, N. (1993). Troubles with functionalism. In A. I. Goldman (Ed.), *Readings in philosophy and cognitive science* (pp. 231–254). Cambridge, MA: MIT Press.

Moxley, R. A. (1992). From mechanistic to functional behaviorism. *American Psychologist*, *47*, 1300–1311.

10

Concepts of Causation in the Behavioral Assessment Paradigm

Introduction

Causation is a central concept of the behavioral assessment paradigm. Causal concepts and causal models of clients strongly affect assessment strategies and intervention decisions. Behavioral interventions are often designed to modify the hypothesized causes of a client's behavior problems and are often based on causal models of the client's behavior problems. The focus of an intervention program is often guided by the results of preintervention assessment, which identifies causal relations that are most likely to be important and clinically useful for a client's behavior problems and treatment goals.

This chapter examines the concepts of causation most closely associated with the behavioral assessment paradigm, and covers causal concepts that have been most useful in accounting for variance in behavior problems across persons and time.

The first section addresses aspects of causal variables and relations that are useful in behavioral assessment: multiple attributes of causal variables, multivariate causality, and multiple causal paths and mediators. The second section addresses classes of causal variables most closely associated with the behavioral assessment paradigm. Contemporaneous environmental causality, learning principles, reciprocal causation, and setting and contextual events are emphasized. Implications of behavioral causal models for assessment strategies are discussed.

We emphasize several aspects of causal variables and relations in the behavioral assessment paradigm:

1. Causal variables have multiple attributes. These include their conditional nature, temporal contiguity with behavior problems, and intrinsic reinforcement properties.
2. A behavior problem can be affected by multiple causal variables.
3. The same behavior problem can be influenced by different permutations of causal variables for different persons.
4. A causal variable may affect a behavior problem through multiple paths.
5. Multiple causal variables can affect a behavior problem through a shared causal mediator.
6. A behavior problem can be influenced through multiple causal paths.
7. Environmental variables and behavior-environment interactions are important determinants of behavior problems, and learning principles can guide the focus of assessment.
8. Response contingencies, antecedent stimuli, and reciprocal causation are important causal factors.
9. Behavior problems can vary across settings and contexts.
10. Behavior problems can be affected by contiguous and noncontiguous causal variables and extended social systems can be particularly important.
11. Change can function as a causal variable.
12. In psychological assessment, we are interested in the phase-space functions of causal variables.
13. Assessment strategies that involve only the administration of several assessment instruments at once are insufficient bases from which to draw causal inferences about a client's behavior problem.
14. Assessment strategies that can be useful for identifying functional relations include the use of causal markers, controlled manipulation in analogue settings, time-series regression analyses, and obtaining specific measures in multiple settings.

15. An empirically informed, broadly focused preintervention assessment is necessary to identify causal variables and functional relations that are relevant for a client.
16. Assessment should focus on reciprocal behavior-environment relations to help identify important causal relations relevant to a client's behavior problems.
17. Assessment should also focus on extended causal chains leading up to a behavior problem, including social systems factors.
18. It is important that assessment methods and foci have a firm empirical foundation: Assessors should be assessment scholars.

Causal Relations and Variables in the Behavioral Assessment Paradigm

Table 10-1 present an overview of concepts of causation emphasized in the behavioral assessment paradigm. Table 10-2 presents an overview of causal variables and relations most closely associated with the behaviors assessment paradigm. These emphases are relative. There is considerable overlap in causal concepts among assessment paradigms. Furthermore, behavioral assessment subparadigms differ in the degree to which they emphasize these concepts and variables. Several concepts from Table 10-1 are discussed below.

Causal Variables Have Multiple Attributes

Causal variables have multiple attributes that can differ in causal properties. Because many attributes of an event can affect its causal properties, the occurrence of a causal variable is insufficient to account for its effects. Important attributes include the temporal relations between a variable and a behavior problem, intrinsic or acquired reinforcement properties, and contextual features associated with the variable.

Table 10-1
Concepts of Causality and Causal Relations in the Behavioral Assessment Paradigm

Multiple causality	Behavior is affected by multiple causal variables
Individual differences in causality	Causal variables and relations can differ across persons with the same behavior problems
Multiple dimensions	Causal variables have multiple dimensions (e.g., rate, magnitude) which can differ in causal effects
Conditional nature of causality	There can be significant variance in causal relations for a behavior problem across situations
Interactive and additive causality	Behavior problems can be a function of the interactive and additive effects of causal variables
Response mode specificity	The effects of a causal variable can differ across the modes and dimensions of a behavior problem
Dynamic nature of causal relations	Causal relations can change over time
Nonlinear causal relations	The relations between causal variables and behavior problems can be nonlinear
Reciprocal causation	Interactions between response modes and between responses and the environment can affect behavior problems
Level of specificity of causal variables	Highly specific, molecular-level causal variables are more useful than less specific, molar-level causal variables
Chains of causal variables	Causal variables for a behavior problem can form chains

Table 10-2
Some Types and Classes of Causal Variables and Relations
Emphasized in the Behavioral Assessment Paradigm

Response contingencies	Social and other environmental contingencies can affect the dimensions of behavior problems
Basic learning principles	Learning processes affect the rate, duration, and magnitude of adaptive behaviors
Contextual and situational factors	Environmental contexts and situations can set the occasion for behavior; behavior problems vary across situations because causal variables covary with situations
Antecedent/discriminative stimuli	Discriminative stimuli affect behavior problems by indicating the probability that particular response contingencies are operating
Compound stimuli	An environment with multiple stimulus components, often with different discriminative functions
Moderator variables	Behavior problems can be affected by variables that affect the relation between two other variables
Mediating variables	A variable that accounts for, or explains, the relation between two other variables
Maintaining variables	Causal variables that maintain a behavior problem (contemporaneous causal variables) are often more clinically useful than causal variables that account for the onset of the problem (historical causal variables)
Multimodal causes	Causal variables can occur across response and stimulus modes (causal variables can be physical environmental, social environmental, cognitive, genetic, physiological)
Behavioral chains	Sequences of behaviors in which each response serves as a discriminative stimulus for the subsequent response
Systems-level variables	Variance in behavior problems may be a function of client, family, or community variables
Change as a casual variable	Causal properties may reside in change in a causal variable
Physiological factors	Can serve as setting events; genetic factors, CNS disorders, head trauma can affect the operation of response contingencies
Observable events	Clinically useful and powerful causal variables may reside in observable events, such as changes in the environment, the behavior of others, or the behavior of the client
Functional response classes and alternative behaviors	Behavior problems can covary inversely with alternative behaviors in the same response class
Reciprocal causation	A person can act on his or her environment in a way that affects that operation of environmental events as causal variables
Contrast	The causal properties of a particular event can be affected by the degree of change in contrast to immediately preceding events

For example, the ***conditional nature*** of a potential reinforcer affects the degree to which it functions as a reinforcer for behavior. Attention from a parent will serve as a reinforcer for a child's oppositional behavior to the degree that it is differentially associated with the behavior. Attention will be a more powerful reinforcer for oppositional behavior if it seldom occurs when oppositional behavior is not occurring.

Temporal contiguity between a variable and behavior also influences the magnitude of causal effect. Although many contingencies are delayed and are still effective (e.g., payment that follows work much later in time; grades that follow by days or weeks the completion of academic work), many common reinforcement relations, such as attention from peers for antisocial behavior and altered physiological states associated with drug use, are most effective when they closely follow a behavior.

The magnitude of causal effects of many variables is affected by the degree to which the variables have intrinsic or acquired reinforcer properties for a person. Persons differ in the

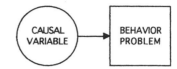

Figure 10-1. Univariate, unidirectional causal relation.

degree to which a particular variable is reinforcing or aversive, and the motivational properties of a variable are affected by many other variables. For example, attention from a parent can affect the rate of oppositional behavior for some adolescents but not others.

These examples illustrate the idiographic and conditional nature of causality in the behavioral assessment paradigm. From this vantage, a particular variable can have a causal relation with a behavior problem for some persons, sometimes, in some conditions.

Multivariate Causality

Figures 10-2 through 10-5 illustrate two important concepts: (a) a behavior problem can be affected by multiple causal variables and (b) the same behavior problem can be affected by different causal variables across persons. Multiple causal variables can act sequentially, additively, or interactively (Haynes, 1992; Kazdin & Kagan, 1994).

Multivariate causal variables have been supported by research on anxiety disorders of children (March, 1995), schizophrenia (Mueser, 1997), substance abuse (Sobell, Breslin, & Sobell, 1997), chronic pain (Turk & Melzack, 1992), sleep disorders (Riedel & Lichstein, 1994), conduct disorders (Phelps & McClintock, 1994), paranoia (Haynes, 1986a), child abuse (Hillson & Kuiper, 1994), eating disorders (Kinder, 1997), fetal alcohol syndrome (Niccols, 1994), personality disorder (Turner, 1994), self-injurious behaviors among developmentally disabled persons (Iwata et al., 1994), and many other behavior disorders (see reviews in Sutker & Adams, 1993). For example, male sexual dysfunctions (e.g., male erectile dysfunctions, dyspareunia) can result from diabetes, hormonal dysfunctions, attention processes, worry, vascular impairment, early learning, environmental contexts, fatigue, relationship distress, and conditioned fear reactions (McConaghy, 1998).

Multivariate causality does not preclude the possibility that a client's behavior problem, or a class of behavior problems, may be significantly influenced by only one causal variable (see Figure 10–1). However, the results of hundreds of published studies suggest that behavior problems are often a function of multiple, concurrently operating causal variables.

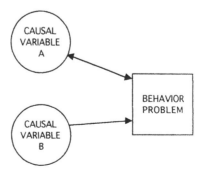

Figure 10-2. Multivariate, unidirectional, and bidirectional causal relations.

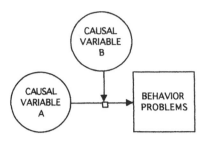

Figure 10-3. Moderating causal variable (B), which affects the magnitude of effect of causal variable A on the behavior problem.

Causal Mediators and Multiple Causal Paths

As illustrated in Figures 10-4 and 10-5, a causal variable may affect a behavior problem through multiple mediators and paths (see Box 10-1). For example, there can be many mediators through which social isolation increases the risk of depressed mood. Social isolation can restrict the opportunity for social reinforcement, increase sensitivity to reinforcement from a few persons, increase the impact of rejection from a friend, and increase negative ruminations.

Although multivariate causal models in psychopathology have been well documented, the mediators underlying multivariate causality, and multiple causal effects, are often unknown and less frequently studied. How can causal variables dissimilar in form have similar effects on a behavior problem? How can hormonal, vascular, interpersonal relationship, and attentional factors all produce sexual dysfunctions? The answer resides with an understanding of the mediators that underlie causal relations.

Multiple causal relations for a behavior can occur when different causal variables operate through the same mediator. Red wine and estrogen levels may both affect platelet-bound serotonin (the mediator) to produce migraine headaches. A causal variable can also affect a behavior problem through multiple mediators. A traumatic life event may affect mood through its effect on interpersonal relations, sleep, and thoughts of self-blame. Also, different causal variables sometimes affect different dimensions of a behavior problem (e.g., the onset and duration of depressive episodes may be affected by different variables).

The identification of causal mediators is important because it can suggest other variables that have not been identified but may operate through the same mediator. Causal mediators can

---

Box 10-1
Causal Paths, Causal Mechanisms, and Mediators

The terms "causal path," "causal mechanism," and "mediator" are often confused. A "causal path" refers to the direction and strength of a causal relation (paths may also be correlational and noncausal). A causal path may or may not include a mediator (e.g., we may know that A and B are associated, but not know what mediates that relation).

A "causal mechanism" refers to the means through which a causal effect is produced. In the language of Baron and Kenny (1986) and Shadish (1996), it is the "mediator" between the independent variable and the outcome. It answers the questions, "How, or why, does X cause Y?" and "What mediates the effects of X on Y?" We use the term "mediator" to refer to the causal mechanism.

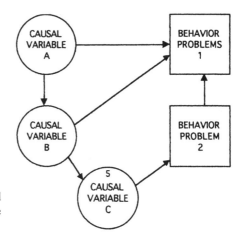

Figure 10-4. Causal chain (A→B→C); multiple causal paths to behavior problem I (note that B and C mediate the effects of A on 2).

also suggest potential intervention foci and strategies that might be effective across a variety of causal variables.

Shared Causal Mediators

Multiple causal variables can affect a behavior problem through a shared causal mediator. Consider physical abuse or neglect of a child (Wolfe & McEachran, 1997). Most models of child abuse and neglect propose multiple, interdependent causal variables and mediators, which also differ in degree of specificity and response mode. Causal variables may include deficient parenting skills, tendencies of the abuser to use aggression as a way to control others, education level, parent anger management skills, parent substance abuse, parent social support, child behavior/misbehavior, frequency and magnitude of daily social/environmental stressors

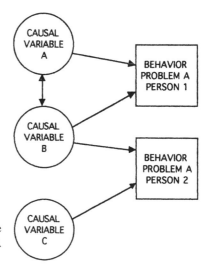

Figure 10-5. Individual differences in causal variables for the same behavior problem (note bidirectional relations between A and B).

in the parents' lives, family financial condition, marital status and distress, and communications skills. If we limit our discussion of child abuse and neglect to one mediator—social/environmental stressors acting on the parent—we can see how multiple causal variables can operate through a common mediator. Because a "stressful social environment" can increase the chance of child abuse, any stressful event for the parent can function as a causal variable. Stressful events triggering abusive behavior may include a noncompliant or frequently crying child, marital conflict, troubles with social service agencies, or conflicts at work.

At a more specific level of analysis we can examine how a stressful social environment affects parenting behaviors (e.g., Wahler & Hann, 1986). Some studies have noted that parents use of appropriate contingency management for their children (e.g., tracking and rewarding good behavior) is adversely affected when the parents are experiencing life stressors. When under stress, parents are less likely to praise their children for good behavior, express affection, or apply negative contingencies systematically. One possible mediator for this causal effect is that social-environmental stressors disrupt a parent's ability to track the behavior of his or her child. When tracking abilities are impaired, the parent cannot apply appropriate contingencies at the appropriate times because his or her attention is focused elsewhere. Positive behaviors by the child go unrewarded and negative behaviors go uncorrected.

This illustrates the clinical utility of identifying causal mediators in psychological assessment. If we can identify a causal mediator, we can predict which events are likely to disrupt the ability of the parent to attend to or track the child and, consequently, which events can increase the chance of child behavior problems or childhood abuse or neglect. One might expect parental substance abuse, parental ill health, and marital distress to be associated with an increased risk to the child.

Multiple Causal Paths and Mediators

Many behavior problems are affected through multiple causal paths, each of which can serve as a conduit for the effects of multiple causal variables (see Figures 10-4 to 10-6). For example, decreased inhibitions for emitting socially disapproved behavior (e.g., aggression toward a child) may be one of several causal mediators for child abuse. Disinhibition of aggressive behaviors (an increased probability of aggression) may be affected through multiple paths—heightened blood alcohol levels, a context in which social contingencies are reduced (e.g., being alone with the child), or in a social/cultural environment in which physical aggression toward children is sanctioned (in which the probability of negative contingencies for hitting are small).

A causal variable can affect a behavior problem through multiple mediators (see Variable A in Figure 10-4; Variables A and B in Figure 10-5). For example, chronic or multiple traumatic life events may result in impaired immune and parasympathetic system functioning (Asterita, 1985) through several mediators. Life stressors may be associated with increased drug use, changes in diet, reduction of lymphocyte levels, reduced production of interferon, and/or sleep disruption.

Multiple paths may also account for the adverse effects of an abusive childhood experience on later adult interpersonal functioning (Brunk, Henggeler, & Whelan, 1987; Harter, Alexander, & Neimeyer, 1988). Experiences with sexual abuse may have long-term effect's on expectancies regarding the consequences of attentive behaviors from others. These experiences may also affect beliefs about the chance of being harmed in intimate interpersonal situations. Early abuse experiences may also produce conditioned fear responses to intimate situations and a tendency to avoid some social situations that resemble the abusive situation. A

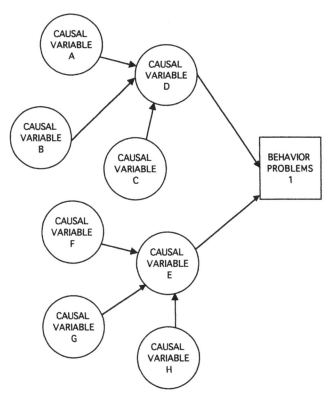

Figure 10-6. Two causal paths, each with three causal variables with a common causal paths to behavior problem; "D" and "E" can represent a mediating variable or causal mechanism shared by "A," "B," "C," and "F," "G," "H," respectively.

child may also develop negative self-labels and become nonresponsive to the positive interpersonal behaviors of others. These are all causal mediators—they may explain *how* a history of sexual abuse can lead to interpersonal difficulties as an adult.

The mediators that account for a causal relation are not always known. For example, Bentall, Haddock, and Slade (1994) proposed a multivariate, nomothetic causal model of hallucinations. They suggested that hallucinations were most likely to occur for at-risk patients when the patient attributes mental events to external sources. This attribution is more likely in the context of anxiety or stress and during conditions of sensory deprivation or unpatterned auditory stimulation. However, the exact cognitive processes that account for the hallucinator's failure to appropriately attribute self-generated mental events, the causal mediators underlying the effects of these attributions, were not identified.

Interactive and Additive Causality

Multiple causal variables can affect a behavior problem additively or interactively. Interactive causality occurs when the causal effects of one variable vary as a function of the values of another variable—the effects of the variables in combination are not a strict function of the sum of their independent effects. Interactive causal models are similar to "vulnerability," "predisposition," "buffering," and "diathesis-stress" causal models, which propose that the effect of a causal variable can vary with the values of another variable.

Data collected by Schlundt, Johnson, and Jarrell (1986) on post-meal purges of bulimic patients illustrate interactive effects. These authors reported that the conditional probability of a purge was elevated with a recent history of purges. However, the conditional probability of purging following a recent history of purges depended on the social context within which eating occurred. The chance of purging was especially higher if the eating occurred in isolation.

There are other possible interactive effects between causal variables: The effects of a particular reinforcer on a behavior may be affected by recent exposure to the reinforcer; the effect of dietary tyramine on the vascular components of migraine headaches may depend on levels of platelet-bound serotonin, which can be affected by life stressors; the effect of time-out from reinforcement may depend on the relative level of reinforcement associated with the natural and time-out environment; and the probability of aggression in a domestic conflict may be affected by substance abuse.

Types of Causal Variables Emphasized in the Behavioral Assessment Paradigm

Within the behavioral assessment paradigm, many classes of variables, such as cognitive and physiological, are presumed to have causal functions. However, the class of causal variables that most distinguishes behavioral from nonbehavioral paradigms derives from the empirical learning literature, especially behavior analysis. Learning principles provide the guiding framework for the focus of behavioral assessment and for the operation of many behavioral interventions.

Learning principles stress the importance of functional relations between behavior and response contingencies, the effects of pairings among environmental events and responses, and the role of discriminative stimuli and contextual factors. For example, an understanding of the concepts of differential reinforcement of other behaviors (DRO, see Glossary) or negative reinforcement schedules inform the assessor about the kind of response contingencies that might be operating to maintain the severe aggressive behavior problems of a child. To construct a functional analysis of an aggressive child, the assessor must understand that aggressive behavior may be a partial function of the fact that aversive tasks are sometimes withdrawn following its occurrence and of the failure to reinforce alternative nonaggressive behaviors.

This section only touches on causal variables in the behavioral assessment paradigm. However, it is essential for a behavioral assessor to be familiar with principles of learning, and there are many sources of information on this topic. The *Journal of Applied Behavior Analysis*, the *Journal of Experimental Analysis of Behavior*, and the *Behavior Analyst* contain hundreds of articles relevant to behavioral causal models for behavior disorders. Several books (Dona-hoe & Palmer, 1994; Eysenck & Martin, 1987; Grant & Evans, 1994; Johnston & Pennypacker, 1993; Nelson & Hayes, 1986; Pierce & Epling, 1999; Plaud & Eifert, 1998) present material relevant to the learning foundations and behavioral causal models of behavioral assessment. An edited book by O'Donohue and Krasner (1995) presents overviews of the matching law, two-factor learning theory, reciprocal inhibition, reinforcement, exposure, conditioning, dyadic exchanges, self-regulation, attribution, information-processing, and other research domains that are useful in causal models of behavior disorders.

Learning principles are important for two reasons: they can be used to account for a substantial proportion of variance in many behavior problems, and they are clinically useful in that they identify functional relations that can be modified in an intervention program. Most learning principles, by definition, address contemporaneous, modifiable factors that could be maintaining a behavior problem.

We provide a general introduction to causal concepts in behavioral assessment but not in sufficient detail to guide behavioral assessment strategies. For example, we do not address the impact of differential reinforcement of incompatible behavior (DRI, see Glossary) or variable ratio schedules of reinforcement, the carry-over effects associated with changes in schedules of reinforcement, stimulus and response generalization, matching laws, contrast effects, time-out from positive reinforcement, compound and multiple discriminative stimuli, the effects of reinforcement history, rule-governed behavior, or multiple factors affecting acquired rein-forcers (e.g., discussions by Timberlake, 1995; and chapters in O'Donohue & Krasner, 1995). Nor do we examine attribution theory (Metalsky, Laird, Heck, & Joiner, 1995), genetics and pathophysiology (Matthysse, 1993), reciprocal inhibition (Wolpe, 1995), two-factor learning theory (McAllister & McAllister, 1995), or paradigmatic behaviorism (Staats, 1995).

Table 10-2 present an overview of some types of causal variables emphasized in the behavioral assessment paradigm. As we noted earlier, many other variables, such as cognitive, genetic, and physiological factors, are recognized as having important causal functions for behavior problems.

Contemporaneous Environmental Causality and Reciprocal Causation

A major contribution of the behavioral assessment paradigm is an emphasis on environmental causality and behavior-environment interactions. Many studies have shown that a significant proportion of variance in many behavior problems can be accounted for by variance in *response contingencies* (see Box 10-2)—what happens following a response affects the future probability or other dimensions of that response. Additional variance in behavior has also been associated with variance in *situational and antecedent stimulus factors*.

The effects of environmental events on behavior are rarely simple main effects. More often, they are a function of complex interactions among multiple variables. The effects of a particular response contingency, such as the effects of praise for a child's good study habits, depend on many interacting parameters, such as schedules of contingencies, temporal parameters of response contingencies, interactions among compound discriminative stimuli, the administrator of the praise, and a history of stimulus and response pairings.

One important element of a model of causality that stresses behavior-environment interaction is *reciprocal causation*—the idea that two variables can affect each other sequentially. In clinical assessment, the principle of reciprocal causation suggests that a client can behave in ways that affect his or her environment that, in turn, can affect the client's behavior. For example, a client's depressive behaviors, such as reduced social initiations and positive talk, slower speech, and lowered affect, may effect a withdrawal by the client's friends. These withdrawals can increase the client's loss of social reinforcement, thereby increasing the client's depressive mood and behaviors, which can further alienate the client's friends.

Reciprocal causation is also congruent with the causal interactions among behavior problems, as noted in Chapter 8. A depressed client may behave less positively and more critically toward his or her spouse and children, which can result in marital distress and child behavior problems, which can also increase depressed mood.

Sensitivity to initial conditions, as discussed in Chapter 9, also has implications for a reciprocal causation paradigm. Small initial differences between young children in their social behavior, interests, and verbal skills can strongly affect their social environment. These envi-

---

Box 10-2
A Taxonomy for Response Contingencies

There are many ways in which response contingencies can affect behavior, and a taxonomy for classifying operant reinforcement processes would help in developing functional analyses for many clients. Woods (1974) developed a taxonomy of 16 operant conditioning procedures. These were refined and expanded by Tryon in 1976 and again in 1996.

In his 1996 article, Tryon presents five tables that organize response contingencies by: (a) emission vs. omission of a response; (b) signaled vs. unsignaled contingencies; (c) accelerative vs. decelerative functions of contingencies, and (d) contingent (emission/omission) vs. noncontingent events. Tryon emphasized the importance of contingencies on response omission. These are contingencies that fail to support the emission of desirable behavior (e.g., positive alternatives to problem behaviors). Response omission contingencies are important in clinical assessment (we often want to know why a person did not develop appropriate social and other coping skills), but the absence of contingencies is difficult to identify in clinical assessment.

Tryon suggested eight diagnostic categories for response contingencies to help guide the focus of clinical assessment, help in the construction of a functional analysis, and help in intervention planning. For example, type 1 is the absence of procedures that increase positive behavior, type 2 is the presence of procedures that decrease positive behaviors, type 3 is the presence of procedures that support negative behavior, and type 4 is the presence of procedures that decrease negative behaviors. This classification system leads to an idiographic and dynamic behavioral case formulation and intervention plan.

---

ronmental changes can affect their behavioral repertoires over time, which, in turn, continues to affect the social environment. Similarly, small differences between persons in the operation of causal variables, such as parent-delivered response reinforcers, can result in large differences between persons in their later behavior.

Clients as Active Participants in Assessment and Intervention

Within a reciprocal determinism framework, clients are considered active participants in the factors that control their behavior and thoughts and feelings, and as active agents of change in intervention. Consequently, clients are encouraged to participate actively in the assessment and intervention process. Informed consent and active participation by clients are essential ingredients of most behavioral assessment and intervention programs. It is important for clients to understand the purpose of assessment methods, how data will be used, how the assessment contributes to their intervention goals, and how their participation is essential to a positive outcome. Clients should also understand the idea of reciprocal causation in behavior problems and in the achievement of treatment goals, as well as their role as active partners in the assessment-treatment process.

The concept of reciprocal causation affects how we label variables in our causal models. The distinction between a "behavior problem" and a "causal variable" becomes fuzzy when bidirectional causation is involved. Either variable in a bidirectional causal relation can be described as a behavior problem or as a causal variable. Both variables have causal properties and either or both can often be considered a behavior problem. Which variable is labeled as "problem" as opposed to "cause" often depends on convention, preferences of the client and assessor, and the focus of subsequent interventions.

The concept of reciprocal causation also promotes a positive, constructional focus on the clients behavioral skills. The assessor attends to the ways that a client may be contributing to his or her behavior problems, and ways he or she can contribute to the attainment of positive intervention goals. Similar to a *task analysis*, and based on the assumptions that behavior problems are a partial function of the client's behavioral repertoire, the assessor may try to identify the skill deficits and the skills necessary to attain intervention goals. For example, within a reciprocal causation framework, behavioral assessment with a socially anxious client might focus on specific behavioral deficits that prevent the client from forming more frequent and rewarding friendships (Beidel & Morris, 1995; Leary, 1991; Stein, 1995).

Although the concept of reciprocal causation has been applied most often to behavior-environment interactions, it is also applicable to reciprocal influences across modes. A client's beliefs, expectancies, attributions, and other thoughts regarding his or her capabilities or expected outcomes of behavior in specific situations (e.g., Linscott & DiGiuseppe, 1998) may affect behavior in those situations. The client's behavior may then affect how the environment responds, which in turn affects behavior and thoughts (see Box 10-3).

Box 10-3
Personality Traits as Causal Variables

Personality traits (e.g., extraversion, conscientiousness, hardiness, neuroticism, emotionality, hostility, shyness) are nomothetically based descriptions of persons. They are dimensions of individual differences. However, personality traits are sometimes used to imply the operation of internal causal processes and can be imbued with circular causal properties. For example, the personality construct "hostility" is sometimes used to explain aggressive behaviors. However, measures of aggressive behavior are often used to infer how "hostile" a person is—items asking about aggressive behaviors are included in a questionnaire whose score is interpreted as an index of "hostility." Used in this manner, a trait label or score implies that a person "possesses" a specified amount of the trait and that this trait amount "causes" behavior. Rather than describing the probability that a person will emit a response from a class of correlated behaviors in particular situation, the trait is used to "explain" behavior.

Traits can be useful in describing and predicting behavior but are often measured in ways that limit their utility. Sometimes a trait measure can suggest the probability that one person, relative to others, will behave in certain ways across time and within particular situations. However, traits often have little explanatory or clinical utility in causal models of behavior disorders. They are not optimally useful causal variables because they usually lack specificity and modifiability. Their utility is also limited by the fact that trait measures often do not reflect important situational sources of variance of behavior (e.g., the situations in which a person is most and least likely to emit aggressive behaviors). Furthermore, behaviors aggregated to form a trait measure sometimes do not strongly covary, suggesting that the elements may not be tapping a homogeneous construct.

The utility of "personality trait" constructs and their role in clinical decision making has been addressed often (e.g., Kendrick & Funder, 1988; McFall & McDonel, 1986). In 1997, Jim Butcher edited a special section in *Psychological Assessment* (Volume 9[4], pp. 331–385) entitled, "Assessment in Psychological Treatment." Two of the six papers discussed the role of personality assessment in treatment planning. Meier (1994) provided a historical and conceptual overview of the situation-trait issue in psychological assessment. A special section on the relations between personality concepts and behavioral assessment was published in *Behavior Modification*, *17*(1), 1993.

Contemporaneous Causal Variables

Causal variables can differ in their temporal relations with a behavior problem. Some antecedent and consequent causal variables are contiguous—they occur immediately before or after the behavior problem. Others are remote—they occur hours, months, or years before or following a behavior problem.

Causal variables across a range of temporal relations can be important in that they can account for a substantial proportion of variance in a behavior problem. The importance of early learning for the development of behavior problems is an important tenet of behavioral construct systems. Many behavior problems result from learning experiences that have occurred for years, or occurred years ago. Additionally, a focus on historical causal variables can help identify patterns, time-course, and the conditional probabilities of behavior problems. A focus on the historical time-course of a behavior problem and associated functional relations may be particularly useful when frequency of occurrence is the main dimension of interest. Such information may help to detect triggering or contextual factors.

Although knowledge about history can have an important explanatory function, a focus on contemporaneous causal variables may provide more clinically useful information. Anorectic eating disorders provide an example of the contrast between remote and contemporaneous causal factors. Most models of anorexia nervosa implicate a long history of peer, family, and cultural influences. These models also emphasize the importance of early learning of associated behavior, such as obsessive-compulsive behaviors, and interactions between environmental and biological predisposition factors (Williamson, Womble, & Zucker, 1998). However, assessment of a client with an eating disorder may more profitably focus on contemporaneous thoughts about eating and body weight, current and ideal body image distortions, food aversions and avoidance behaviors, specific eating behaviors, dieting strategies, contextual factors associated with restricted food intake, and thoughts regarding the outcomes of increased eating and weight gain (Allison, 1995). A focus on contemporaneous causal factors is especially important in advanced cases of anorexia nervosa because patients are often malnourished. Following stabilization of caloric intake and weight to more healthy levels, assessment might also examine contemporary functional relations involving depressed mood (which can be a consequence of malnutrition) and other behavior, such as obsessive and compulsive behaviors, overgeneralization, and personalization.[1]

Paranoid personality styles are also probably learned at an early age (Haynes, 1986b). For example, a tendency to view ambiguous events in self-referent terms and as threats can undoubtedly be learned from parents. They may instruct a child not to trust others, to suspect hidden meanings in other persons' behaviors, or that the behavior of others is often directed at the child. There may also be biological predispositions to paranoid attributions. However, despite the explanatory importance of early parent-child experiences, they are difficult to measure in assessment and address in intervention. Thus, it may be more effective to focus assessment and intervention efforts on contemporaneous causal variables for paranoid thoughts and actions. Social isolation can reduce corrective feedback to the paranoid person

[1] In contrast, psychodynamic models of eating disorders emphasize the importance of unconscious conflicts originating in early developmental periods. Conflict themes may center on individuation from the parent, denial of sexuality and sexual maturity, an approach-avoidance search for power over one's behavior and body, fears and avoidance of personal responsibility. Note that some of these are molar, nonspecific causal variables but are not necessarily incompatible with a behavioral causal model. One could develop a causal model that emphasized reciprocal interactions among family members regarding eating and weight, fears regarding sexuality, the client's effectiveness in obtaining rewards from others through alternative behaviors.

about his or her thoughts, social skills deficits can contribute to social isolation and interpersonal difficulties, and selective attention or hypersensitivity to ambiguous social stimuli can increase the chance of paranoid interpretations of events.

It is also important to understand that historical causal variables are unmodifiable. However, their sequelae often can be modified. Spinal cord damage may not be modifiable, but some cognitive and behavioral sequelae that lead to interpersonal, self-help, and occupational difficulties associated with spinal cord damage can be modified.

Sequelae to unmodifiable causal variables are important elements of the functional analysis. We can sometimes change the way a client thinks about a historical event, modify the social behaviors learned in the context of historical events, and change emotional responses to contemporaneous discriminative stimuli.

Situations, Contextual and Setting Events, and Systems Factors as Causal Variables

As we noted in Chapter 8, behavior problems are presumed to be conditional—the probability, magnitude, or duration of a behavior problem will vary across situations, settings, and as a function of transient eliciting and discriminative stimuli. The conditional nature of behavior problems has important implications for their causation. The contexts and eliciting stimuli that are reliably associated with a behavior problem serve as markers for the differential operation of causal variables. For example, the fact that a clients' self-injurious behavior, marital conflict, social anxiety, nightmares, or depressed mood are more likely to occur in some situations than in others suggests that the causal variables for those problems historically or currently covary with those situations. The differential occurrence of behavior problems across situations alerts the assessor to the possibility that variables that differ across those situations may have causal functions for the behavior problem.

The contextual and situational model is congruent with a person × situation "interactional" perspective (McFall & McDonel, 1986), which is a refinement of traditional, primarily trait-based models of behavior and behavior problems. As we noted earlier, personality trait models often fail to reflect important environmental sources of variance in behavior problems and fail to reflect the changing nature of behavior across time.

An emphasis on situational factors does not preclude the possibility that some behaviors, for some persons, occur reliably across situations. The degree of cross-situational consistency of behavior can vary across different behaviors, individuals, and situations. Some persons have paranoid delusions or extreme social anxiety across most social situations, while others are delusional or anxious only in some situations.

A person x situation interactional model suggests that we can best predict how a person will behave, and understand the causes of this behavior, if we know something about his or her dispositions, something about the situations in which the dispositions are most likely to be manifested, and something about the characteristics of situations in which we are attempting to predict behavior.

The behavioral assessment paradigm emphasizes situational factors but provides little specific guidance for conducting situational assessments. A taxonomy of situations associated with variance on dimensions of specific behavior problems would help the assessor focus on important situational variables in assessment and when constructing a behavioral case formulation (see Box 10-4). It would also help the clinician identify and anticipate high-risk situations for the client and organize preventive strategies. However, situation taxonomies for behavior

---

Box 10-4
The Concept of "Setting" in Ecological Psychology

A book by Schoggen (1989), a revision of Barker's original work on ecological psychology, illustrates the complexity of constructing a classification system for behavior settings. He noted that settings are defined by their structure and their dynamic characteristics (consider the structure, changing social stimuli, and complex role expectations associated with a social gathering in a person's home). He noted eight possible sources of behavior-environment interactions: (a) physical forces such as the shape of a room, (b) social forces such as the behavior of a teacher in a classroom, (c) physiological processes, such as drowsiness triggered by an overheated room, (d) physiognomic perception such as the effect of open-spaces on the motor behavior of children, (e) prior learning associated with settings, (f) the selection of settings by persons such as the selection of social environments by those who find social activity reinforcing, (g) the effect of the person on the setting milieu (similar to the principle of reciprocal causation), such as when a gregarious persons enters a social gathering, and (h) the selection of persons by settings such as age requirements for sports activities.

---

disorders have not been developed and validated. Consequently, the assessor is forced to rely on idiographic methods.

Context

Context (i.e., contextual and situational stimuli, setting, extant conditions; see Glossary) is congruent with the idea that there are situational sources of variance for behavior problems. It refers to the stimulus conditions in a particular time and setting or when a particular response occurs. Context includes the situational conditions, often dynamic and involving the behavior of others, associated with a behavior or that form the background when discriminative stimuli are presented or training occurs. Context affects, or sets the occasion for, behavior because there is a learning history associated with its elements. Consequently, each setting will contain unique discriminative and consequential stimuli. These stimuli will have different effects on a person's behavior, depending on intraindividual, temporal, and social contexts.

Context can refer to a range of conditions and stimuli, from complex social/environmental situations, the recent history of reinforcement, and the arrangement of questionnaire items. Responses to a questionnaire and interview items can be influenced by the sequence and content of previous items; a child's response may be affected by whether the mother or father is present and depend on the "mood" of each parent; the chance of domestic violence, bingeing and purging, and a panic episode may be affected by the social context. Thus, context can serve as an important domain for functional relations.

Social Systems Factors

Despite the importance of contiguous causal variables in the behavioral assessment paradigm, noncontiguous variables are frequently necessary for a functional analysis of a client's behavior problems. In particular, *extended social systems* are important (Alessi, 1988; Kanfer, 1985; Mash & Terdall, 1997; Nezu & Nezu, 1993; Ollendick & Hersen, 1993a).

Given that many contiguous causal variables involve the behavior of others (e.g., parents, spouses), variables that affect the behavior of these persons are important elements in a functional analysis. It may not be possible to adequately account for variance in a client's behavior problems, and it may be difficult to develop powerful predictive, explanatory, and intervention models for behavior problems unless we consider factors within the extended social systems in which the behavior problem is imbedded. Consider the case of a seven-year-old child who is brought to a clinic by his mother because of multiple, severe, persistent noncompliant, aggressive, and oppositional behaviors. An assessment of the contingencies on the child's behavior reveals high rates of maternal reinforcement for negative behaviors, inconsistent negative contingencies for problem behaviors, infrequent reinforcement for positive alternative behaviors, and infrequent noncontingent reinforcement by his mother.

Is the identification of these immediate and important response contingencies sufficient for a behavioral case formulation? Can we plan an intervention based on these identified functional relations alone? There are data from multiple sources indicating that with an appropriately instituted contingency management program, the child could probably be taught to increase positive and decrease negative behaviors. However, would one expect quick, positive, long-lasting effects from a behavior management training program for the mother? The usual answer is "it depends." The likelihood of effective intervention depends on the functional relations relevant to the mother's behavioral management strategies (Alessi, 1988, called these concerns "metacontingencies"—contingencies on those who deliver contingencies to the target person). If the mother is facing multiple and severe difficulties in her life, beginning a behavior management training program for her might be ineffective. She might not attend sessions, attend to learn new skills in sessions, practice skills at home, or carry out and maintain skills once they were acquired. Decisions about the best intervention strategy would be helped by a behavioral case formulation that included information about the relationship between the mom and dad, the role of the father in the family, the mother's work load, medical and physical problems of family members, and economic issues.

Figure 10-7 illustrates a case in which there are significant social systems-level factors impinging on a mother seeking assistance for her child's behavior problems. The implications for this model are clear—many variables affect the degree to which the parent will attend to, and appropriately consequate, the child's behavior. Failure to assess these systems variables will result in a case formulation with low content validity: The behavioral case formulation will have omitted variables that have an important effect on the behavior of the child.

Systems variables have been implicated in many behavior problems. For example, Craske and Waikar (1994) suggested that in the treatment of clients with panic disorders, problems with persons close to a client's can affect the client's co-occurring problems and progress in intervention. The character of social interactions in a group home for individuals with developmental or central nervous system disabilities may affect the rate at which they learn adaptive self-help, cognitive, and physical skills. Sobell, Toneatto and Sobell (1994) noted that chronic alcohol and other substance abuse can have important effects on a client's family, marital, friendship, and occupational relationships. Some of these interactions can serve as triggers and maintaining variables and can be important components of intervention.

Degree of Change of a Variable Can Have Causal Properties

Variance in behavior problems and the magnitudes of causal relations can sometimes be strongly associated with the dynamic attributes of a variable; causal effects can sometimes be associated with the degree and/or rate of change of a variable. For example, presume that there is a causal relation between the frequency of positive social exchanges and mood (see general review in Coyne & Downey, 1991). For two persons with an identical rate of positive social

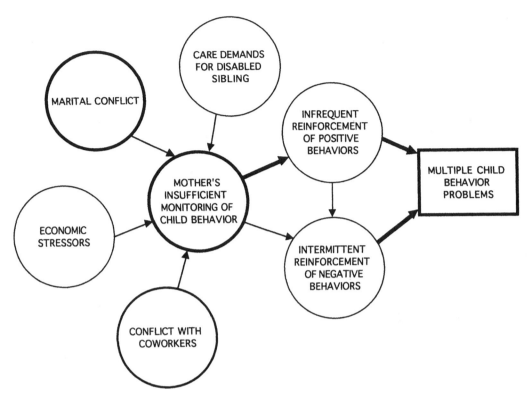

Figure 10-7. A model illustrating extended systems variables affecting a child's behavior problems. Note that multiple life stressors affect the mother's ability to attend to and effectively respond to the child. This model suggests that a treatment program that focuses solely on teaching the mother behavior management skills would not be optimally effective because it does not address variables that affect the mother's ability to appropriately monitor the child. For example, this model suggests that regular respite care would increase the chance that the mother could attend to and appropriately consequate the child's behavior (A complete functional analysis would include many more variables and causal paths).

exchanges at a particular measurement point, the magnitude of depressed mood at that time is likely to be greater for the person who has experienced greater and more recent loss of social support. We might observe similar causal effects associated with the magnitude and recency of change of other causal variables for depressed mood, such as loss of a friend or spouse, functional impairment associated with health problems, and the rate of negative self-evaluations.

The self-monitoring study by Schlundt, Johnson, and Jarrell (1986) provides another example of causal properties associated with the dynamic qualities of a variable. These authors found that the probability of vomiting by a bulimic client was significantly associated with the magnitude of mood changes before eating: Vomiting after a meal was moderately correlated with the client's negative mood state but even more strongly correlated with recent changes in the client's mood.

Degree of change is another element of the conditional and contextual nature of causal relations. Here, we are suggesting that the direction and magnitude of effect of a causal variable can be affected by the value of the causal variable, in relation to its previous values. Three

---

Box 10-5
Reinforcement Contrast Effect

One contextual concept in behavior analysis, consistent with our discussion of "change" as a causal variable, is *reinforcement contrast* (Sidman, 1960). This construct suggests that the effect of a schedule of reinforcement is a partial function of its degree to which it contrasts with previous schedules of reinforcement. Some studies have reported an immediate effect of a change in reinforcement rate followed by a parabolic "contrast effect" (a recovery beyond baseline levels, then a return to baseline). The magnitude of the contrast effect is often a function of the magnitude of contrast between the two schedules of reinforcement—extinction following a "lean" schedule of reinforcement (e.g., 1:5 ratio of reinforcement to responses) would likely to be associated with a smaller contrast effect than would extinction following a "rich" schedule of reinforcement (e.g., 1:3 ratio of reinforcement to responses).

---

interrelated dimensions of change in a causal variable can have implications for the focus and methods of psychological assessment: (a) the magnitude of change, (b) the rate of change, and (c) the recency of change (see Box 10-5).

Phase-Space Functions

As described in Chapter 5, a phase-space function is a value of any dimension of a variable plotted over time. The value of a variable (its state) coupled with the current direction and rate of change of the variable (its phase), at a single measurement point, is its phase state. In psychological assessment, we are interested in the phase-space functions of causal variables, such as rate of reinforcement, aversive social interactions, and daily hassles. A single measure of a variable captures it at a particular state and at a particular phase.

The vertical axis in Figure 5-3 could represent any dimension of a causal variable such as frequency of positive social interactions, minutes of exercise, or subjective magnitude of daily stressors. If the vertical axis represents "frequency of positive social interactions," at measurement point 10, the frequency is identical for all persons—they have the same absolute value; they are in an identical state. However, the dynamic context of the causal variable differs across persons. Each person is in a different phase of positive social interactions: decreasing for Person A, increasing for Person B, and stable for Person C. Most important, given the hypothesized functional relations noted earlier, mood is likely to be higher for Person B than for person A. The main point is that any effects of positive social interactions are going to be significantly associated with the phase and the state of a causal variable.

Implications for Psychological Assessment

The necessary conditions for causal inferences discussed in Chapter 9 and the multivariate, idiographic, contemporaneous environmental, reciprocal, nonlinear, and dynamical causal models of behavior problems associated with the behavioral assessment paradigm discussed in this chapter affect the strategies and focus of behavioral assessment. These conditions and models support the use of causal markers, manipulation, and multivariate time-series regression analyses; support a focus on functional relations in the natural environment of the client;

support systems-level assessment; support a scholarly orientation to assessment; and indicate the kind of data that are necessary for an assessment of functional relations.

Detecting Causal Relations in Clinical Assessment

Assumptions about the necessary conditions for inferring causal relations, the characteristics of causal models for client behavior problems, and limitations on causal inferences have important implications for psychological assessment and causal inference in clinical assessment contexts. The necessary conditions for causal inference means that contiguous elevation of measures of behavior problems and hypothesized causal variable and contiguous co-occurrence of a behavior problem and hypothesized causal variable are insufficient to infer a causal relation.

A frequent error in causal inference is interpreting concurrent elevation of measures as an indication of causal relations (e.g., a high marital distress score and a high depression score). Concurrent elevation between two measures, especially when prior research has supported a possible causal relation between them, marks, but does not confirm, a possible causal relation. However, covariation is insufficient for causal inference because it cannot address two criteria for causation: Two measures may be concurrently elevated for a client without covarying across time and without the necessary temporal precedence relation. Co-occurrence should alert the assessor to possible causal relations but, ultimately, such judgments should be based on data from follow-up evaluation of functional relations, such as multivariate time-series assessment, analogue observation, or functionally oriented interviews. In sum, assessment strategies that involve only the administration of several assessment instruments at once are an insufficient basis to draw causal inferences about a client's behavior problem.

The emphasis on contemporaneous behavior-environment interactions and reciprocal causation underscores the importance of obtaining data about the client in his or her natural environment. Whether the assessment strategies include naturalistic observation, analogue observation, interviews, questionnaires, or self-monitoring assessment methods, the focus is on current behavior-environment interactions, contrast effects, and changes across time in causal variables, in the natural environment.

Strategies for Detecting Causal Relations

The Use of Causal Markers

A causal marker is a measure that covaries with the strength of a causal relation. Causal markers are not causal variables. They are variables that are highly correlated with functional (and hypothesized causal) relations. An example of a causal marker is a client's psychophysiological response to a brief stressor presented in a laboratory situation. The measure, the degree of response to the laboratory stressor, is presumed to be a marker for the degree to which the client responds to similar stressors in his or her natural environment.

Causal markers are cost-effective indices of functional relations in the natural environment. For example, measuring the psychophysiological responses of the client in the natural environment can often be difficult, expensive, and time consuming, compared to laboratory assessment. Consequently, causal markers are particularly useful when a causal relation is difficult to measure.

Causal markers are difficult to validate and are only estimates of the functional relations of interest. To be clinically useful, the correlation between a causal marker and the predicted functional relation must be substantial. A causal marker that correlates .7 with the strength of a functional relation in the natural environment would still underestimate or overestimate the strength of the relation for many clients.

Manipulation in Analogue Settings

A powerful method of testing causal hypotheses is the systematic manipulation of the hypothesized causal variable and observation of the effect on the targeted behavior problem while holding possible confounding sources of variance constant. Manipulation strategies, particularly in ABAB interrupted time-series designs, are often used in experimental and applied behavior analysis (Kazdin, 1998).

For example, the effect of the topic of discussion on the delusional talk of a hospitalized psychiatric patient could be investigated by having a staff member systematically vary the topic of conversation: five minutes of talk on a neutral or positive topic, five minutes of talk on an anxiety-provoking topic, five minutes of talk on a neutral or positive topic, five minutes on an anxiety provoking topic. This strategy allows the assessor to examine covariance and precedence between the behavior problem and hypothesized causal variable. Replication of effects also allows the assessor to control some alternative explanations for the covariance.

Manipulation can address most of the requirements of causal inference. It can provide information on the strength of covariance between two variables and the precedence of the hypothesized causal variable is controlled (because the hypothesized causal variable is systematically manipulated). Many alternative explanations for the covariance can also be controlled.

As with all assessment strategies, there are limitations on the inferences that can be drawn from analogue manipulation assessment. This assessment strategy can be time-consuming, intrusive, and cumbersome, and the generalizability of some inferences to clients in the natural environment is often suspect. The assets and limitations of analogue manipulation studies are discussed in greater detail in Chapter 12.

Multivariate Time-Series Regression Analyses

With multivariate time-series regression measurement strategies, a behavior problem and one or more hypothesized causal variables are measured concurrently and frequently (e.g., 40 or more measurements) across time. With many time samples, it is possible to estimate the magnitude of covariation among multiple variables. Temporal precedence can be controlled through time-lagged correlations, and it is also possible to control for trends and autocorrelation in the data sets.

Although time-series measurement methods have disadvantages, particularly the amount of data necessary for estimating functional relations, it is a powerful and underused assessment strategy. It is also amenable to a variety of methods: time-series regression strategies can be used with data from questionnaires, behavioral observation, self-monitoring, and psychophysiological instruments. For example, using self-monitoring assessment methods, Hazelett and Haynes (1992) measured life stressors, sleep quality, and pain in 11 chronic pain clients for 40 to 80 days. The goal of this study was to estimate the degree to which each client's nighttime sleep quality was affected by the previous day's stressful events, which, in turn, affected the client's pain the next day. The authors found that, for some patients, increased life stressors were associated with impaired sleep patterns and, consequently, with pain affect and mobility.

Consider a client who has reported severe, chronic difficulty falling asleep and who has been unresponsive to standard behavioral treatments. The client could self-monitor sleep-onset latency along with several potential causal and moderator variables, such as caffeine and alcohol intake, presleep activities, pain, and presleep worry, over several weeks (these might have been identified as potential causal variables during interviews). With such time-series data, it would be possible to examine the degree to which each hypothesized causal variable covaries with sleep-onset latency, to examine the time-lagged covariation among them (e.g., to examine the relative magnitude of the correlations between presleep worry and sleep-onset latency on the same night vs. sleep-onset latency and the subsequent nights presleep worry). It would also be possible to examine interaction and additive effects of the causal variables (e.g., perhaps presleep worry is aggravated when the client drinks too many diet colas just before bedtime).

Time-series regression analysis, conditional probability analysis, and Markov chain analysis can help estimate functional relations from time-series data. Time-series analysis, with multiple regression, can help estimate the degree of covariation between variables across time for a client while controlling for the effects of trend and autocorrelation in a set of measures across time.

Obtaining Specific Measures across Settings and Informants

The conditional nature and limited domain of causal relations suggests that the assessor should be aware of possible interaction effects. The strength of a causal relation can vary across settings, the state of the individual, or another source of variance. Consequently, assessment should involve measurement of causal relations in different settings and conditions and use of multiple sources of information. These assessment goals can often best be approached through multiple methods with multiple informants.

The conditional nature of causality reaffirms the emphasis on the use of highly specific measures in psychological assessment. Because of the conditional nature of causal relations, the assessor must carefully specify the response mode, the dimension of the behavior problem, and the environmental context. Is assessment attempting to account for the onset or duration of the problem, for behavioral or cognitive facets of the problem, and in which situation? In what context were the measures obtained?

Discordance among components of higher-level causal variables can impede the identification of clinically useful causal relations. Many assessment instruments (e.g., "life stressor" questionnaires, observed rates of "positive interactions" among family members, "autonomic lability" scores) give a summary "score" for a person on a higher-level causal variable that has multiple components. For example, Schmidt (1994) used the Schema Questionnaire and the Schema Avoidance Questionnaire, which measured constructs such as "disconnection," "overconnection," "emotional deprivation," "emotional inhibition," "vulnerability," and "enmeshment." These constructs are composed of so many lower-level components with undermined magnitudes of covariance that the role of more specific and clinically useful causal variables cannot be inferred. Consequently, the use of nonspecific causal constructs impairs our ability to identify clinically useful causal relations.

The assessment implications of a contextual and systems perspective are consistent with the emphases of the behavioral assessment paradigm on the use of specific, lower-level variables and on the use of validated multimethod assessment strategies. Assessment methods should be situation-specific. Interviews should ask about behavior problems and strengths in multiple situations; self-monitoring data should reflect the situations in which the data were obtained; questionnaires should contain situation-specific items; and analogue observation methods should involve systematic manipulation or control of situational factors. It is particularly important for the assessor to examine functional relations involving specific eliciting stimuli and the differential response contingencies that may be associated with different settings. Are there differences across situations in the contingencies for aggressive behavior, in the rate of positive interactions, in the performance demands, in reinforcement rate and quality?

Assessment Strategies that Are Sensitive to the Dynamic Qualities of Causal Relations

Psychological assessment strategies should be sensitive to the dynamic qualities of variables. Measures of change and of contrast in causal variables can sometimes be very helpful in accounting for variance in behavior problems. The estimated magnitude of variance accounted for in a behavior problem will be attenuated if dynamic dimensions of the causal variable and behavior problems are subjected to static measurement strategies, such as single-point or infrequent measurement (see Box 10-6).

A Note on Client Estimates of Functional Relations

It can be difficult to estimate the magnitude, recency, and slope of change of a causal variable in clinical assessment situations and to determine if those changes are functionally related to a behavior problem. We are often restricted to retrospective self-reports of change. However, causal relations are difficult for clients to validly report (Kleinmuntz, 1990). Several types of errors and biases can affect client reports of the causes of their behavior problems. Clients may overestimate or underestimate the relative importance of dispositional factors, clients may forget important causal events, their causal attributions of current behavior problems may be affected by recent experiences, causal attributions may be self-serving, magnitudes of covariation may be difficult to estimate, and it is often difficult for clients to make retrospective judgments about change. Some self-report methods, such as the *timeline followback procedures* (e.g., Sobell, Toneatto, & Sobell, 1994), may help avoid the biases associated with retrospective estimates.

Box 10-6
Times Series Measurement and the Dynamic Characteristics
of Measured Variables

The utility of time-series measurement and the best rate and duration of time sampling will depend on the rate of change of the measured variable. Time-series measurement may be useful with variables that are changing rapidly over time but less useful with variables that change slowly or irregularly. Time-series measurement can provide accurate information about the phase of a variable only to the degree that the sampling rate is sufficient to capture its time-course (see Suen & Ary, 1989, for a more detailed discussion of time sampling).

In many studies that have used time-series assessment methods, the sampling rate and the number of samples obtained have been determined more by convenience than by the characteristics of the measured variables. Many behavior problems and causal variables (e.g., headaches, mood, stressors) are sampled on a daily basis, which may not be sufficient to capture the phase state of the variable.

The Focus of Assessment

The focus of behavioral assessment is most often on functional relations, rather than confined to attributes of behavior problems. For most clients, an empirically informed, broadly focused preintervention assessment is necessary to identify causal variables and functional relations that are relevant for a client (see Box 10-7).

We have frequently noted the types of functional relations emphasized in the behavioral assessment paradigm: contemporaneous, behavior-environment interactions. Although the importance of proximal causal variables and functional relations is stressed, assessment should also attend to noncontiguous variables and extended social systems.

Because a causal variable can affect a behavior problem through multiple paths, it is also important to identify the mediators for causal action. An important question to be addressed in preintervention assessment is, "In what ways does this causal variable affect the behavior disorder?" The identification of causal paths and mediating variables is particularly important with unmodifiable causal variables. It may be possible to moderate the impact of a historical variable by identifying the mediators through which it currently affects the client's behavior problems.

The assessor should also attend to extended causal chains leading up to a behavior problem. As with our emphasis on extended social systems, it can be helpful to examine sources of variance in contiguous causal variables. Given that we often treat clients by changing causal variables, we must understand the factors that control contiguous causal variables before initiating intervention. To omit this important step increases the chance that we will develop incomplete functional analyses and ineffective interventions, or that intervention effects will not be maintained over time.

A Scholarly Approach to Clinical Judgments

Given the extensive research on the causal relations for many behavior problems, it is important that assessment methods and foci have a firm empirical foundation. Assessors should be assessment scholars—well versed in the empirical literature about the behavior problems of their client, possible causal variables and relations, and the methods of assessment. A scholarly approach helps the assessor address the most difficult-to-satisfy condition of causal inference— the reasonable exclusion of alternative explanations for covariance between two variables.

The experimental psychopathology and intervention literature is a rich source of hypoth-

---

Box 10-7
Observations of Functional Relations During Client-Assessor Interactions

In *Functional Analytic Psychotherapy*, Kohlenberg and Tsai (1991) suggested that ongoing observations of the interpersonal behaviors of the client, while interacting with the assessor/therapist, are a rich source of hypotheses about the antecedent and consequent factors that affect the client's behaviors. Kohlenberg and Tsai emphasized the identification of clinically relevant behaviors that occur in the natural environment, which can occur during client-assessor interactions (e.g., negative self-statements; the absence of self-expressive behaviors; insight into behavior chains).

eses about possible causal variables for a client's behavior problems. Once a client's behavior problems have been identified, the clinician often has a vast base of studies on possible causal variables. Knowledge of this literature is necessary for a scholarly approach to clinical assessment.

One source of nomothetic information is the literature about a client's psychiatric diagnosis. However, as indicated in Chapter 8, a diagnosis is insufficient for identifying causal relations for a particular client because it is often based on invalid assessment methods and can be imprecise and unreliable. Furthermore, diagnosis is based only on nomothetically based inferences about the form and assumed covariances among problem behaviors (symptoms). A diagnosis may suggest an array of possible causal variables for a client's behavior problems, but additional assessment data are necessary to identify those causal factors relevant for a particular client.

Because of the idiographic nature of causation, assessors should avoid biases and premature assumptions regarding the causal variables relevant to a particular client or a particular behavior problem. Also, because the identification of an important causal relation does not preclude other important causal relations and may be in error, the assessor should not suspend the search for causal relations when an important causal variable has been identified.

Summary

Causal models of behavior disorders are metajudgments involving hypotheses about which events may have causal functions for a particular behavior problem and the nature, strength, and boundaries of those causal relations. Assumptions about necessary conditions for inferring causation and hypotheses about the particular causes of a client's behavior problems affect decisions about the best assessment strategies, the content of the behavioral case formulation, and the intervention and psychopathology research strategies used with a client.

Some of the assumptions and characteristics of causal models in the behavioral assessment paradigm include: (a) multivariate causality, a behavior problem can be the result of different permutations of multiple causal variables; (b) a causal variable may affect a behavior problem through multiple paths and mediators; (c) multiple causal variables can affect a behavior problem through a shared causal mediator; (d) the particular causal factors affecting a behavior problem will often be different across clients with the same behavior problem; (e) causal variables that span a range of temporal relations are important, but a focus on contemporaneous variables often provides more clinically useful information; (f) historical causal variables are often important but unmodifiable, whereas their contemporaneous sequelae often can be modified; (g) causal variables can affect a behavior problem in an additive or interactive fashion; (h) most behavior problems are conditional in that the dimensions of a behavior problem will vary across contexts; (i) functional analyses often must address less noncontemporaneous causal variables, particularly those involving extended social systems; (j) the best degree of specificity will vary across assessment occasions, but causal models often err by including excessively high-level variables.

The behavioral assessment paradigm includes many classes of causal variables. The paradigm incorporates functional relations between behavior and response contingencies, the effects of pairings among environmental events, and the role of discriminative stimuli and contextual factors. Cognitive factors, psychophysiological and neurophysiological, and developmental and genetic variables have also been implicated as important causal variables. Many causal variables in the behavioral assessment paradigm involve multiple elements, such as temporal contiguity, and intrinsic or acquired reinforcer potential for a person. Persons differ in the degree to which a particular variable is reinforcing or aversive.

The behavioral assessment paradigm emphasizes the importance of environmental causality and behavior-environment interactions. The effects of environmental events on behavior depend on many interacting factors, such as schedules of contingencies, temporal parameters, and multiple arrays of stimulus and response pairings. An important element of this behavior-environment interaction model of causality is reciprocal causation—the idea that two variables can affect each other.

Behavioral causal models reflect the dynamic nature of behavior problems and functional relations. Nonlinear functions are also acknowledged. Sensitivity to initial conditions is one type of nonlinear causal relation. Other forms of nonlinear functions include sensitive periods, causal discontinuity, functional plateaus, critical (threshold) levels, parabolic (hyperbolic) functions, and log-linear functions.

The direction and strength of a causal relation can change across time. Changes in causal relations can be a result of repeated exposure to a causal variable (e.g., extinction, habituation, and sensitization), changes in moderating or mediating variables, unpredictable changes in the occurrence of causal variables, changes in contextual factors, or new causal relations triggered by another causal relation.

Causal effects can be a function of the dynamic and relative attributes of the causal variable, such as the degree and rate of change from prior to current values of a variable. The magnitude of change, the rate of change, and the recency of change have important implications for psychological assessment.

Causal models in a behavioral assessment paradigm have several implications for psychological assessment: (a) clients are considered active participants in problem identification and goal assessment and are encouraged to participate actively in the assessment-intervention process, (b) differences between "behavior problem" and a "causal variable" designations become less distinct, (c) a constructional focus on the client's behavioral skills and a task analysis is promoted, (d) analogue and naturalistic observation and self-monitoring are well suited for estimating contemporaneous functional relations, (e) the best assessment strategies will often involve the use of multiple informants, assessment in multiple settings, and attention to causal chains, (f) a comprehensive preintervention assessment is important, (g) psychiatric diagnosis is an insufficient basis for identifying causal relations, (h) assessors should avoid premature assumptions regarding the causal variables relevant to a particular client, (i) assessment should be ongoing, (k) it is important to identify mediators of causal action, (l) the identification of causal paths and mediating variables is particularly important when important causal variables are unmodifiable, and (m) psychological assessment strategies should be sensitive to the dynamic qualities of variables.

Suggested Readings

Behavioral Paradigms of Behavior and Behavior Problems

Donahoe, J. W., & Palmer, D. C. (1994). *Learning and complex behavior*. Boston: Allyn & Bacon.
Grant, L., & Evans, A. (1994). *Principles of behavior analysis*. New York: HarperCollins.
O'Donohue, W. (Ed.). (1998). *Learning and behavior therapy*. Boston: Allyn & Bacon.
Pierce, W. D., & Epling, W. F. (1999). *Behavior analysis and learning*. Upper Saddle River, NJ: Prentice-Hall.
Plaud & G. H. Eifert (Eds.). (1998). *From behavior theory to behavior therapy*. Boston: Allyn & Bacon.

Identifying Causal Relations in Clinical Assessment

Haynes, S. N., Spain, H., & Oliviera, J. (1993). Identifying causal relationships in clinical assessment. *Psychological Assessment, 5,* 281–291.

Models of Causality for Behavior Problems

Haynes, S. N. (1992). *Models of causality in psychopathology.* Boston: Allyn & Bacon.

Nonlinear and Dynamic Causal Relations

Haynes, S. N., Blaine, D., & Meyer, K. (1995). Dynamical models for psychological assessment: Phase-space functions. *Psychological Assessment, 7,* 17–24.
Vallacher, R., & Nowak A. (Eds.). (1994). *Dynamical systems in social psychology.* San Diego, CA: Academic Press.

Systems Perspectives for Behavior Problems

Mash, E. J., & Terdal, L. G. (1997). Assessment of child and family disturbance: A behavioral-systems approach. In E. J. Mash & L. G. Terdal (Eds.), *Assessment of childhood disorders* (3rd ed., pp. 3–68). New York: Guilford.

11

Psychometric Foundations of Behavioral Assessment

Introduction

Previous chapters emphasized that clinical judgments are influenced by the validity of data available to the assessor. This chapter examines principles of validation—how psychological assessment instruments can be evaluated on the degree to which they provide valid and useful information.

The evaluative processes applied to psychological assessment is called ***psychometry***, or ***psychometrics***. Psychometrics is concerned with the evaluation of data from assessment instruments and the judgments based on those data; it is the science of psychological measurement. Geisinger (1987) suggested that there are two divisions of psychometrics. The first division is ***psychometric theory***, which is concerned with mathematical models and principles that can be used to evaluate assessment instruments and data. The second division is ***applied psychometrics***, which is concerned with the applications of psychometric theory and principles to the evaluation of assessment instruments and data. This chapter deals with both divisions—psychometric principles and their application to behavioral assessment.

Although psychometric principles have been used for centuries (e.g., applied to "psychophysical measures" in the eighteenth century; McReynolds, 1986), modern psychometry has evolved primarily from early efforts to measure intelligence and personality traits (Anastasi & Urbina, 1997; McReynolds, 1986; Rust & Golombok, 1989). In these early applications, an emphasis was placed on validity and reliability to estimate the degree to which an assessment instrument provided a good measure of the construct it was intended to measure.

As the field evolved, psychometrics also focused on identifying and estimating the impact of sources of variance in the obtained measures, such as response biases and rater errors. Psychometry has guided the development, refinement, application, and interpretation of thousands of psychological assessment instruments.

Psychometrics addresses several important evaluative dimensions of psychological measurement and the clinical inferences that can be drawn from assessment data. The essential questions include: Are data from an assessment instrument valid measures of the targeted events and constructs? Are data from an assessment instrument relevant to, and representative of, the targeted events and constructs? Could data reflect some facets of the construct more than others, or could data reflect the influence of extraneous constructs or events? Are data and inferences from an assessment instrument generalizable across individuals, groups, time, assessors, settings, behaviors, and response modes? What are the sources of variance in data obtained from an assessment instrument? What are the methods of developing, evaluating, and refining an assessment instrument that are best for a particular application?

These questions focus on a supraordinate question that is central to clinical judgments—How confident can we be that data from an assessment instrument are appropriate for the clinical judgments we must make? Psychometric evaluations help us estimate the degree of confidence that can be placed in our data and in the clinical inferences influenced by those data. For example, do reports from a particular teacher or data from a particular observation instrument, provide an accurate estimate of the rate of aggressive behaviors of this child at school? Is the estimated rate of aggressive behaviors a valid estimate for this child in other classrooms, or at recess, or at home, or on other days in the same classroom? Would this child's other teachers or parents provide the same estimate? Did we define "aggressive behaviors" appropriately?

Our approach to psychometric principles and evaluations, and on the clinical judgment implications of psychometric evaluation, is consistent with that espoused by Messick (1991, 1993, 1995) and with a functional approach to psychological assessment. We presume that each psychometric evaluative dimension, such as temporal stability, is differentially useful for estimating the validity of obtained measures, depending on the goals of assessment, the assessment settings, the methods of assessment, the characteristics of the measured variable, and the inferences that are to be drawn from the obtained measures. We examine the conditional applicability of psychometric principles across instruments, purposes, settings, and variables.

We provide a framework for evaluating and constructing behavioral assessment instruments, for selecting the best assessment strategy, for interpreting published assessment data, and for drawing inferences from clinical assessment data. Although we define and discuss many psychometric concepts, we presume that the reader has a basic knowledge of psychometric principles, such as validity and reliability. There are many excellent books on psychometry (see Suggested Readings at the end of this chapter and the Glossary for definitions of terms used in this chapter.)

We emphasize several concepts about psychometry and behavioral assessment:

1. Psychometrics helps us estimate how confident we can be in drawing inferences from measures obtained in psychological assessment.
2. Measures are only estimates of an attribute and reflect both extraneous and relevant sources of variance.
3. Validation indices provide information about the construct validity of an obtained measure and about the clinical judgments based on that measure.
4. Validity coefficients are conditional. They can vary across populations, settings, foci, and goals and are not generalizable attributes of an assessment instrument.
5. Validity indices are not stable over time.
6. Behavioral assessment instruments, measures, and inferences are subject to multiple dimensions of psychometric evaluation.
7. The applicability of various psychometric dimensions depends on the degree to which a measure is considered a sign of a higher-order construct or a sample of the primary event of interest.
8. Idiographic measures decrease the importance of some dimensions of psychometric evaluation but increase the importance of accuracy and content validity.
9. Judgments about the consistency of behavior across situations and time, and the importance of temporal consistency estimates, are affected by the ways situations and behaviors are defined and measured.
10. Estimates of the stability of behavior or traits are influenced by the degree to which the measure is aggregated and the statistical methods that are used to estimate change.
11. The appropriateness of the elements of an aggregate is an element of its content validity.
12. Content validity and internal consistency are important considerations with aggregated measures.
13. Psychological assessment measures can be evaluated on dimensions of clinical utility, such as treatment validity, sensitivity to change, cost-effectiveness, and incremental validity.
14. Assessment data that have been shown to be reliable and valid in many ways may not be incrementally useful for treatment planning or evaluation.
15. Content validity, the degree to which elements of an assessment instrument are relevant to and representative of the targeted construct, for a particular assessment purpose is one of the most important psychometric evaluative dimensions in behavioral assessment.

16. Population sampling and expert review are two of the most important methods of increasing the content validity of a new assessment instrument.

Psychometrics and Measurement

In Chapter 5, we noted that measurement is the process of applying quantitative values to an attribute of a person, event, or construct. We emphasized that the validity of clinical judgments can often be increased if we acquire quantitative measures of important variables. Psychometrics helps us estimate how confident we can be in drawing inferences from these measures.

We also noted several important caveats in drawing clinical inferences from psychological assessment measures: (a) measures are only estimates of an attribute, (b) different estimates of an attribute will be obtained from different assessment instruments, (c) single measures seldom capture all aspects of an attribute, (d) the measurement process can have reactive effects, (d) not all important constructs lend themselves to quantification, (e) clinical judgments can also be aided by qualitative information, and (f) measures always reflect phenomena superfluous to the attribute being measured.[1]

Psychometrics addresses the correspondence between attributes and the obtained measures of attributes. Psychometrics provides multiple indices that can help the clinician decide to what degree measures reflect attributes of interest. In turn, more adequate judgments about a client or attribute can be rendered.

Psychometric evaluation of assessment data is a judgment based on the integration of multiple indices. As we discuss later, most aspects of psychometrics address the ***construct validity*** of a measure and the inferences and actions based on the measure. For example, inferences about the effects of treatment on a client's depressive behaviors, or inferences about the best treatment strategy for a depressed client, depend on how validly the depressive behaviors were measured. Similarly, inferences about the degree to which response-contingent attention affects self-injurious behavior of a client with developmental disabilities depends on how accurately attention, self-injurious behavior, and their functional relation were measured. Invalid measures of depressive behaviors can lead to erroneous functional analyses and erroneous inferences about treatment effects.

Dimensions of Psychometric Evaluation

There are multiple dimensions upon which measures and assessment instruments can be evaluated. These have been discussed in many books and we recommend several at the end of the chapter. Table 11-1 presents a brief overview of some psychometric dimensions that are particularly relevant to behavioral assessment methods.

The dimensions of validation outlined in Table 11-1 provide information about the multiple aspects of construct validity of an obtained measure and the validity of the clinical judgments based on that measure (Haynes, Richard, O'Brien, & Grant, 1999; Messick, 1995) (see Box 11-1). Construct validity of psychological assessment measures and associated inferences is important for: (a) selecting the best assessment instrument to use with a client or

---

[1]The inferences that can be drawn from measures, and the permissible methods of manipulating the obtained measures, are affected by the level of scales used. Nominal, ordinal, interval, ratio, and other scales are briefly described in the Glossary and in the readings recommended at the end of this chapter. As Sarle (1995) noted, the scale of measurement from an assessment instrument may not correspond precisely to any of these levels.

Box 11-1
What Is a Construct?

A "construct" is a created attribute or variable, usually higher-order, that is the target of measurement and is invoked to organize and account for data. Examples of constructs are intelligence, hitting, positive marital interaction, attention-deficit disorder, and negative outcome expectancy.

Constructs can differ in their level of specificity. Most are molar-level constructs such as "conscientiousness," "depression," "social skills," "stress," and "intelligence." Lower-level constructs, such as "interruptions" or "pushing/hitting/slapping," are less inferential.

Some authors have argued that molecular variables such as "hitting," or "heart-rate" are not constructs because they are not indirectly measured latent variables. Lower-level variables are often considered "samples" or "categories" of events. However, lower-level variables can also be synthesized and measured in different ways.

Regardless of their level of specificity, all targets of measurement are rationally defined attributes of people or events and can be considered "constructs." Consequently, principles of construct validation apply to all behavioral assessment measurements.

---

for research, (b) drawing inferences from research results, (c) drawing inferences from clinical assessment data, and (d) developing and validating an assessment instrument.

Construct validity is a metajudgment—a judgment that integrates multiple indices about the degree to which an obtained measure reflects the targeted attribute and the validity of judgments based on assessment data. For example, judgments of the construct validity of measures from a self-report questionnaire are based on an integration of (a) coefficients of covariance with other instruments that measure the same or similar constructs, (b) the degree to which the factor structure of a multielement instrument matches the factor structure expected for the construct, (c) qualitative and quantitative estimates of content representativeness and relevance (i.e., content validity), (d) the degree to which obtained measures are replicable or generalizable, (e) the internal consistency of the instrument, and (f) the degree to which the instrument reflects changes when hypothesized causal variables for the construct are manipulated.[2]

Validity indices can vary across methods of evaluation. For example, an assessment instrument with inadequate content validity (e.g., an observational system for marital communication that omits important nonverbal and paralinguistic behaviors such as shrugs, and sarcastic tones) can be valid in other ways. It could still accurately measure the observed verbal behaviors, exhibit excellent interobserver agreement, provide temporally and situationally stable measurements, and have excellent discriminative validity and internal consistency.

One of the more difficult dimensions to approach is *discriminant validity*—the degree to which measures from an assessment instrument reflect variance in the target but not other constructs. Discriminant validity is difficult to address because alternative explanations for score variance cannot be excluded. Furthermore, many constructs are imprecisely defined and overlap with others. Out of 328 manuscripts submitted to *Psychological Assessment* in 1998, 33% examined convergent validity while only 10% examined discriminant validity.

---

[2]Construct validation can have implications for the validity of the targeted construct (Smith & McCarthy, 1995), especially when multiple instruments that purport to measure the same construct are evaluated. Evidence about the validity of instruments designed to measure a construct provides evidence about the utility, domain, facets, boundaries, and predictive efficacy of the construct. Low indices of construct validity can indicate problems with the assessment instrument and problems with the construct.

Table 11-1

Dimensions of Psychometric Evaluation

Reliability: The part of a test result that is due to systematic effects and therefore persists from sample to sample, or the stability of measures obtained under constant conditions.

Homogeneity: The conceptual similarity of a set of assessment instrument (or scale) elements (e.g., questionnaire items, behavior codes).

Internal consistency: The degree of consistency among items or elements within an assessment instrument. Can be reflected by split-half reliability, Kuder-Richardson 20 formula, coefficient alpha (Kazdin, 1998).

Interobserver (interrater) agreement: The extent of agreement between scores (or ratings, diagnoses, behavior rates) obtained from different assessors evaluating the same events at the same time.

Temporal stability (test-retest reliability): The stability of obtained scores over a specified time; it can be reflected by correlations or degree of agreement between scores obtained at different points in time.

Validity: Close in meaning to "construct validity": An integrated evaluative judgment of the degree to which empirical evidence and theoretical rationales support the adequacy and appropriateness of inferences based on data acquired from an assessment instrument.

Accuracy: The extent to which obtained measures approximate the "true" state of nature.

Agreement: The degree of correspondence between the output of two or more assessment instruments. The degree of overlap between two more independently obtained measures.

Concurrent: Any index of validity obtained when different measures of the same construct are administered on the same assessment occasion.

Construct: Comprises the evidence and rationales supporting the trustworthiness of assessment instrument measures and inferences, in terms of explanatory concepts that account for both the obtained data and relations with other variables.

Content: The degree to which elements of an assessment instrument are relevant to and representative of the targeted construct, for a particular assessment purpose. The "relevance" of an assessment instrument is the degree to which its elements are appropriate for measuring the targeted construct, for a given assessment purpose. The "representativeness" of an assessment instrument is the degree to which its elements proportionately sample the facets of the targeted construct. It is important to specify the construct that the instrument is intended to tap and to match the content of the instrument to that construct.

Convergent: The degree to which data from an assessment instrument are coherently related to other measures of the same or similar constructs. The magnitude of covariance among scores from two assessment instruments that measure the same or similar constructs.

Criterion-referenced: (criterion-related validity; criterion validity) The degree to which measures from an assessment instrument correlate with scores from previously validated instruments that measure the construct of interest or with criterion of practical value.

Discriminant (divergent): The degree to which data from an assessment instrument are distinct from measures of dissimilar constructs.

Discriminative: The degree to which measures from an assessment instrument can differentiate individuals in groups, formed from independent criteria, known to vary on the measured construct.

Incremental: The incremental value of acquired data for clinical judgment. The degree to which additional assessment data increase the power, sensitivity, specificity, and predictive efficacy of judgments.

Postdictive: The degree to which scores from an assessment instrument correlate with scores from another validated assessment administered at a previous point in time, or the degree to which scores predict historical events.

Predictive: The degree to which measures from an assessment instrument correlate with measures from another validated assessment administered at a later point in time (the time frame of measurement is less important than the criterion in determining if validation is predictive).

Treatment: The degree to which data from an assessment instrument(s) contribute to enhanced treatment outcome.

Power and Sensitivity (of an assessment instrument): The predictive accuracy of measures from an assessment instrument. The overall proportion of persons accurately classfied on the basis of obtained measures.

Negative predictive power: The proportion of individuals indicated as not having a disorder or behavior who truly do not.

Positive predictive power: The proportion of individuals identified by an instrument as having a disorder or emitting a behavior who truly have the disorder or emit the behavior.

Sensitivity: The probability that a person with a particular attribute will be so identfied by a particular assessment instrument. The probability that a test will yield a positive result among persons with a disorder or attribute.

Table 11-1 (*Continued*)

Sensitivity to change: The degree to which measures reflect true changes in (the dynamic aspects of) the targeted variable.

Specificity: The probability that a person without a particular attribute will be so identified by a particular assessment instrument. The proportion of negative cases so identified by an assessment instrument.

Note: See Glossary for expanded definitions and supporting citations.
An alternative taxonomy of validation principles was proposed by Messick (1995; p. 745). He suggested that construct validation could be labeled as: (1) *content* (the relevance, representativeness and technical quality of an instrument and obtained measures), (2) *substantive* (the theoretical rationales for observed consistencies and their underlying mechanisms), (3) *structural* (assessment items and scoring that should reflect the internal structure of the construct), (4) *generalizability* (the degree to which measures and inference generalize across groups and settings), (5) *external* (similar to convergent and discriminant validity as in Table 11-1), and (6) *consequential* (the social and policy implications of inferences from measurements).

The construct validation process is susceptible to many sources of error. For example, patterns of covariance between an assessment instrument and convergent measures is affected by the degree to which obtained coefficients of covariance reflect common method variance (Meier, 1994). Strong correlations between two anxiety questionnaires can partially reflect the fact that both are self-report methods, both are paper-and-pencil questionnaires, and both use similar response formats (e.g., both have a four-point Likert scale). The correlation between two instruments can also reflect item contamination, in which two instruments share identical elements.

An influential strategy for construct validation has been the "multitrait-multimethod" approach outlined by Campbell and Fiske (1959). These authors and many others (e.g., Kenny & Kashy, 1992; Meier, 1994) have suggested that estimates of construct validity should be based on patterns of covariance with theoretically related constructs (convergent validation) and theoretically unrelated constructs (discriminant validation). High correlations among instruments that measure similar constructs provide strong evidence for construct validity, especially if measures are obtained from instruments that use different methods.

The Integrative, Conditional, and Dynamic Nature of Validation

Validity Is Estimated from Multiple Evaluations

Validity and reliability indices provide information about the construct validity of an obtained measure and of the clinical judgments based on that measure. The degree to which an obtained measure reflects the targeted attribute and the judgments that are permissible from those measurements are inferred from multiple indices of temporal stability, the representativeness and relevance of the items, predictive power, and other evaluative dimensions as outlined in Table 11-1.

Often, validation data provide an inconsistent portrait of construct validity. For example, scores from a self-report questionnaire of social anxiety may have correlated strongly with self-monitored ratings of daily social exchanges and discomfort while subscales showed low magnitudes of internal consistency or temporal stability.

Consistent with a functional approach to assessment, the degree to which each source of validity data contributes to judgments about the construct validity of the assessment instrument depends on the assessment method and the intended use of the assessment instrument. Given the divergent validity indices for this social anxiety questionnaire, the total score may be useful for initial screening at health clinics. However, because of low internal consistency and temporal stability, the subscale scores may not be valid measures of social anxiety in specific problematic situations, or valid measures of specific facets of social anxiety.

Validity Inferences Are Conditional

The magnitude of covariance among measures, which is the basis for most validity inferences, is affected by many conditions. Because of their conditionality, validity indices may not be generalizable across important sources of variance. Conditions associated with variance in validity coefficients and inferences are outlined in Table 11-2.

For example, we may be interested in the degree to which an analogue clinical observation system is a valid measure of social skills. The observation instrument could involve behavioral observations of the client while interacting with confederates in several situations. Does this instrument provide a valid measure of social skills? Can it be used as a preintervention assessment instrument with a client or for research on social skills? As is so often the case, it depends on the characteristics of the assessment occasion and on the inferences that are to be drawn.

The validity of this analogue assessment instrument can be estimated by examining the degree to which obtained measures correlate with measures from home or clinical observation of social interaction and other previously validated instruments (e.g., a self-report questionnaire measure of social anxiety, peer reports of social skills and anxiety, other analogue observation instruments). These correlations would provide indices of convergent or criterion-related validity.

However, the obtained validity indices are likely to vary across many dimensions. This analogue assessment instrument might be a valid measure for college students but not for persons randomly selected from the community, or for white but not for Chinese-American

Table 11-2
Conditions that Affect the Generalizability of Inferences
About the Construct Validity of an Assessment Instrument

Assessment Setting and Context: An assessment instrument may provide valid measures in outpatient but not inpatient environments, or when the client is alone but not in the presence of others. Valid measures may be obtained in some client states but not others (e.g., the validity of self-reports of substance use may vary according to the intoxication level of the client).

Facets, Dimensions, and Modes of a Variable: An instrument may provide valid measures of cognitive but not behavioral aspects of depression, or educational but not emotional facets of social support, of frequency but not duration of oppositional behavior.

Goals of Assessment/Clinical Judgments to be Made: An assessment instrument may provide valid measures for initial screening but not for a behavioral case formulation; for assessment of ultimate but not immediate treatment goals. An analogue observation instrument may provide a valid measure "skill" under high demand situations but not a valid measure of the client's typical performance in his or her daily life.

Measures Derived: An instrument may provide valid scale scores but not a valid total score; it may provide a valid index of conditional probabilities (e.g., response contingencies) but not of the rate of the events.

Population and Individual Differences: The validity of an instrument may vary across ethnicity, age, clinical status, and other factors.

Type of Validation: An instrument may demonstrate excellent discriminative validity and poor predictive validity and positive predictive power.

Note: Modified from table 2 in Haynes, Nelson, and Blaine (1998).

students, or for volunteer but not for court-referred clients. It may also provide valid measures of general social skills in treatment outcome evaluation, but provide less valid measures for preintervention identification of specific socials skills deficits of the client. It may also be valid for measuring behavioral skills of a client but not for measuring the client's typical behavior in naturally occurring social situations.

These examples reiterate a point made earlier in this chapter—validity coefficients are conditional; they are not generalizable attributes of an assessment instrument. An instrument is not "valid" or "invalid." The degree of validity of an instrument varies across many conditions, as outlined in Table 11-2. The assessor should consider and differentially weight the different sources of validity data when judging the applicability of an assessment instrument for an assessment occasion and when drawing clinical inferences from assessment data.

Suppose that we are considering whether to use an assessment instrument that has undergone multiple reliability and validity evaluations. The degree to which data from those validity evaluations are applicable to our assessment goals is constrained by the congruence between the characteristics of the original validation procedures and our assessment occasion. We must carefully consider the match between the conditions, populations, settings, target variables, and goals of our assessment occasion and those of the validation studies.

Most constructs have multiple facets. Consider the multiple facets of assertive skills (e.g., initiating conversations with strangers, asking for favors, refusing unreasonable requests, communicating needs) and post-traumatic stress disorders (e.g., intrusive images and thoughts, avoidance of trauma-related stimuli). An assessment instrument can provide a valid measure of some but not other facets of a construct. Additionally, aggregated scores from an assessment instrument may either over- or underrepresent facets of a construct.

When deciding whether to use an assessment instrument, the assessor should consider other aspects of the validation research: (a) the degree to which the characteristics of the samples and population used in the validation studies are similar to those of the client or current sample; the characteristics of validation samples are particularly important when clinical judgments are nomothetically based, such as when affected by norms; (b) the context and setting of the validation assessment (for example, the validity of observation measures of coercive parent-child interactions could vary as a function of whether they were obtained in the home or clinic), (c) the judgments that were validated (e.g., diagnosis vs. sensitivity to change); (d) the response mode and dimensions targeted by the assessment instrument; (e) validity inferences may be constrained by interactions among the conditions listed in Table 11-2; (f) an assessment instrument may provide valid measures for one population in one context but not for the same population in another context.

These considerations also guide the process for developing and validating a new assessment instrument. In the initial phase of development, the developer should specify: (a) the goals of the assessment instrument (the judgments that will be made from it), (b) the populations for which it will be used, (c) the facets, modes, and dimensions of the constructs to be measured, and (d) the setting and context in which it will be administered.

Social Consequences of Measures and Judgments

Messick (1995) stressed the adverse social consequences when assessors failed to consider the conditional nature of validity indices, obtained measures, and permissible judgments. Although he was concerned mainly with adverse social consequences of educational testing (e.g, intelligence testing of children with disabilities or social disadvantages), clinical assessment measures can also have adverse consequences for clients. Consider the potential negative consequences of data that suggest neuropsychological impairment for a psychiatric inpatient, a psychiatric diagnostic label applied to a school child, and personality testing of job applicants.

It is particularly important that psychological assessment measures and judgments not reflect unfair disadvantages of a person or group. Important decisions made from assessment instrument measures and influences from superfluous variables should be minimized. For example, if a school-readiness or grade-level placement test included items that covaried with race or ethnic experiences, some groups would be disadvantaged over others in terms of academic placement.

Validity Inferences Are Unstable

Validity indices are not stable over time. Assessment instruments are developed and evaluated in the context of contemporaneous ideas about the targeted construct. The definition of the measured construct and ideas about the domain and facets of a construct can evolve over time. Consider the evolution of ideas about PTSD, eating disorders, personality disorders, and cardiovascular disorders. Consequently, inferences about the validity of measures from an instrument are unstable and are likely to decrease over time. For example, a behavior observation instrument for "marital communication" developed in the 1960s would have diminished content validity 30 years later if the original observation instrument failed to include para-linguistic and nonverbal elements of dyadic communication that have more recently been shown to be important facets of communication efficacy and satisfaction (Floyd, Haynes, & Kelly, 1997; O'Leary, 1987; Weiss & Heyman, 1990). Similarly, a structured interview that was a valid diagnostic instrument for a disorder listed in DSM-III may be less valid for diagnosing the same disorder in DSM-IV if diagnostic criteria had changed.

Summary and Implications

In summary, the integrative, conditional, and dynamic nature of validity has several implications for selection and development of assessment instruments and for drawing inferences from obtained measures:

- Validation studies should be conducted and interpreted in a manner congruent with the intended application of the instrument in terms of samples, contexts, and clinical judgments.
- Validation indices may vary as a function of the assessment method used in the validation instruments, and validation should involve multiple methods, sources, and instruments.
- The applicability and utility of extant validity indices for an intended application of an assessment instrument depend on the degree to which the current assessment occasion matches the validation occasion on important sources of measurement variance.
- Estimates of the validity of an assessment instrument can vary as a function of many conditions and dimensions. Validity inferences are not necessarily generalizable across populations, settings, and assessment goals.
- Inferences involving revised constructs may be in error when drawn from unrevised assessment instruments.
- Assessment instruments should be applied and interpreted cautiously in conditions, for persons, or for judgments outside of their domain of validation.

- Congruent with a functional approach to assessment, assessment instruments should be selected and constructed congruent with the intended conditions of assessment.
- The validity of an assessment instrument can diminish across time, and past indices of validity may overestimate current validity.
- The construct validity of psychological assessment instruments should be periodically examined, and assessment instruments should be revised to reflect revisions in the targeted construct.

The Applicability of Psychometric Principles to Behavioral Assessment

The applicability of psychometric principles to behavioral assessment has been controversial (e.g., Cone, 1988, 1998; Silva, 1993). As we discussed previously, behavioral and nonbehavioral assessment paradigms differ on many dimensions, such as (a) the types of variables, units of analysis, and parameters measured, (b) methods of assessment, and (c) their underlying assumptions about the conditionality of behavior. There are also differences in the relevance of norms and idiographic assessment data in making clinical judgments. Furthermore, behavioral and nonbehavioral paradigms often differ in the level of aggregation. Measures from traditional nonbehavioral psychological assessment instruments more often use higher-level, aggregated, hypothetical, and latent-variable constructs, which are presumed to be more stable across situations. Given these differences in paradigms and the historical association between psychometry and traditional psychological assessment instruments, it has been reasonable to question the applicability of psychometric principles to the behavioral assessment paradigm.

Despite paradigm differences, psychometric principles have an important role in behavioral assessment. Measures obtained from behavioral assessment instruments can vary in their validity, accuracy, stability, generalizability, consistency, and meaning. Psychometry is a set of principles and tools to help understand the validity, usefulness, and sources of error in assessment data. Psychometric principles are indispensable guides to the clinical judgments that can be derived from behavioral assessment data. In this section we examine the applicability of psychometric principles to the behavioral assessment paradigm.

Level of Inference and Measures as Behavior Samples or Signs of Higher-Order Constructs

Validity and Accuracy Dimensions

Measures obtained from psychological assessment instruments vary in the degree to which they are considered a *sign* of a higher-order construct or a *sample* of the primary event of interest (Hartmann, 1982; Ollendick & Hersen, 1993a; Suen & Ary, 1989). The placement of a measure on the sign-sample dimension reflects the level of inference involved in interpreting obtained measures.[3]

For example, in psychophysiological assessment "heart rate" is rarely sampled as an independent measure of primary interest (e.g., when measuring heart rate responses to trauma

---

[3]This is similar to the issue of whether items on a questionnaire are considered effect or causal indicators of an underlying construct (latent trait). In some cases (e.g., a survey of traumatic life events) items would not be expected to covary highly. Consequently, indices such as internal consistency are not valid measures of the validity of the instrument/scale (see discussion in Fayers & Hand, 1997).

scenarios of persons with PTSD).[4] We are usually interested in heart rate because it serves as a sign of a higher-order construct, such as "cardiovascular stress response," or an even higher-order construct, such as "anxiety" (see reviews in Cacioppo & Tassinary, 1990).

However, a sample of heart rate measures can also be of primary interest. We may be interested in the effects of medication and cognitive-behavioral treatments on heart rate. In these cases we do not consider heart rate a sign of some higher-order construct, it is considered a sample of the phenomena of primary interest.

We can make similar sign-sample distinctions with behavioral observation measures. For example, we can record the rate of "critical comments" during a 10-minute analogue clinic observation session with a distressed married couple while they are talking about a problem in their relationship. "Critical comments" would be a primary event of interest if we considered this class of behaviors as a cause of the couple's problem-solving difficulty. Alternatively, we could consider "critical comments" as a sign of a higher-order construct, such as "marital distress," or "negative problem-solving strategies." In such cases, several behaviors might be aggregated to form a measure of "negative interactions."[5]

These examples lead to three principles. First, the sign vs. sample attributes of a measure fall on two related continua. The sign and sample attributes of a measure are neither discrete nor incompatible, and a measure can be described as high or low on both dimensions, depending on how the obtain measure will be interpreted. Consider self-monitored data on sleep-onset latency. It can be treated as an independent sample of an important phenomena (e.g., an important measure of outcome measure in a sleep or trauma treatment program) and, concurrently, it can be treated as a sign of "depression."[6]

Second, psychometric evaluative dimensions are important, regardless of where a measure falls on the sign and sample dimensions. Psychometric evaluation is necessary in order to know which inferences can be drawn from assessment data. With either a sign or a sample approach to measurement, it is important to estimate the degree to which data (a) accurately represent the targeted phenomena, (b) were affected by the measurement procedures and other sources of error (i.e., demonstrated reactive effects), and (c) were affected by and generated measures that were stable over time or situations.

Third, the applicability of each dimension of psychometric evaluation depends on where a measure falls on the sign and sample continua. For example, if "critical comments" during marital problem solving are measured as a sign of "distressed communication," two evaluative dimensions become paramount: (a) content validity—the degree to which the variable "critical comments" is relevant to, and representative of, the construct of "distressed communication," and (b) convergent validity—the degree to which measures of "critical comments" correlate with other signs (e.g., "interruptions," physiological arousal during problem-solving episodes, subjective reports of distress) of distressed communication. The importance of these evaluative dimensions is diminished, however, if "critical comments" is taken as a

---

[4]There are a number of cardiovascular disorders for which heart rate (or patterns, activity, rhythm) is a primary measure of interest (Andreassi, 1995).

[5]As we introduced in previous chapters, variables such as "marital distress," "paranoia," "extraversion," and "depression" can be considered *"latent" variables*. They are usually unobserved variables presumed to explain the relation between obtained measures. In latent variable modeling, an obtained measure, such as "critical comments," is presumed to be an imperfect index of the latent variable (see Loehlin, 1998, for an in-depth discussion).

[6]Some authors (e.g., Cone, 1998; Suen & Ary, 1989) have persuasively suggested that molecular variables such as "hitting," "interruptions," or "heart-rate" are not constructs because they are not markers of latent variables (they should be considered as samples or "categories" of events). Although they are highly specific and narrow, we consider them "constructs" because they can be synthesized and measured in different ways.

sample. If "critical comments" is considered a sample, we are more interested in accuracy, interobserver agreement, and temporal stability.

Idiographic Assessment Strategies: An Emphasis on Accuracy and Content Validity

As we discussed in Chapter 6, an idiographic approach to assessment decreases the importance of some, but increases the importance of other, dimensions of psychometric evaluation. With nomothetic approaches, when our clinical judgments are influenced by comparing measures with norms, we must consider the fit between the normative sample and our client. For example, inferences regarding a client's educational achievement, intellectual and cognitive abilities, and behavioral dispositions, measured from standardized questionnaires, can be affected by ethnic and cultural characteristics of the normative samples (Okazaki & Sue, 1995; Suzuki, Meller, & Ponterotto, 1996).

With idiographic assessment, such as goal-attainment scaling or criterion-related assessment, we noted that it is important that judgments be based on measures that are reliable, accurate, content valid, and appropriately scaled. The **accuracy** and content validity (see Glossary) of idiographic measures are particularly important (Cone, 1982, 1988; Suen, 1988).

Consider the psychometric issues involved in developing a strategy for measuring the positive social interactions of a shy client. First, there are many methods of measuring positive social interactions in the natural environment. We could interview the client and ask about the type, frequency, duration, and satisfaction and thoughts associated with social interactions. We could also ask the client to respond weekly to a brief questionnaire about social interactions since the previous session. A weekly questionnaire might also be used for the client to estimate the degree to which goals for social interaction were achieved that week. Alternatively, we could ask the client to self-monitor social interactions daily. Self-monitoring could be facilitated with a timer-watch to intermittently signal the client to write down contemporaneous or recent social activities.

We described six methods of measuring a shy client's social interactions. All methods were idiographic in that our clinical judgments about the client would not depend on normative comparisons, as would be the case if we used any of a number of social anxiety, distress, and avoidance questionnaires (e.g., Leary, 1991). However, several psychometric dimensions are relevant in evaluating these idiographic assessment methods: How accurately do the obtained measures estimate the client's social interactions in the natural environment? What are the sources of measurement error associated with each method? How sensitive are the obtained measures to the dynamic characteristics of the targeted phenomenon? Do the instruments adequately sample the domain of interest? If we obtain several measures of social interactions, how strongly do they covary? Confidence in our clinical judgments (e.g., Are the client's treatment goals being met?) based on the obtained data depends on the degree to which we can address these psychometric evaluative dimensions.

Person × Situation Interactions and Reliability Estimates

In Chapter 8, we noted that the degree to which persons behave consistently across situations and the factors affecting the degree of cross-situational consistency have been controversial topics. Judgments about the consistency of behavior across situations and time are affected by the ways that situations and behaviors are defined and measured. These estimates are particularly affected by the degree to which measures are aggregated.

We defined a "trait" or "disposition" as a behavior, or a set of co-occurring behaviors upon which people differ, that exhibit a meaningful (i.e., predictively useful) magnitude of temporal and/or situational stability. We also commented on the conditional nature of "traits" and the fact that traits differ in their level of specificity.

Estimates of the stability of behaviors or traits across time or situations are influenced by the degree to which a measure of them is aggregated and the statistical methods that are used to estimate change (Alder & Sher, 1994; Costa & McCrae, 1994). A composite, higher-order measure is less likely to demonstrate variation across situations and time because changes in any element have a proportionately small effect on the composite. Furthermore, changes in one direction in any element of the composite may be canceled out by changes in the other direction of other elements. The result can be stability of the aggregate measure even though the behaviors, attitudes, and emotions that constitute the aggregate change. Consistent with our functional approach to assessment, the assessor must determine if changes in the elements are sufficiently important to warrant individual measurement, or if an aggregated measure of the elements is important, or both.

Methods of statistical analysis also affect judgments of consistency. For example, test-retest analyses essentially evaluate relative ranking of scores on a measure across time. High correlations may be obtained if the mean level changes significantly across time or situations as long as the change is consistent across persons and their relative ranking is not substantially changed in the sample. The high correlations could be mistakenly construed as an index of consistency.

A person $\times$ situation interaction model suggests that we can best predict behavior by knowing something about the person (i.e., measuring a person's "traits") and also knowing something about the situation in which the behavior is occurring. However, the degree of person $\times$ situation interactions is also conditional—there are important differences in behavioral stability across persons, behaviors, situations, and measurement strategies. Some persons behave more consistently than others across some situations, depending on how behaviors are measured; some situations exert more powerful affects on behavior than do others; and some behaviors are more situationally stable than are other behaviors. The impact of these considerations for clinical assessment were discussed in Chapters 8 through 10.

The assumption that behavior can change across time and situations affects the meaning of reliability coefficients. Most important, instability of behavior across time or situations makes it difficult to separate variance associated with measurement error (or unmeasured variance) from variance associated with true changes in the measured behavior. Differences in measures of presumably stable variables acquired in close temporal proximity (e.g., differences in scores obtained on an IQ or an "ego strength" test obtained two weeks apart) can indicate the magnitude of error, or precision, of the measure because changes in the measured event or construct would not be expected to occur within that testing interval.[7]

When differences in obtained measures might reflect true changes in the target behavior, "true" and "error" variance cannot easily be partioned. Consider the difficulties in interpreting significant differences between observations of the social initiation behaviors of our shy client in two different role-playing scenarios, or, differences in the client's social behaviors in the same role-playing scenarios administered three weeks apart. On the former occasion, the

---

[7]In traditional psychometric theory, there are three sources of variance in obtained scores: (a) common variance (or true variance, due to variance in the targeted construct), (b) systematic error variance (or specific variance—reliable variance that is not due to variance in the targeted construct), and (c) random error variance (unreliable variance).

client emits five positive initiations, evidences low levels of heart rate increases during the initiations, and is rated as "very skilled" by observers. On the latter occasion the client emits only one positive initiation, shows large heart rate increases, and is rated as "very unskilled" by observers. Low test-retest agreements may reflect measurement error or true changes in the client's behavior. Regardless of source of variance, unreliable measures place limits on the inferences that can be made from them. In particular, judgments about the *generalizability* of measures across time or situations is diminished.

There is only one strategy to separate true from error variance in unreliable measures of presumably unstable events—*concurrent convergent validity assessment*. We must obtain two or more concurrent measures of the variable at the same time and setting. For example, we would have greater confidence that discrepant estimates of social initiation behaviors in two role-playing situations represented true differences in behavior between the situations if two independent observers evidenced a high level of agreement about those behaviors in both situations. High interobserver agreement reduces the chance that the observed differences were attributable to observer error.

Our attention is again drawn to the functional nature of behavioral assessment: The goals of an assessment occasion affect the implications of low reliability coefficients. If the assessor is interested in estimating the general disposition for (e.g., cross situation probability of) "delusional speech" by a psychiatric inpatient, and there is considerable variability in the behavior across situations (e.g., lunch time vs. recreation time), multiple situations must be sampled in order to derive a useful estimate. The probability of an valid estimate from a single sample varies directly with the degree of cross-situational stability of the measure. However, if the assessor is interested only in delusional speech in narrow situations, such as socially provocative situations with other patients, a low rate of agreement between socially provocative and socially neutral or positive situations is irrelevant to the clinical judgments. In the latter case, variability in delusional speech across time in the same socially provocative situations suggests the need for more samples in order to derive good estimates of the behavior.

Interobserver agreement provides estimates of reliability, observer accuracy, precision of a measure, and it indicates the degree to which the obtained measures reflect true variance. Measures of interobserver agreement indicate the degree to which data can be expected to be *generalizable* across observers. Inferences that variance in obtained observation data reflect true variance in behavior would also be strengthened if data from observers were in agreement with data from alternative methods, such as the client's or participant's observer reports of his or her social initiations.

Low levels of agreement among multiple measures of the same event suggest that one or more measures are invalid. If two "equivalent" instruments provide inconsistent measures we cannot presume that either measure is valid. If nonequivalent instruments provide inconsistent data (e.g., discrepancies among measures of a child's aggressive behavior from a teacher, from the child's self-report, and from a parent), there are two possible explanations: (a) one or more measures are invalid, or (b) one or more may be valid measures of different facets of the targeted construct. However, in either case the unsatisfactory validity indices indicate that acquired data must be interpreted with caution.

In the case of behaviors that can vary across time, their time-course must be considered when examining the temporal stability of a measure. The test-retest interval must be one in which significant changes would not be expected in the measured event. Therefore, test-retest reliabilities can be a useful index of validity only if the intervals selected are appropriate for the expected changes in the behavior across time.

Aggregated (Composite) Measures and Estimates of Temporal Stability and Internal Consistency

We noted that aggregated measures often provide a more stable estimate of a variable than that provided by the individual elements of the aggregate. Aggregated measures are most often used in the assessment of higher-order constructs that are presumably composed of multiple, functionally related facets. Multiple items are often necessary to capture all important facets of higher order constructs (e.g., consider a one-item question on PTSD). Aggregation can occur across time samples, questionnaire items, assessment situations, responses, and response modes. If we assume that the aggregate measure has been correctly constructed (e.g., that the elements are highly intercorrelated and relevant to the domain of the targeted construct), estimates of temporal and cross-situational consistency, predictive validity, and criterion-related validity are usually higher for aggregated than for nonaggregated measures.

For example, the agreement between spouse reports and external observer reports of marital interactions will usually be higher if the measures are based on aggregation across several hours rather than 15 seconds of observation (i.e., time-sample aggregation). The increased robustness associated with aggregation occurs because each element (in this case, individual 15-second time samples) is associated with idiosyncratic sources of measurement error that often cancel out when multiple elements are combined. Additionally, many behaviors are emitted in irregular patterns and short time samples are unlikely to result in generalizable measures.

Although aggregation can increase the reliability of estimates, it can hinder clinical judgments when it excessively reduces the specificity of assessment inferences and predictions. Aggregation can mask important sources of behavior variability and introduce new sources of inferential error. For example, the hyperactive behaviors of an elementary school-child may vary substantially from day to day and from hour to hour within days because of changes in classroom stimuli and learning environments (i.e., because of changes in causal variables). Aggregation of observation data across time or settings could reduce the ability to identify important sources of variance.

Aggregation across important sources of behavioral variance when that source of variance is relevant for clinical decision making is inconsistent with the functional approach of behavioral assessment. Because there are often clinically meaningful differences in behavior across time and situations, composite measures that involve temporal and situational aggregation can result in the erroneous inference that the behavior is stable and can diminish the clinical utility of the assessment data. In sum, the assessor must consider the goal of the assessment and whether use of an aggregated measure facilitates that goal.

Aggregation and Content Validity

The appropriateness of aggregation to the goals of the assessment occasion and the appropriateness of the elements of an aggregate are relevant to the *content validity* of the assessment strategy (Haynes, Richard, & Kubany, 1995). The content validity of the aggregated measure is the degree to which the aggregate or the dimension of aggregation (e.g., time samples, situations, questionnaire items) is relevant to and representative of the targeted construct. For example, content validity would be reduced if we formed a composite measure of classroom social activity of a child that included observed rates of academic activity and if we formed a composite self-monitor measure of panic-related thoughts that included elements of depressive mood. In these cases the aggregated measure would involve behaviors extraneous to the targeted construct.

Aggregation and Internal Consistency

Aggregation also increases the importance of ***internal consistency***. Internal consistency refers to the magnitude of covariance among elements of an instrument (or factor, subscale, other composite) that are intended to measure the same construct. For example, we presume that 10 items of a self-report "social anxiety" questionnaire should be strongly correlated if the items are summed to provide an estimate of the social anxiety construct. Low magnitudes of covariation suggest that some elements of the items may be poorly constructed or that they tap constructs other than social anxiety. Composite measures with low internal consistency among their elements can impair clinical judgment because the judgments would be based on measurement error and irrelevant sources of variance (see Box 11-2).

For many behavioral assessment instruments, covariance among elements is not presumed, aggregation to form a composite measure of a construct is not appropriate, and internal consistency is not a relevant psychometric evaluative dimension. Consider a sources of trauma scale (the Trauma Related Events Questionnaire; Kubany, 1999). This is a self-report questionnaire that asks respondents to indicate whether they have experienced any of a list of 23 traumatic events, such as rape, auto accidents, sexual abuse as a child, or the death of a loved one. There is no reason to expect self-reports of rape and auto accidents to covary, and elements are not aggregated to measure a higher-order construct. Therefore, indices of low internal consistency do not compromise the validity of the instrument.

Similarly, internal consistency is not usually an important evaluative dimension in time-sample observations, because the degree of correlation between samples is not an index of the validity of the observation system. Internal consistency is important only when obtained data

---

Box 11-2
Internal Consistency and Number of Elements in an Aggregate

The effect of increasing or decreasing the number of elements on estimates of internal consistency is estimated by the Spearman-Brown formula:

$$r_{nn} = \frac{nr_{tt}}{1 + (n - 1)r_{tt}}$$

r_{nn} = the estimated reliability coefficient (for an instrument with more or fewer elements)
r_{tt} = the obtained coefficient (e.g., coefficient alpha for the existing instrument)
n = the number of times the length of the aggregate is increased or decreased

However, the Spearman-Brown prophecy formula is valid only when the additional items tap the same construct.

The reliability of an element of an aggregate would be lower than the reliability of the aggregate because each element is associated with unique or random sources of variance. For example, individual time samples in observation data (e.g., 15-second samples of behavior) are likely be unreliable because they will reflect natural variability in behavior across time. The impact of each specific source of variance on overall estimates would be expected to diminish when multiple elements are combined.

Strategies for evaluating internal consistency include Cronbach's alpha, split-half reliability, average interitem correlation, Kuder-Richardson 20 formula, item-total correlations, and item-factor loadings.

are aggregated to form a composite measure of a higher-order construct (e.g., summing several behavior codes in marital interaction to estimate "positive dyadic exchanges").

Clinical Utility

Psychological assessment measures can be evaluated on dimensions of clinical utility, such as treatment validity, sensitivity to change, cost-effectiveness, and incremental validity. These dimensions are outlined in Table 11-3.

Treatment Validity and Utility

Behavioral assessment measures are often used to help clinicians design cognitive-behavioral intervention programs. The degree to which assessment strategies and measures contribute to treatment planning is **treatment validity**, or **treatment utility**. **Treatment sensitivity** (a special case of sensitivity to change) is the degree to which measures can be used to judge treatment effects.

As Hayes, Nelson, and Jarret (1987) and Silva (1993) noted, there are many aspects of treatment validity. In examining the treatment validity of clinical assessment data, the assessor is asking the questions: To what degree will this information contribute to the design of a more effective treatment program for the client? How likely is treatment outcome to be improved with the use of this assessment instrument and data?

Assessment data that have been shown to be reliable and valid in many ways may not be incrementally useful for treatment planning and evaluation. For example, measures of intellectual functioning may be valid but may not affect our decisions about how to treat an adolescent with substance abuse problems. In many treatment settings all participants receive a standardized set of assessment instruments that provide data unrelated to the treatment they will receive. As we discuss below, these assessment protocols often lack content validity for the goal of treatment planning. Consequently, they are not cost-efficient, in that the amount of useful information may not warrant the cost of assessment.

Like other types of validity, the treatment validity of an assessment instrument falls on a continuum. A measure, such as verbal IQ, may have some impact on the treatment of a child

Table 11-3
Dimensions and Concepts of Clinical Utility

Treatment utility/ validity	The degree to which data from an assessment instrument contribute to clinical case conceptualization, treatment outcome, or the measurement of treatment process and outcome.
Incremental utility/ validity	The degree to which data from an assessment instrument aid clinical judgment. The degree to which acquired assessment data increase the power, sensitivity, specificity, and predictive efficacy of judgments, beyond that associated with other assessment data.
Functional analysis utility	The degree to which data from an assessment instrument assist in the construction of a functional analysis for a client.
Sensitivity to change	The degree to which data from an assessment instrument reflect changes in the targeted construct.
Cost-effectiveness	The cost of deriving information with an assessment instrument relative to the contribution of that information to a clinical judgment.
User-friendliness	The ease with which an assessment instrument can be administered and data obtained and interpreted.
Power and sensitivity	See Table 11-1.

with self-injurious behaviors, but it probably has significantly less treatment validity than measures of the response contingencies maintaining those behaviors.

The treatment validity of assessment data often reflects the degree to which the obtained measures are relevant to the variables targeted in treatment. For example, treatment of self-injurious behaviors often involves manipulation of situations, task demands, and response contingencies. Assessment data specifically focused on these variables will have higher treatment validity than data based on general intellectual functioning, educational achievement, and neuropsychological functioning. Similarly, in the treatment of a rape survivor with PTSD symptoms, treatment may involve exposure to rape-related cues; modification of automatic thoughts, negative beliefs, and personal schema; use of anxiety reduction coping strategies; and education. Assessment data on these variables will have significantly higher treatment utility than data on general personality traits, intellectual functioning, and ego strength.

A number of issues relevant to treatment validation were discussed by Silva (1993). Inferences about the treatment validity of an assessment instrument are constrained by (a) other aspects of the instrument's validity (e.g., content and construct validity), (b) a lack of rigorous research demonstrating the differential efficacy of specific treatment programs; (c) insufficient research on the mechanisms responsible for treatment outcome; (d) the quality of measures used to evaluate treatment outcome; and (e) the fact that there are multiple indicators of treatment outcome and efficacy.

Incremental Validity and Utility

Construct validity is a necessary condition for the adoption of an assessment instrument for a particular assessment occasion (Foster & Cone, 1995). However, it is an insufficient criterion and the assessor should also consider the degree to which acquired assessment data increase the power, sensitivity, specificity, and predictive efficacy of judgments (see Table 11-3).

As noted in Haynes, Richard, and Kubany (1995), the decision about whether to use an assessment instrument should be based on several considerations of its incremental validity: Will measures from the assessment instrument capture the targeted construct more specifically and validly than those from other instruments? Will the obtained measures increase the validity of the behavioral case formulation? Will the obtained measures facilitate the measurement of the treatment process and outcome?

Incremental validity is related to the relative *cost-effectiveness* of an assessment instrument. Cost-effectiveness is the amount of useful information obtained from an assessment instrument, the degree to which it contributes information beyond that available from other instruments, and the cost of the incremental information.[8]

Content Validation in Behavioral Assessment

Concepts and Elements of Content Validity

One of the most important psychometric evaluative dimensions for behavioral assessment is content validity—the degree to which elements of an assessment instrument are relevant to,

---

[8]Judgments about the clinical significance of treatment effects can be aided with the use of multiple outcome measures, statistical criteria, and decision-making algorithms (see review in Kazdin, 1998; Ogles, Lambert, & Masters, 1996). Judgments of clinical significance of treatment effects can be guided by the use of effect size estimates, norms and standard deviations of outcome measures of persons with and without a behavior problem or disorder, the identification of socially important impacts of treatment (e.g., social validity), and multiple sources of outcome data.

and representative of, the targeted construct for a particular assessment purpose. Content validity is important in behavioral assessment because obtained measures are most often considered as behavior or event samples, rather than as signs of higher-order constructs. It is thus important to estimate the degree to which a measure adequately samples the targeted construct.

Content validation includes all aspects of the assessment process and associated clinical judgments (Haynes, Richard, & Kubany, 1995). For example, content validation of a behavioral observation system requires consideration of the definitions of codes, instructions to participants, time-sampling parameters, and the situations and scenarios in which observation occurs, and the method of data reduction analysis. More broadly, content validation applies to the following elements of an assessment instrument and strategy:

- The *definition and domain* of the measured construct
- The *criterion or goal* against which obtained measures are compared
- The *array of items/behaviors* selected or sampled by an assessment instrument
- The *specificity of items*
- *Format* of obtained measures (e.g., response scale on questionnaire; dimension, such as frequency, duration) in observation system
- The *situations sampled*
- The *order or sequence* of items and other stimuli
- The *instructions to participants*
- The *temporal parameters* of responses (e.g., the interval of interest, such as "today" or "in the past week" when reporting on sleep patterns)
- The *components* of an aggregate/factor/response class (the degree to which the components sample the domain of interest)
- The *method of administration or presentation*
- The *scoring and data reduction*
- The *time-sampling parameters* (e.g., whether a client self-monitors mood daily or four times per day)
- *Assessment method-response mode match* (e.g., is participant observation the best method of measuring "internal" events such as mood?)
- *Assessment goal-instrument/method match* (e.g., given that there are multiple instruments and methods for measuring social anxiety and performance, which is the best, given that the purpose of the assessment is to assist in the behavioral case formulation of a client)
- The *array of assessment instruments* selected for an overall assessment strategy; the instruments that compose an assessment battery.

The content validity of an assessment instrument is conditional. An instrument may have satisfactory content validity for one assessment application but not for another. For example, an analogue assessment instrument for measuring social skills may have satisfactory content validity for treatment outcome evaluation but not for behavioral case formulation.

Methods of Initial Instrument Development and Content Validation

There are many ways to err in the development of an assessment instrument. One of the most common is to include elements that tap constructs outside the domain of the targeted construct (i.e., the inclusion of irrelevant elements). Another common error is the failure to measure all relevant facets of a multifaceted construct, or to measure them disproportionately (i.e., the elements are unrepresentative of the targeted construct). "Proportionate" sampling refers to the degree to which variance in aggregate measures of a construct is affected by the facets of a construct (e.g., using 3 mood items and 10 cognitive items to form an aggregated measure of depression would be disproportionate unless the construct of depression was so defined).

DeVellis (1991) and Haynes, Richard, and Kubany (1995) discussed methods of assessment instrument development to strengthen and evaluate its content validity. Although content validation has been applied primarily in the construction of self-report questionnaires, it is particularly important for naturalistic and analogue observation and self-monitoring. It is important to reiterate that all elements of a behavioral assessment instrument that can affect obtained data and the clinical inferences that can be drawn from data are subject to content validation. For behavioral assessment instruments, these include elements such as instructions to participants during role play and psychophysiological assessment, the audiotaped and videotaped scenes presented during analogue assessments, the behavior codes used in analogue and naturalistic observation, and response formats on participant report instruments.

Table 11-4 outlines methods of content validation that promote the development of assessment instruments that include relevant and representative measures of the targeted

Table 11-4

The Content Validation Process: Guidelines for Determining and Evaluating
the Elements of an Assessment Instrument During Its Initial Instrument Development

---

1. *Specify the construct(s)* to be measured
   A. Specify the domain of the construct (the boundaries of the construct; what is to be included and excluded)
   B. Specify the facets, dimensions, response modes of the construct
2. Specify the *contexts* (settings, situations) for the measures
3. Specify the *intended functions* of the instrument
4. Select *items* (e.g., questionnaire items, individual behavior codes) congruent with decisions in 1–3 above. Use a table of facets of construct multiple items for each facet (DeVellis, 1991). Methods of item generation include:
   A. Rational deduction
   B. From clinical experience
   C. From theories relevant to construct
   D. From empirical literature relevant to construct
   E. From other assessment instruments
   F. From suggestions by experts
   G. Population sampling: generate items from suggestions by target population
5. *Match all other elements to facets, dimensions, response modes, goals*
6. Examine each item for *construction* (grammar, reading level, form)
7. Establish *quantitative parameters* of instrument (e.g., response formats, scales, time-sampling parameters)
8. Develop specific and relevant *instructions* to participants
9. Have multiple *experts review* all elements of assessment instrument (1–8 above). The review can include quantitative ratings (e.g., five-point scale) of the precision, relevance, and representativeness of elements as well as qualitative evaluations.
10. *Population review*: In some cases, it is helpful to have elements reviewed by persons from the targeted population.
11. *Refine elements* on the basis of 9 and 10, and repeat process.
12. *Pilot test* the instrument and gather quantitative and qualitative data on each element of the instrument.
13. Proceed with additional psychometric evaluation.

Note: Adapted from Haynes, Richard, and Kabany (1995). The applicability of these strategies will vary across assessment methods.

construct. As illustrated, content validation involves a careful sequence of multiple quantitative and qualitative methods. The purpose of content validation is to minimize potential error variance associated with an assessment instrument and increase the probability of obtaining supportive construct validity indices in later studies. Consequently, content validation begins early in the development of an assessment instrument. The exact methods of content validation will vary across assessment methods and instruments because sources of content invalidity vary with the targeted construct, the method of assessment, and the function of assessment.

Most developers use a rational and clinical-experience–based approach to construct elements of a clinical assessment instrument, determining elements on the basis of theoretical considerations, their experience with clients, and relevant published research. Less frequently used but very important methods are ***population sampling*** and ***expert review***. The chance that the instrument captures important facets of the domain can be increased by using carefully structured, open-ended interviews with persons from the targeted population and experts in the domain of the assessment instruments. For example, in the development of an analogue observation method for assessing the verbal and psychophysiological responses of male batterers to high-risk situations, interviews with batterers and professionals who work with battering men about situations that are especially provocative for this population could help ensure that the best scenarios are included.

Summary

Psychometrics is the quantitative and qualitative evaluation of data and inferences from assessment instruments. It is the science of psychological measurement and has an important role in the behavioral assessment paradigm. Psychometry helps us decide how confident we can be that data from an assessment instrument are appropriate for the clinical judgments we must make.

Psychometry relies on measurement. We apply numbers to an attribute of a person or an event to permit us to draw inferences about the attribute. Measurement allows us to estimate how much an attribute changes over time, how a person stands relative to other persons on that attribute, and the relation between different attributes.

There are many dimensions of psychometric evaluation. All are relevant to the construct validation of an assessment instrument. These dimensions include concurrent, construct, content, convergent, discriminant, discriminative, predictive, postdictive, and criterion-referenced validity; accuracy, temporal stability, and internal consistency; power and sensitivity/specificity.

Validity is not a generalizable attribute of an assessment instrument. The applicability of validation data to an assessment occasion are constrained by the congruence between the characteristics of the original validation and the assessment occasion. The construct, facets measured, samples, populations, contexts, and goals of assessment are some of the factors that affect the relevance of validation data.

Validity is an unstable characteristic of measures and past indices of validity for an assessment instrument that may not pertain to current conditions. The validity of psychological assessment instruments should be periodically revised to reflect revisions in the targeted construct.

It is important that behavioral assessment instruments, measures, and inferences be subject to psychometric evaluation. Measures obtained from behavioral assessment instruments can vary in their validity, accuracy, stability, generalizability, and meaning. Evaluative psychometric dimensions are indispensable guides to the clinical inferences that can be drawn from behavioral assessment data.

Idiographic assessment strategies affect the relevance of the various dimensions of psychometric evaluation. Regardless of the idiographic/nomothetic attributes of an assessment instrument, judgments should be based on valid measures. The accuracy and content validity of the measures obtained from idiographic instruments are particularly important.

Estimates of stability across time or situations are influenced by the degree to which a measure is aggregated and the statistical methods that are used for estimating change. A composite, molar-level measure is less likely to demonstrate changes across situations and time because changes in any element have a proportionately smaller effect on the composite. The assumption that behavior can change across time and situations renders more difficult the separation of variance associated with measurement error from variance associated with true changes in the measured behavior. True and error variance in measures of unstable events can be separated through concurrent validity assessment.

Aggregation can also hinder clinical judgments when it reduces the specificity of assessment inferences. The appropriateness of aggregation to the goals of the assessment is an element of the content validity of the assessment strategy. Aggregation also increases the importance of indices of internal consistency but for many behavioral assessment instruments covariance among elements is not presumed.

Content validity acquires special importance in behavioral assessment because obtained measures are most often considered as behavior samples rather than signs of higher-order constructs. The "elements" of an assessment instrument and strategy amenable to content validation include all attributes of the assessment instrument and process that can affect the obtained data and associated clinical judgments. Many methods are helpful in content validation; expert and population sampling review are among the most important.

Suggested Readings

General Psychometric Principles and Concepts

Anastasi, A. & Urbina, S. (1997). *Psychological testing* (7th ed.). Englewood Cliffs, NJ: Prentice-Hall.

Haynes, S. N., Nelson, K., & Blaine, D. C. (1998). Psychometric foundations of assessment research. In J. N. Butcher, G. N. Holmbeck, & P. C. Kendall, *Handbook of research methods in clinical psychology*. Boston: Allyn & Bacon.

Linn, R. L. (Ed.). (1993). *Educational measurement* (3rd ed.). Phoenix, AZ: The Oryx Press.

Messick, S. (1995). Validity of psychological assessment: Validation of inferences from persons' responses and performances as scientific inquiry into score meaning. *American Psychologist, 50*, 741–749.

Nunnally, J. C., & Bernstein, I. H. (1994). *Psychometric theory*. New York: McGraw-Hill.

Psychological Assessment. Special Issue: Methodological Issues in Psychological Assessment Research, 7(3) (1995): 227–241.

Wainer, H., & Braun, H. I. (Eds.). (1988). *Test validity*. Hillsdale, NJ: Lawrence Erlbaum Associates.

Psychometrics in Behavioral Assessment

Cone, J. D. (1998). Psychometric considerations: Concepts, contents, and methods. In A. S. Bellack & M. Hersen (Eds.), *Behavioral Assessment: A practical handbook* (4th ed.). Boston: Allyn & Bacon.

Haynes, S. N., & Waialae, K. (1994). Psychometric foundations of behavioral assessment. In R. Fernández-Ballestros (Ed.), *Evaluacion conductual hoy: Behavioral assessment today*. Madrid: Ediciones Piramide.

Silva, F. (1993). *Psychometric foundations and behavioral assessment*. Newbury Park, CA: Sage.

Suen, H. K., & Ary, D. (1989). *Analyzing quantitative observation data*. Hillsdale, NJ: Lawrence Erlbaum Associates.

Tomarken, A. J. (1995). A psychometric perspective on psychophysiological measures. *Psychological Assessment, 7,* 387–395.

Interesting Reading on Measurement

Darton, M., & Clark, J. (1994). *The Macmillan dictionary of measurement*. New York: Macmillan.

III

Observation and Inference

12

Principles and Strategies
of Behavioral Observation

Introduction

Behavioral observation is the systematic recording of behavior by an external observer. The systematic nature of behavioral observation is characterized by carefully detailed procedures that are designed to collect reliable and valid data on client behavior and the factors that control it (Barrios, 1993; Tryon, 1998). For example, nursing staff in a hospital setting might record the number of times that a patient yells or acts aggressively so that the effects of a behavioral management program can be evaluated. Similarly, a clinician may request that the parents of a child with enuresis record the time, date, and location of incontinent occurrences so that the timing of prompts and bathroom trips can more effectively be arranged in an intervention. Finally, observers may be stationed in a classroom to record the extent to which a child with behavioral problems exhibits on-task and off-task behaviors.

Behavioral observation can be aided by automated recording where specialized instruments are used to record facets and dimensions of behavior that produce measurable changes in photic, mechanical, thermal, electrochemical, and electromagnetic energy. For example, a clinician may choose to record reaction time as an index of attention arousal for a client with traumatic brain injury. In order to accomplish this, the clinician could use a computerized measurement device that detects the amount of time that occurs between the onset of a stimulus presentation and a button press by the client.

The use of systematic observation methods as a means for measuring behavior and functional relations is firmly rooted in empiricism, where minimally inferential measurement procedures and quantitative evaluation of event sequences are posited to be the best strategy for learning about cause-effect relations. Behavior modification, behavior therapy, and behavioral assessment methods emerged out of the empirical tradition. Consequently, behavioral observation has often been cited as the hallmark of a behavioral approach to assessment (cf., Foster, Bell-Dolan, & Burge, 1988; Haynes, 1978; Suen & Ary, 1989).

As basic and applied science in behavioral psychology evolved, so too have behavioral observation methods. Currently, behavioral observation is one of the most frequently used, and extensively evaluated, methods of behavioral assessment for children, families, and adults (Hops, Davis, & Longoria, 1995). For example, Elliot, Miltenberger, Kaster-Bundgaard, and Lumley (1996) conducted a survey in which they evaluated the assessment and therapy practices among practitioners (operationally defined as doctoral level psychologists who spent 50% or more of their worktime in clinical practice) and academics (operationally defined as doctoral level psychologists who spent 50% or more of their worktime in research and/or teaching) who were members of the Association for the Advancement of Behavior Therapy. The results of their survey indicated that 76.5% of the practitioners and 82.1% of the academics reported that they used behavioral observation methods in their clinical work. Additionally, these same respondents reported that they respectively used behavioral observation methods for 52.3% and 51.9% of their clients. When these data are compared against survey data collected 18 years earlier (Swan & MacDonald, 1978), the use of behavioral observation appears to have slightly increased. Behavioral observation has also been extensively used in the published treatment outcome literature. For example, our review of treatment outcomes research published in the *Journal of Consulting and Clinical Psychology* (*JCCP*) in 1968, 1972, 1976, 1980, 1984, 1988, 1992, and 1996 (also described in Chapter 2) indicated that behavioral observation methods were used to assess behavior in 31% of the 194 studies (see Table 12-1). No clear temporal trends were apparent in these data, although the years 1996 and 1984 represented atypically low percentages (7% and 16% respectively) while the year 1968 was an atypically high percentage (56%).

Table 12-1
Percentage of Treatment Outcome Studies
Published in the *Journal of Consulting and Clinical Psychology*
that Used Behavioral Obervation Methods

Year	Number of Treatment Outcome Studies	% Used Behavioral Observation
1968	9	56
1972	23	35
1976	34	44
1980	21	33
1984	37	16
1988	21	24
1992	21	33
1996	28	7

In an additional review of the literature, we surveyed single subject treatment studies covering the first six months of 1998 in the leading behavioral journals (*Behavior Modification, Behavior Research and Therapy, Behavior Therapy, Journal of Applied Behavior Analysis, Journal of Behavior Therapy and Experimental Psychiatry*). Each article was coded according to client age group, presenting problems targeted for assessment and treatment, and assessment methods used to evaluate behavior. Results indicated that behavioral observation was used in 56% of these treatment outcome studies.

Taken together, the aforementioned surveys and reviews of the literature indicate that behavioral observation is commonly used in clinical settings, single subject designs, and treatment outcome studies. The difference in frequency of reported use between *JCCP* and the behavioral journals supports the argument that behavioral observation is more strongly associated with the behavioral assessment paradigm. It may also reflect the possibility that behavioral journals tended to conduct assessments on a higher percentage of children and persons with developmental disabilities who are less able to participate in interviews, questionnaire, and self-monitoring methods.

In this chapter, a primary goal is to provide readers with essential information about the principles, diversity, and utility of behavioral observation methods in clinical settings. We also aim to communicate details about the advantages and disadvantages of various observational strategies, and about the techniques that can be used to evaluate observational data. To accomplish these goals, we first review the assumptions that underlie behavioral observation and describe the common and differentiating elements of behavioral observation strategies. We then review techniques that can be used to collect and evaluate observational data. Finally, we examine psychometric issues that are relevant to behavioral observation.

Caveats

Highly sophisticated observation strategies and quantitative techniques (e.g., marital interaction coding systems) have been described and reviewed in the behavioral assessment literature (e.g., Heyman, Weiss, & Eddy, 1995; Quera, 1990). While these techniques are critical in research applications that require observational measures (e.g., parent-child interaction research, marital interaction research, group process interaction research), they require extensive resources (e.g., trained coders, elaborate coding, and reliability analyses systems) and are time consuming. It is not surprising then, that highly sophisticated observation systems are very rarely used in clinical settings.

This book is designed to provide guidance on behavioral assessment principles that are most relevant to the design of the functional analysis, which in turn, guides treatment design for an individual client. Consequently, our coverage of behavioral observation will emphasize conceptual issues, data collection strategies, and data analysis techniques that are most relevant for the design and evaluation of interventions in clinical settings. Detailed presentation of conceptual issues, data collection techniques, and data analysis methods that are more relevant for research applications of behavioral observation can be found in Gottman (1995) and Suen and Ary (1989).

We stress several principles and strategies of behavioral observation:

1. The systematic recording of behavior can yield valid information that is useful for the goals of behavioral assessment.
2. The definition of behavior codes is an important element in the validity of the observation instrument.
3. Operationalization and quantification of behavior and causal variables can guide diagnostic judgments, normative comparisons, judgments of social significance, and the identification of functional relations.
4. Decisions about the operationalization and quantification of variables are affected by training and experience, published literature, and preliminary assessment data on the client.
5. An important element of behavioral assessment is a strategy for behavior sampling, time sampling, and situation sampling that partitions ongoing behavior, time, and/or settings into discrete categories.
6. Naturalistic observation permits evaluation of naturally occurring functional relations, but can be cost-inefficient.
7. Analogue observation, particularly functional analytic experimentation, permits the clinician to test and evaluate casual relations.
8. Observation methods are used across a diverse set of populations, behaviors and events, and settings.
9. There are three classes of instruments for behavioral observation: written forms, audiovisual recordings, and computerized data entry instruments.
10. There are two approaches to data evaluation: intuitive judgement and statistical testing.
11. Interobserver agreement is an important psychometric dimension of behavioral observation.

Assumptions in Behavioral Observation Strategies

Behavioral observation strategies are founded on the assumption that the systematic recording of carefully defined, quantifiable, and publicly accessible behaviors will yield information that has maximal utility for the goals of behavioral assessment including the most important goal which is the functional analysis. In turn, this assumption is primarily based on the position that direct observation of behavior requires less inference, and as a result, is less prone to error.

There are several additional arguments that have been forwarded in support of the assumption that observation yields valid and useful information. First, it has been argued that the link between the observed behavior and treatment selection is more easily made when observational measures are used. Second, it has been argued that observational measures more readily permit evaluation of behavioral sequences and interactions between environmental events (e.g., antecedents and consequences) and target behaviors. Third, observation methods can be designed to be highly specific and sensitive measures of behaviors and contingencies for a specific client (Hops, Davis, & Longoria, 1995). Fourth, the quantitative data obtained from observation methods can be more readily analyzed for the purposes of testing hypotheses about the function of client behaviors. Fifth, evaluation of public events makes it possible to empirically evaluate the reliability and validity of coding systems and observational measures. Finally, observational methods permit the clinician to evaluate behavior in context.

These assertions about the utility of observation methods have not gone unchallenged. In particular, arguments have been advanced that observation methods carry unique sources of error (e.g., reactivity, observer bias, sampling error) that affect the validity of observations (cf., Barrios, 1993; Mann, Ten Have, Plunkett, & Meisels, 1991; Tryon, 1998). Further, it has been argued that some observation methods do, in fact, require substantial inference when an observed behavior is interpreted as an index of a higher order variable or construct (cf., Greenberg, 1995; Jacobson, 1985).

Common Functions of Behavioral Observation

Operationalizing and Quantifying Target Behaviors

The goals of all behavioral observation strategies are to measure behavior and identify functional relations. To realize these goals, the behavior clinician must first construct operational definitions of critical target behaviors. These operational definitions must be designed so that they capture and classify the most relevant and essential characteristics of the targeted behaviors. Definitions must be developed that maximize the content and construct validity, and reduce measurement errors, of the observation instrument (Bramlett & Barnett, 1993; Foster, Bell-Dolan, & Burge, 1988; Krejbeil & Lewis, 1994; Smith & McCarthy, 1995). Subsequent to target behavior operationalization, the clinician must construct operational definitions of causal variables that are hypothesized to exert nontrivial effects on the target behaviors. Again, the operationalization of these putative causal variables requires that the clinician carefully consider the validity of the operational definitions.

Because there are an infinite number of ways that target behaviors can be operationalized, simplification strategies are needed. One simplification strategy is to sort target behaviors into three main modes (the assets and limitations of various mode categorization strategies were discussed in Chapter 8): verbal-cognitive behaviors, physiological-affective behaviors, and overt-motor (nonverbal) behaviors (Hollandsworth, 1986).

Because observational methods are restricted to the codification of publicly accessible responses, the verbal-cognitive and affective/physiological modes of responding must be operationalized in a manner that permits direct observation and quantification. For example, an affective-physiological response such as "anxiety" could be operationalized as motor trembling, rapid breathing, facial flushing, or pacing. Similarly, a verbal-cognitive response such as hopelessness could be operationalized as verbal statements that the future is bleak and uncertain. Although the three modes of responding can be evaluated along many different dimensions, most behavioral observation strategies in clinical settings emphasize the measurement of frequency, intensity, duration, and/or latency of responding (see Chapter 8 for further discussion of response dimensions).

As an example, in behavioral medicine settings, we often receive consultation requests from staff members who report that an inpatient appears to be "manipulative." Under these circumstances we first operationally define what constitutes "manipulative" behavior. Using the aforementioned simplification strategy of trichotomizing behavior into modes, we typically seek to articulate specific verbal-cognitive responses (e.g., complaints to staff members about quality of care, verbal reports of feeling helpless), physiological-affective responses (e.g., anxious arousal, tearfulness), and overt-motor responses (e.g., use of the call light, requests for specialized meals or caregiving routines) that are identified by staff as representing "manipulative" behaviors. Following operationalization of the problem behavior, we will then determine which dimensions of responding (i.e., frequency, intensity, duration, latency) are most relevant to the assessment question.

Operationalization and quantification of behavior serves very important purposes in behavioral observation:

- *They can help the clinician to establish a diagnosis.* While the advantages and disadvantages of using diagnostic language in behavioral assessment have been argued extensively in many articles, it is important to note that the consolidation of multiple behaviors into a single diagnostic category promotes enhanced communication about a behavior problem and simultaneously permits the clinician to access research literature on causation, assessment, and/or treatment.
- *They allow the clinician to make normative comparisons.* Specifically, the clinician can evaluate the client's behavior in terms of published normative data and/or make comparisons with other persons in the client's cohort.
- *They allow the clinician to establish social significance or personal importance of the behavior problem.*
- *They allow the clinician to establish the presence of potential functional response classes or behaviors that appear to covary in particular contexts.*
- Most importantly, *operationalization can help the clinician and client clarify their thinking about problem behaviors.* Such careful consideration of behavior content and the construct(s) that the behavior represents can correct what might otherwise be an oversimplified, biased, and nonscientific description of the behavior problem.

Generating Operational Definitions of Causal Variables and Relations

Once the target behaviors are adequately described in terms of modes and dimensions, we are in a position to define operationally potential causal factors. Causal factors, like behavior, can be described in an infinite number of ways. Thus, simplification strategies are also needed for their operationalization. At a basic level, controlling factors can be divided into social/interpersonal events and nonsocial/environmental events (O'Brien & Haynes, 1997). Social/interpersonal controlling factors subsume interactions with other people or groups of people. Nonsocial/environmental controlling factors are situational events or characteristics that exert an influence on behavior outside of social interactions. Examples of nonsocial/environmental causal factors include temperature, noise levels, lighting levels, food, and room design. These latter nonsocial/environmental causal factors can exert a significant effect on behavior, and unfortunately, have not been extensively researched nor cataloged in the field of behavior therapy. Further, clinicians do not appear to routinely evaluate the effects of nonsocial environmental factors. Like target behaviors, frequency, duration, intensity, and latency are the more commonly measured dimensions of social/interpersonal and nonsocial/environmental controlling factors.

Returning to the aforementioned example, once the manipulative behavior is operationally defined, we would seek to identify and operationally define hypothesized causal factors. Relevant social/interpersonal events might include staff member responses to patient behavior (e.g., Are staff members inadvertently reinforcing specialized requests or frequent call light use?), staffing patterns (e.g., Are the patients medical needs being adequately addressed when appropriate requests are made?), or proximity of nursing staff. Potentially relevant nonsocial/environmental events might include room location, time of day, meal composition, or medication administration schedule. These causal factors can be measured along multiple dimensions such as frequency, duration, intensity, or latency. Consequently, the assessor would select the dimension that is most relevant to achieving the goal of the assessment.

Operationalization and quantification of causal variables serve important purposes in behavioral observation. First, like operationalization of target behaviors, the process of carefully defining and quantifying causal variables may permit the clinician to establish a diagnosis. For example, if an anxiety response only occurs in the presence of a discrete environmental stimulus, it would be classified as a specific phobia according to DSM-IV criteria. Alternatively, if the anxiety responses occur in multiple situations, then other diagnoses such as panic disorder or generalized anxiety disorder would be considered.

Second, the operationalization of causal variables helps the clinician think about the possible function of the target behavior—its relations with antecedent and consequent environmental events. In turn, these hypotheses about behavioral functions guide the process of treatment design. Finally, and again most importantly, careful consideration of a broad array of social/interpersonal and nonsocial/environmental causal factors can help the clinician adopt a scholarly approach to the nature of the problem behavior and the possible factors that control it.

In summary, two important and common functions of all observation strategies are to generate operational definitions of target behaviors and causal variables. Operational definitions of target behaviors can be simplified by sorting responses into three modes and measuring these modes of responses on dimensions of frequency, intensity, duration, and/or latency. Causal variables can also be partitioned into modes and measured on dimensions of frequency, duration, intensity, and/or latency.

Identifying Functional Relations

After the target behaviors and causal variables have been operationalized, the behavior clinician will then collect information about functional relations among causal variables and target behaviors. As can be seen in Figure 12-1, there are many ways that these variables can interact and it is not possible for even the most ambitious behavior clinician to design an observation system that will collect data on these numerous possible interactions. Consequently, a priori decisions must be made regarding which variables and interactions may be most relevant to the design and evaluation of an intervention program. These a priori decisions are analogous to the concept of "presuppositions to the causal field," as described by Einhorn (1988), or "observation windows," as described by Barrios (1988).

As noted in Chapter 3, the nature of a priori decisions used by assessors to reduce the complexity of assessments has not been adequately researched (Hayes & Follette, 1992). Consequently, little is known about the utility, accuracy, and/or factors governing these decisions. Drawing from the general decision-making literature, however, we propose that there are at

Interactions Among Response Modes, Parameters of Responses, and Classes of Causal Variables

Response Modes	Response Parameters	Causal Variable Class	
		Social/Interpersonal	Nonsocial/Environmental
Cognitive/Verbal	Frequency		
	Intensity		
	Duration		
	Latency		
Affective/Physiological	Frequency		
	Intensity		
	Duration		
	Latency		
Overt/Motor	Frequency		
	Intensity		
	Duration		
	Latency		

Figure 12-1. Depiction of the Multiple Interactions among Causal Variables and Target Behaviors. Note that if a single target behavior is operationalized according to a minimum of three response modes, and four parameters are measured for each mode, then there are at least 24 combinations of possible interactions among causal variables, response mode, and response parameter.

least three major sources of influence: training and experience, published literature, and the client.

Information gained through training (e.g., courses, supervision, research), professional supervision, workshops, and personal experience with clients can exert a significant effect on presuppositions. For example, a behavior clinician with training and experience in biofeedback may presume that a client's pain symptoms are caused by problematic muscle tension levels that occur in response to lifting requirements at work. Logically, the clinician's observational system would emphasize the operationalization and quantification of physiological-affective responses (e.g., muscle tension levels), nonsocial/environmental causal factors (i.e., the weight of objects to be lifted at work), and the functional relations among these variables. Alternatively, a behavior clinician with training and experience in operant conditioning may presuppose that social reinforcement is the primary cause of pain complaints. Her observational system would thus emphasize social/interpersonal causal factors (e.g., solicitous behaviors from a spouse), verbal-cognitive target behaviors (e.g., verbalization of pain complaints), and/or overt-motor target behaviors (e.g., posturing, guarding, pained facial expressions).

A second major factor guiding presuppositions is the published literature. For example, Durand (1990) developed a conceptualization of self-injurious behavior in which he posited that the behavior is maintained by social attention, tangible reinforcement, intrinsic sensory reinforcement, and/or escape from aversive contexts. A behavior clinician who is familiar with Durand's work may opt to narrow his or her range of causal factors to these crucial causal factors when conducting an assessment of self-injurious behavior.

A third important factor that may influence presuppositions is preliminary assessment data gathered from the client and other informants. This information is typically gathered through interviews and other more broadly focused assessment methods such as questionnaire administration, ratings scale completion, and informal observation.

While presuppositions to the causal field are necessary for simplifying the complex task of generating an observational system, clinicians should avoid using an excessively narrow set of presuppositions because important and relevant assessment information could be lost under these circumstances. As noted in Chapter 3, to guard against acquiring an excessively limited set of presuppositions, the clinician should (a) evaluate his or her own assessment strategies and collect data on the accuracy or treatment utility of clinical predictions and decisions; (b) discuss cases with colleagues and/or supervisors; and (c) update his or her knowledge of causal fields by reading the published literature, conducting clinical research, attending conferences, and participating in professional workshops.

Once the operational definitions have been generated and the causal field has been narrowed through presupposition, the clinician will need to design an observation system that will permit the identification and measurement of functional relations among causal events and target behaviors. As noted in Chapter 10, covariation between a controlling event and some dimension or facet of a target behavior is an essential condition for identifying functional relations. Covariation among variables, however, may imply causality or covariation with a common third variable. Thus, in order to separate causal and noncausal functional relations, the clinician will minimally need to design an observation method that will permit establishment or evaluation of temporal order. Additionally, the assessor will need to extrapolate from the clinical research literature a plausible argument supporting the potential presence of a causal relation between two variables.

In summary, the primary functions of observation systems are to generate precise and quantifiable operational definitions of target behaviors and causal factors. Following operationalization of these critical sets of variables, the assessor will then need to develop strategies for collecting data on functional relations among target behaviors and causal factors that are initially identified through preliminary data collection and presuppositions.

As noted throughout this book, the process of operationalizing variables and generating estimates of functional relations is complex and poorly understood. We recommend, however, that the clinician attempt to abide by the multiple recommendations and precautions presented in earlier portions of this book. Specifically, the assessor should strive to recognize that multiple behaviors may be influenced by multiple causal factors in a dynamic and context-specific manner. In turn, efforts should be made to systematize the decision-making process so that it can be reconstructed and dissected at a later point for self-education purposes.

Elements of Behavioral Observation Methods

Humans are continuously behaving within ever changing internal and external environments that contain critical antecedent, co-occurring, and consequating events. Completely understanding the complex interactions that occur among multiple behaviors within these continuously changing contexts can be considered the ultimate goal of behavioral assessment. An assessor cannot, however, conduct continuous observations of all relevant modes and dimensions of behavior across all relevant contexts. Consequently, a coherent strategy for behavior sampling, time sampling, and context sampling must be developed.

When designing a sampling strategy, a primary goal is to select methods that will generate data that are generalizable to relevant constructs (construct validity) and settings (external validity). Additionally, the assessor will need to balance concerns for psychometric integrity (e.g., reliability and validity) against practical constraints that invariably arise in clinical settings. Finally, an evaluation of the ratio of information gained by a particular methodological feature must be weighed against the costs involved in implementing the procedure. In this section, we will present the most commonly used methods of sampling in behavioral observation.

Sampling Strategies

Sampling systems partition subset of ongoing behavior, time, and/or settings into discrete categories. Observation systems are commonly classified according to the sampling strategy that is used to collect data. The major strategies used to sample behavior, time, and settings are described in this section.

Event sampling is a data collection strategy where target behavior occurrence is systematically sampled. Specifically, the observer records whether the targeted behavior has been exhibited by a client during an observation interval. Other, nontargeted behaviors that occur during the observation session are not recorded. Figure 12-2 provides an example of an event sampling form.

Most often, event sampling yields frequency or rate measures, which are calculated by summing the number of target behavior occurrences across a relevant time interval. Returning to the manipulative client example, each occurrence of call-light use could be recorded by nurses during the day, evening, and night shifts. The total number of calls could then be divided by the number of hours under observation to derive a measure of calls per hour.

Event sampling can be used most effectively for target behaviors that have clear onsets and endpoints. That is, the observer must be able to clearly determine when the behavior has started and when it has stopped so that each instance of target behavior occurrence can be accurately recorded. Event sampling is also more useful when the observer is assessing target behaviors that do not occur at either very high or very low frequencies. Finally, the targeted behavior should be sufficiently salient so that it is easily recognized by observers.

Duration measures quantify the amount of time that elapses between the beginning and end of target behavior occurrence. Duration sampling is most useful when the clinician is concerned with the length of responding (e.g., the duration of time of a compulsive ritual for a client with obsessive-compulsive disorder can often be an important target of assessment). An example of a duration sampling form is provided in Figure 12-3.

Similar to event sampling, duration sampling requires that target behaviors have clearly observable onset and termination points. It is also more effectively used for behaviors that are not extremely brief and for behaviors that do not occur at a high frequency. Returning to the

	Setting A	Setting B	Setting C	Total
Behavior 1 Hitting				
Behavior 2 Kicking				
Behavior 3 Throwing				
Behavior 4 Screaming				
Total				

Recordng Instructions:

1.   Place a tick mark in the appropriate box every time James hits, kicks, throws objects at another person, or screams.   More than one tick mark can go in each box.

Figure 12-2. An Example of an Event Recording Form

case of the manipulative client, we may wish to obtain data on the length of time the patient calls out for assistance during the evening shift.

Interval sampling divides an observation session into discrete observation intervals that can last from a few seconds to hours. In partial interval sampling, an entire interval is recorded as an occurrence of the target behavior if it is observed for some proportion of the interval (see Figure 12-4 for an example of a partial interval recording form). In whole interval sampling, the behavior must be present for the entire interval before the interval is scored as an occurrence of the targeted behavior (see Figure 12-5 for an example of a whole interval form). Event-within-interval sampling is a third commonly used sampling strategy (Hartmann et al., 1988). In this case, the observer records the number of times the target behavior occurs (event sampling)

	Monday	Tuesday	Wednesday	Thursday	Friday	Saturday	Sunday	Total
7:30 - 7:35								
7:35 - 7:40								
7:40 - 7:45								
7:45 - 7:50								
7:50 - 7:55								
7:55 - 8:00								
8:00 - 8:05								
8:05 - 8:10								
8:10 - 8:15								
8:15 - 8:20								
8:20 - 8:25								
8:25 - 8:30								
8:30 - 8:35								
8:35 - 8:40								
8:45 - 8:50								
8:50 - 8:55								
8:55 - 9:00								
9:00 - 9:05								
9:05 - 9:10								
9:10 - 9:15								
9:15 - 9:20								
9:20 - 9:25								
9:25 - 9:30								
9:30 - 9:35								
Total								

Recordng Instructions:

1.   Place a "B" in the interval when the behavior began, then place an "E" in the interval when the behavior ended.   Draw a vertical line between the "B" and the "E" to indicate the total amount of time that occurred between the beginning and end of the behavior.

Figure 12-3. An Example of a Duration Recording Form

within each interval (see Figure 12-6 for an example of an event-within-interval form). With this method, the observer is able to determine variation in target behavior occurrence across relevant time units. Returning to the manipulative client example, the clinician could request that nursing staff record call-light use using event sampling during a one-hour interval.

Sampling strategies should match the goals of assessment and the characteristics of the observed events. Partial and whole interval sampling strategies are well suited for target behaviors that do not have discrete onset and termination points. They are also appropriate when the target behavior occurs at such a high rate of frequency that observers could not be expected to accurately or reliably record the beginning and endpoints of each response.

	Monday	Tuesday	Wednesday	Thursday	Friday	Saturday	Sunday	Total
7:30 - 8:00								
8:00 - 8:30								
8:30 - 9:00								
9:00 - 9:30								
9:30 - 10:00								
10:00 - 10:30								
10:30 - 11:00								
11:00 - 11:30								
11:30 - 12:00								
12:00 - 12:30								
12:30 - 1:00								
1:00 - 1:30								
1:30 - 2:00								
2:00 - 2:30								
2:30 - 3:00								
3:00 - 3:30								
3:30 - 4:00								
4:00 - 4:30								
4:30 - 5:00								
5:00 - 5:30								
5:30 - 6:00								
6:00 - 6:30								
6:30 - 7:00								
7:00 - 7:30								
7:30 - 8:00								
8:00 - 8:30								
8:30 - 9:00								
Total								

Recordng Instructions:

1. **Place a check mark in the appropriate box if James hits or kicks another person.**

Figure 12-4. An Example of a Partial Interval Recording Form

Returning again to the manipulative patient example, we may determine that the patient is frequently complaining about the quality of care. Under these circumstances it would be impractical to use event or duration sampling strategies because observers could not be able to reliably and accurately code each instance of the frequently occurring behavior. As an alternative, we could design an interval recording strategy where the day is divided into 30-minute intervals. If the patient is observed to exhibit the complaining behavior at any point during that interval, the nurses would simply record the interval as an occurrence of the target behavior. They would not need to record the number or duration of target behavior responses that occur during the interval.

One of the principal difficulties with interval sampling is related to the misestimation of behavior frequency and duration when partial or whole interval sampling is used (Mann, Ten

	Monday	Tuesday	Wednesday	Thursday	Friday	Saturday	Sunday	Total
7:30 - 7:35								
7:35 - 7:40								
7:40 - 7:45								
7:45 - 7:50								
7:50 - 7:55								
7:55 - 8:00								
8:00 - 8:05								
8:05 - 8:10								
8:10 - 8:15								
8:15 - 8:20								
8:20 - 8:25								
8:25 - 8:30								
8:30 - 8:35								
8:35 - 8:40								
8:45 - 8:50								
8:50 - 8:55								
8:55 - 9:00								
9:00 - 9:05								
9:05 - 9:10								
9:10 - 9:15								
9:15 - 9:20								
9.20 - 9:25								
9:25 - 9:30								
9:30 - 9:35								
Total								

Recordng Instructions:

1.   **Place a check mark in the appropriate box if James exhibits hitting or kicking behavior for the entire observation period.**

Figure 12-5. An Example of a Whole Interval Recording Form

Have, Plunkett, & Meisels, 1991; Quera, 1990; Tryon, 1998). Unless the duration of a response exactly matches the duration of the observation interval and the behavior begins and ends simultaneously with the observation interval, these sampling strategies will, by definition, either underestimate or overestimate duration and frequency (see Figure 12-7).

Suen and Ary (1989) provided an extensive discussion of how the mismatch between interval timing and behavior timing will yield overestimations and underestimations of behavior frequency and duration. Quera (1990) offered some potential remedies for these problematic misestimations of frequency and duration. Other researchers, such as Mann, Ten Have, Plunkett, and Meisels (1991), argued that interval-only sampling procedures (this excludes event-within-interval sampling) are so problematic that they should be avoided.

	Monday	Tuesday	Wednesday	Thursday	Friday	Saturday	Sunday	Total
7:30 - 8:00								
8:00 - 8:30								
8:30 - 9:00								
9:00 - 9:30								
9:30 - 10:00								
10:00 - 10:30								
10:30 - 11:00								
11:00 - 11:30								
11:30 - 12:00								
12:00 - 12:30								
12:30 - 1:00								
1:00 - 1:30								
1:30 - 2:00								
2:00 - 2:30								
2:30 - 3:00								
3:00 - 3:30								
3:30 - 4:00								
4:00 - 4:30								
4:30 - 5:00								
5:00 - 5:30								
5:30 - 6:00								
6:00 - 6:30								
6:30 - 7:00								
7:00 - 7:30								
7:30 - 8:00								
8:00 - 8:30								
8:30 - 9:00								
Total								

Recordng Instructions:

1.   **Place a tick mark in the appropriate box every time James hits or kicks another person. More than one tick mark can go in each box.**

Figure 12-6. An Example of an Event-Within-Interval Recording Form

Mann and associates also noted that the increased availability of audiovisual equipment has increased the feasibility for an assessor to record behavior and then more accurately code observational data using event and/or duration recording.

Real-time sampling involves having the observer record clock time at the onset and offset of the target behavior. This method of sampling can yield event-sampling information (target behavior frequency), duration-sampling information (length of target behavior occurrence), and interval-sampling information (number of time units where the behavior was observed to occur). In the manipulative client example, trained observers could be instructed to record real time at the moment that a verbal complaining bout is initiated. They would then record the time when the verbal complaints stop. Estimates of the frequency of verbal

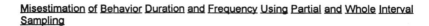

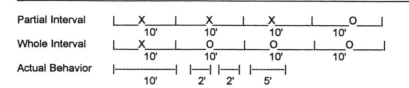

Actual Frequency of Behavior = 4 Bouts
Estimated Frequency From Partial Interval Sampling = 3
Estimated Frequency From Whole Interval Sampling = 1

Actual Duration of Behavior = 19'
Estimated Duration Using Partial Interval Sampling = 30'
Estimated Duration Using Whole Interval Sampling = 10'

Figure 12-7. Misestimation of Behavior Frequency and Duration Using Whole and Partial Interval Sampling

complaints could be obtained by summing the number of onset points that were recorded across a relevant time interval (e.g., a daily rate). Duration information would be derived by subtracting each onset time from each offset time. Interval information could be obtained by segmenting the day into relevant time units (e.g., 30-minute intervals) and subsequently recording the number of intervals where one or more target behavior onsets were recorded.

Observers using real-time sampling must be able to reliably, accurately, and consistently record time at the beginning and end of a target behavior occurrence. Thus, this method of sampling cannot be effectively used when the behavior occurs at a high rate of frequency or when the behavior has unclear beginning and endpoints. Recently, this method of sampling has become more feasible in clinical settings with the introduction of computerized devices that automatically record real time whenever the observer presses keys that represent target behavior onset and offset (e.g., Dumas, 1987; Greenwood et al., 1994).

Momentary-time sampling is a specialized form of interval recording where observation occurs only for a very brief interval (no more than a few seconds) and occurs at present times during a day (e.g., once every hour). During each brief observation interval, the observer records whether the target behavior is being exhibited by the client at that exact moment. Paul (1986) developed an elaborate momentary–time-sampling system that was used to evaluate the behavior of patients in psychiatric settings. In this system, observers were trained to successively observe each of several inpatients for a two-second interval and record whether specific behaviors were being emitted. These momentary-time samples were collected many times throughout the day. Thus, at the conclusion of a relevant time interval (e.g., a shift), observers were able to record the number of momentary intervals when the target behaviors were observed (event sampling) and the time of target behavior onset (real-time sampling).

Once again returning to the manipulative client example, a momentary–time-sampling system could be devised where an observer, stationed near the patient's room, would systematically scan for the occurrence of one or more target behaviors during a brief observation interval every 30 minutes.

Types of Observers

Observations are conducted by nonparticipant and participant observers. In this section each observer type will be briefly described.

Nonparticipant Observation

Nonparticipant observation systems use trained observation technicians to record target behavior and causal variable. In the research literature, professional observers, research assistants, and volunteers have been used to collect data on a wide array of behaviors and causal variables. Nonparticipant observers can also collect data using any of the aforementioned sampling methods. Finally, nonparticipant observers can conduct observations in a wide variety of naturalistic or analogue settings.

One of the principal advantages of nonparticipant observation is related to the quality of collected data. Because nonparticipant observers have no alternative responsibilities, they can concentrate on observation activities and, as a result, collect data on more complex behaviors and causal variables. Additionally, given equivalent training, nonparticipant observers, relative to participant observers, would be expected to collect observational data that are more reliable and accurate.

Although nonparticipant observation is a versatile and sound assessment method, it is rarely used in clinical settings. This lack of use is a function of its principal drawback—cost. In most clinical settings, the assessor will have limited resources for recruiting, training, and employing nonparticipant observers to collect data for most clients. Additionally, compared to participant observation, nonparticipant observation may be more reactive—it may alter the behavior of the persons being observed.

Participant Observation

Participant observers are persons who are normally part of the client's natural environment and have alternative responsibilities. In most cases, participant observers will be recruited from a client's family, workplace, academic setting, or clinic setting. Subsequent to recruitment, the participant observers are oriented to the observational system. This orientation involves familiarizing them with the operational definitions, sampling strategies, data-collection strategies, and the rationale and goals of the assessment.

The main advantage of participant observation is cost related. Because participant observers are typically persons who either report an interest in helping the client change his or her behavior, or who are employed to provide other types of services (usually therapeutic services or care-giving services), it is often not necessary to provide payment for conducting observations. Thus, this form of observation is less costly. Additionally, because participant observers are typically stationed in the client's home, work, or therapeutic environments, there is an increased opportunity for collecting data in a wide variety of settings, which, in turn, enhances the ecological validity of observations. Participant observation may be particularly cost-effective in the assessment of low-rate behaviors (e.g., seizures).

The major drawbacks associated with participant observation are related to the quality of recording. Specifically, because participant observers have responsibilities outside of conducting observations, it is necessary to limit the number of behaviors and causal variables that are to be observed. It is also typically necessary to use less complex sampling methods.

In summary, participant observers can record target behaviors and controlling factors in many naturalistic settings. The lower costs of participant observation and the potential for collecting data in naturalistic settings are two of the more important characteristics of this method. However, it is likely that data collected by participant observers may be more prone to error because observers have multiple responsibilities. As a corrective strategy, the assessor will typically need to develop a less complex sampling and recording system.

Observation Settings

One of the most important conceptual foundations of behavioral assessment is the position that behavior can be strongly influenced by context. This situational specificity of behavior has been observed repeatedly in clinical settings and across various behavior disorders. Because is its assumed that behavior will vary in relation to context, many behavioral assessment authors recommend that observations be conducted in multiple settings.

There are innumerable settings within which observations can be conducted, so again, a simplification strategy is needed. Rather than attempt to sort observation settings into discrete categories. It is more reasonable to view assessment settings on a continuum that ranges from unstructured naturalistic settings to controlled analogue observation settings.

Naturalistic Observation

On one end of the continuum is naturalistic observation. Naturalistic observation settings can be thought of as situations where variation in target behaviors and causal variables arises out of naturally occurring (i.e., nonmanipulated) functional relations and contingencies. Observational data collected in naturalistic observation is designed to provide information that more adequately generalizes to real-world settings.

One of the principal drawbacks of naturalistic settings, however, is that the lack of control over target behavior or causal variables makes it difficult to accurately measure behaviors that occur only in the presence of discrete and rarely occurring stimuli. For example, a client may exhibit social anxiety only when he or she is confronted with a requirement for public speaking (which may be vigorously avoided). If a naturalistic setting was selected to observe social anxiety, there would be few opportunities to collect data and the opportunity to examine functional relations and the form of the client's social anxiety would be limited.

To address some of these problems, the environments in naturalistic observation are often constrained. For example, a family may be required to remain in two rooms during an observation when naturally they might go to different parts of the house and not interact. These constraints reduce the ecological validity of the observation but increase its cost-effectiveness.

Analogue Observation

At the other end of the continuum of setting structure is analogue observation. In analogue observation, the assessor systematically varies some aspect of one or more hypothesized causal variables while observational measures of the target behavior(s) are collected. A number of single subject design strategies (e.g., ABAB, changing criterion, multiple baseline across persons) can then be used to evaluate the direction and strength of the relationships between the causal variables and target behaviors in analogue observation. There are many different types of analog observations including role playing, marital interaction assessments, behavioral approach tests, and functional analytic experiments. In the following section, functional analytic experiments will be emphasized because: (a) it is a methodological element of behavioral observation that is particularly well suited for establishing causal relations between target behaviors and causal variables, (b) it has been much more extensively evaluated as a tool for generating functional analyses and interventions, and (c) it can be readily incorporated into clinical settings.

Functional analytic experiments have received renewed interest in the recent years. As noted above, functional analytic experiments involve the systematic manipulation of hypothesized causal variables in order to observe their effects on target behaviors. For example, Iwata and colleagues (1994) and Durand and colleagues (e.g., Durand, 1990; Durand & Crimmins, 1988) developed a standardized protocol for conducting functional analytic experiments to identify the function of self-injurious behavior.

In their protocols, a client with self-injurious behavior is evaluated under controlled analogue observation conditions so that the function of the behavior can be identified. One condition involves providing the client with social attention contingent upon the occurrence of self-injurious behavior. Specifically, a confederate carefully ignores that client until the self-injurious behavior occurs. At that point, the confederate provides social attention (e.g., verbally and/or physically redirecting the client to another activity). A second condition involves providing tangible rewards (e.g., an edible reinforcer, a magazine) contingent upon the occurrence of self-injurious behavior. A third condition involves providing the client with an opportunity to escape from a negative or aversive task (negative reinforcement) contingent upon performance of self-injurious behavior. Finally, in the fourth condition, the client's level of self-injurious behavior is observed while he or she is socially isolated. It is presumed that rates of self-injurious behavior in this setting occur as a function of intrinsic reinforcing mechanisms such as opioid release, tension reduction, and/or nocioceptive feedback.

Iwata et al. (1994) summarized data from 152 functional analytic experiments that used the aforementioned analogue observation protocol. Using visual-data-inspection procedures, they determined which of the four types of consequences was most closely associated with increased rates of self-injurious behavior occurrence. Information about these causal relations was then used to assign the client to treatment procedures that corresponded to assessment data. For example, if a client was shown to display higher rates of self-injurious behavior in the social attention or tangible reinforcement conditions, a matching intervention would use procedures such as noncontingent attention, differential reinforcement of other behavior (e.g., providing attention or access to preferred materials/activities when self-injurious behavior was not observed), or time-out. If a client exhibited higher rates of self-injurious behavior during the negative reinforcement conditions, a matching treatment would use procedures that capitalized on negative reinforcement principles such as noncontingent negative reinforcement (providing breaks from the aversive task independent from self-injurious behavior) and/or differential reinforcement of other behavior (providing breaks from the aversive task contingent upon performance of nonself-injurious behavior occurrence). Finally, if a client exhibited higher rates of self-injurious behavior during intrinsic reinforcement conditions, the matching intervention would use access to alternative sources of self-stimulation, differential reinforcement of other behavior (sensory stimulation delivered contingent upon performance of non-SIB behaviors), and/or response interruption procedures.

Results from Iwata et al.'s (1994) study indicated that 80% of the treatments based on functional analytic experiment results were successful (operationally defined as achieving self-injurious behavior rates that were at or below 10% of those observed during baseline). Alternatively, interventions not based on the functional analytic experiment results were described as having minimal effects.

Other researchers supported the general findings reported by Iwata et al. (1994). For example, Carr, Robinson, and Palumbo (1990) summarized the results of a literature review of 96 studies that evaluated the outcomes of interventions for self-injurious behavior that used functional analytic experiments to identify the function of the target behavior. They concluded that success rates (defined as 90% or more suppression in the level of behavior problems relative to baseline) were "much lower for procedures not based on functional analysis than it was for procedures based on such an analysis" (p. 365). Unfortunately, no statistical or quantitative information was provided about the magnitude of outcome differences between interventions based on the functional analytic experiment relative to intuitively derived or prepackaged interventions.

Similar to Iwata et al. (1994) and Carr et al. (1990), Derby and associates (1992) evaluated the treatment utility of functional analytic experimentation on 79 outpatient cases. They reported that the goal of their project was to adapt this analogue observation technique for self-injurious behavior to a more standard clinical setting. Essentially, they wanted to create a time-efficient and clinically useful analogue observation strategy that would conform to the pragmatic requirements of an outpatient setting. They also evaluated the treatment utility of this technique for aggressive behaviors and stereotypical behaviors.

Clients were assessed using multielement single-subject analogue observation designs in which different stimulus conditions were presented while target behavior occurrence was recorded. Drawing from the research literature on analogue observation, an emphasis was placed on evaluating variation in target behavior under conditions of contingent social attention, contingent tangible reward, contingent negative reinforcement, and intrinsic reinforcement conditions. All assessments were conducted in a classroom setting that had a one-way observation mirror.

Each stimulus condition was presented for 10 minutes and two independent observers recorded whether target behaviors occurred during consecutive six-second observation intervals using a partial interval recording system. Data were subsequently plotted on an interrupted time-series graft and evaluated using visual inspection procedures.

In total, 83 functional analytic experiments were conducted across a three-year period. All clients were diagnosed with mild, moderate, or severe mental retardation, and a sizable minority were diagnosed with either a seizure disorder or sensory disability. Target behaviors included self-injurious behavior, aggressive behavior, and stereotypical behavior. Complete data were available for 79 of the 83 clients. Results indicated that 63% of the clients exhibited target behaviors during the analogue observation and that a specific stimulus condition elicited higher rates of problematic behavior in 74% of the cases.

The authors concluded that the functional analytic experiment methodology was an effective strategy for identifying specific stimulus conditions that may reinforce problematic behavior. They also demonstrated that functional analytic experiments can be effectively used in a standard clinical setting. Finally, they noted that the results of the functional analytic experiments yielded information that was very helpful in intervention design.

Horner (1994) reviewed a number of functional analytic experimental studies and generated a commentary about the efficacy and future directions of this methodology. First, he noted that it is important to consider analogue observation in general, and functional-analytic experiments in particular, as ongoing assessment procedures that do not need to be restricted to the initial consultation. Second, he suggested that the procedures should be extended so that antecedent variables and conditions could be more fully evaluated. Third, he argued that the ultimate clinical utility of these procedures should be based on their ability to contribute meaningful clinical information while simultaneously balancing the increment in knowledge against the costs involved. Finally, Horner suggested that procedures and decisional strategies for evaluating analogue observational data and translating it into intervention design needed to be more fully developed.

In summary, the assessment procedures developed and evaluated by Iwata et al. (1994), Durand (1990), and Derby et al. (1992) are excellent examples of how analogue observation can be used to estimate causal relations. This is particularly true for self-injurious behavior, aggressive behavior, and stereotypical behavior. However, many questions about the treatment utility of analogue observation remain unanswered. First, the psychometric properties (e.g., reliability, validity) of analogue observation are largely unexplored. Second, an estimate of the incremental contribution of analogue observation to treatment outcomes has not been determined. Finally, most demonstrations of the treatment utility of analogue observation have been limited to a restricted population of clients who were presenting with a restricted number of behavior problems. Thus, the degree to which the apparent treatment utility of this procedure for identifying functional relations generalizes to other client populations, problem behaviors, and settings has not been evaluated.

Summary of Common Elements and Differentiating Elements

Observation systems are common to the extent that they require the establishment of operational definitions of target behaviors and causal variables. Additionally, observational systems commonly collect data on functional relations. Observational systems differ, however, in methods used to sample behavior, the settings where observation occurs, and the types of observers used to collect data. Each of the differentiating elements has unique advantages and limitations. Naturalistic observation permits evaluation of naturally occurring casual variable—target behavior interactions. Because the observations are uncontrolled, however, causal inferences cannot be firmly established. Analog observation, particularly functional analytic experimentation, permits the clinician to test and evaluate casual relations. This method is also well suited for establishing the function of a target behavior in clinical settings. The extent to which analogue observation data generalizes to other settings, however, is frequently unknown. In designing an observation system, the clinician must weigh relative advantages and disadvantages of using various combinations of sampling strategies, observer types, and observation settings so that data most relevant to the goal of assessment can be collected.

Applications of Behavioral Observation

As noted earlier in this chapter, we reviewed all of the single subject treatment studies published during the first six months of 1998 in several leading behavioral journals. As can be seen in Table 12-2, a wide variety of observation methods were used to evaluate clients of many different ages, with many different sorts of presenting problems, using many different types of observation sampling methods.

In addition to supporting the notion of diverse applicability of observation methods, a more detailed evaluation of the information contained in Table 12-2 suggests that the most commonly evaluated modes of behavior fell into the overt/motor dimension. Further, in 68% of the studies, event sampling was used to collect observation data. The next most commonly used sampling strategy was interval sampling (26%). Duration (11%) and momentary time sampling (5%) were rarely used, and no instance of real-time sampling was observed.

Table 12-2

Summary of Assessment Methods Used in Cased Studies as Published in Major Behavioral Journals in 1998

Authors	Client Population	Client Diagnosis	Target Behavior	Method Used to Assess	Type of BO
Ashbaugh, R. & Peck, S. M.	Child	No diagnosis	Disturbed sleep	BO, awake or asleep	I
Bennett, K. & Cavenaugh, R. A.	Child	Learning disability	Performance on test when given change to correct often versus only at test's tend	OTHER, arithmetic skills OTHER, correct/incorrect answer	
Botella, C., Banos, R. M., Perpina, C., Villa, C., Acaniz, M., & Rey, A.	Adult	Claustrophobia	Fear, anxiety, inability to undergo testing for lesion in spine	SR, self efficacy SR, fear and avoidance SR, functional impairment	
Boutelle, K. N.	Adult	Anorexia nervosa	Fear of/refusal to maintain normal body weight, body image disturbance, compulsive exercise	Int, cognitions SR, distress OTHER, weight OTHER, eating foods in session SM, daily intake of food	
Cordon, I. M., Lutzker, J. R., Bigelow, K. M., & Doctor, R. M.	Adult	No diagnosis reported for child abuse	Home safety, child health care, mother-child interacting	BO, verbal aggression	ER
Cuvo, A. J., Lerch, L. J., Leurquin, D. A., Gaffaney, T. J., & Poppen, R. L.	Adolescent	Mental retardation (MR), and each client holds various additional diagnoses	Performance under fixed ratio schedules, on more less desirable work tasks	OTHER, intellectual functioning BO, silverware sorting BO, beanbag throwing BO, jumping over hurdles	ER ER ER
Dixon, M. R., Hayes, L. J., Binder, L. M., Manthey, S., Sigman, C., & Zdanowski, D. M.	Adult	MR, each had additional diagnoses	Failure to complete day's activity, failure to stay in seat 5 minutes, exercise with arm bands	BO, for target behavior	I, DUR

Author	Population	Diagnosis	Target	Methods	
Eisen, A. R., & Silverman, W. K.	Child	Overanxious disorder	Anxiety symptoms "cognitive and somatic"	SR, cognitive errors; SM, daily diaries for anxiety; SI, anxiety disorders; SR, generalized anxiety; SR, somatic forms of anxiety; PHYS, heart rate; RS, internalizing and externalizing of anxiety; RS, parent ratings of child impairment due to anxiety	ER
Ervin, R. A., DuPaul, G. J., Kern, L., & Friman, P. C.	Adolescent	ADHD, oppositional defiant disorder	Problem behaviors in classroom	OTHER, intelligence; RS, assessed for ADHD; SI, diagnostic interview; RS, teacher and guardian ratings for problem behaviors; BO, off task behavior; SR, satisfaction ratings, teacher; Int, with teachers to determine antecedents	DUR
Farmer-Dougan, V.	Child	Diagnosis	"On task behavior" among normal children and children with developmental delay, language and/or behavioral delays	OTHER, language, behavioral, developmental abilities; OTHER, on task component; BO, on task vs. off task	
Farrell, S. P., Hains, A. A., & Davies, W. H.	Child	PTSD	Maladaptive thoughts, affective concerns, PTSD symptoms	OTHER, level of intelligence; RS, level of certainty of sexual abuse; SR, PTSD symptoms; SR, depression; SR, anxiety	
George, M. S., Huggins, T. A., McDermut, W., Parekh, P. I., Rubinow, D., & Post, R. M.	Adult	Bipolar affective disorder	Ability to recognize facial emotions, as function of depression	OTHER, report emotion cognition	
Hanley, G. P., Piazza, C. C., Keeney, K. M., Blakely-Smith, A. B., & Worsdell, A. S.	Child	Profound MR, self injurious behavior (SIB)	Self injurious behaviors	BO, positive behaviors; BO, self injurious behavior	ER; ER

(continued)

Table 12-2 (*Continued*)

Authors	Client Population	Client Diagnosis	Target Behavior	Method Used to Assess	Type of BO
Harris, T. A., Peterson, S. L., Filliben, T. L., & Glassberg, M.	Adult	No diagnoses, all had children with autism	Spousal feedback effects on teaching their children	BO, performance topics covered in instructional program BO, teaching of children BO, 4 step spousal feedback	ER DUR DUR
Kelly, S., Green, G., & Sidman, M.	Child	Autism	Visual identity matching	OTHER, vocabulary ability OTHER, expressive language OTHER, auditory comprehension OTHER, difficulty with auditory comprehension OTHER, level of intelligence OTHER, score on comprehension test	
Kerwin, M. E., Ahearn, W. H., Eicher, P. S., & Swearingin, W. C.	Child	None	Food refusal, SIB	BO, occurrence of SIB OTHER, latency of SIB BO, occurrence of food refusal OTHER, weight of food	MT MT
Krantz, P. J. & McClannahan, L. E.	Child	Autism	Social interaction skills	OTHER, intelligence level BO, words spoken, scripted and unscripted interaction, elaborations	ER
Lalli, J. S. & Kates, K. Lane, S. D. & Critchfield, T. S.	Child Adolescent	Developmental delays Down syndrome	SIB, aggression, disruption Improving acquisition of new skills	BO, for SIB, aggression, disruption OTHER, assess mental age OTHER, computer program that tested ability to match stimuli to various options	ER
McComas, J. J., Wacker, D. P., & Cooper, L. J.	Child	Developmental delays, SIB, short bowel syndrome	Failure to follow medical instructions, touches sterile wound, rips out tubes	BO, compliance with "hold still" request BO, request delivered (ER), compliance (ER), social reinforcement (I)	I ER, I

					"% DUR"
Miltenberger, R. G., Long, E. S., Rapp, J. T., Lumley, V., & Elliott, A. J.	1 child, 1 adult	Trichotillomania (both), adult also with MR, depression	Hair pulling thumb sucking, finger manipulation	BO, percentage of hair pulling in each session	
Pantalon, M. V. & Motta, R. W.	Adult	PTSD	Intrusive war memories, avoidance of stimuli reminiscent of war	Int, intrusions and avoidance; SM, intrusions and avoidance; SR, level of combat exposure; SR, combat related PTSD; SR, impact of events	
Peine, H. A., Darvish, R., Blakelock, H., Osborne, J. G., & Jenson, M. R.	Adult	Moderate MR, bipolar affective and oppositional defiant disorder	Reduction of maladaptive behaviors associated with cigarette consumption	BO, verbal aggression; BO, all other maladaptive behaviors	ER ER
Piazza, C. C., Fisher, W. W., Hanley, G. P., LeBlanc, L. A., Worsdell, A. S., Lindauer, S. E., & Keeney, K. M.	2 children 1 adolescent	Pica	Eating nonfood items	BO, eating nonfood items	I
Rapp, J. T., Miltenberger, R. G., Long, E. S., Elliott, A. J., & Lumley, V. A.	Adolescent	ADHD, depression, hair pulling	Hair pulling with noticeable hair loss	BO, hair pulling	I
Reid, D. H., Parsons, M. B., & Green, C. W.	Adult	Severe multiple disabilities, severe physical impairment	Identifying work preferences prior to entering supported jobs	OTHER, preference assessments; BO, choosing favorite tasks on job site	ER
Saper, Z. & Brasfield, C. R.	Adult	Panic disorder with agoraphobia, PTSD	Panic disorder symptoms and then PTSD symptoms	SR, intrusion and avoidance; SR, personality assessment; SR, personality; Int, subjective feelings	
Stromer, R., Mackay, H. A., McVay, A. A., & Fowler, T. Part 1	1 child 1 adolescent 1 adult	MR for all three	Ability to remember objects with and without a list	OTHER, reading and writing; OTHER, mental age equivalent; OTHER, ability to do the focus of research tasks	

(continued)

Table 12-2 (*Continued*)

Authors	Client Population	Client Diagnosis	Target Behavior	Method Used to Assess	Type of BO
Stromer, R., Mackay, H. A., McVay, A. A., & Fowler, T. Part 2	1 child 1 adolescent	MR for both	Ability to discriminate between situations when writing a list is beneficial and when it is not	OTHER, reading and writing OTHER, mental age equivalent OTHER, ability to do the focus of research tasks	
Thompson, R. H., Fisher, W. W., Piazza, C. C., & Kuhn, D. E.	Child	Severe MR, pervasive developmental disorder, hemophilia	Aggression	BO, frequency of aggressive behavior BO, aggressive behavior	ER
Weems, C. F.	Adult	None	Study of heart rate control, biofeedback	PHYS, heartrate PHYS, skin conductance	
Werle, M. A., Murphy, T. B., & Budd, K. S.	Child	None, except #3 had failure to thrive and mild motor delay	Chronic food refusal	BO, parent behaviors, child behaviors, food groups OTHER, parent monitoring	ER
Williams, K. E., Chambless, D. L., & Steketee, G.	Adult	OCD	Excessive washing, contamination, need to hoard	SI, check for psychosis I, cognitions about disorder SI, obsessive compulsive behavior RS, fears, obsession, rituals RS, avoidance	
Woods, D. W., & Wright, L. W.	Adult	None, stutters	Stutters in first and second languages	RS, stuttering difficulties BO, stuttering	ER
Zanolli, K., & Daggett, J.	Child	One had autism, others had no formal diagnosis	Failure to initiate social interaction	BO, initiations of interactions with others	ER

Note: SR = self-report inventory; SM = self-monitoring; RS = rating scale; Int = interviewing; SI = structured interview; BO = behavioral observation; Other = other method of assessment; I = Interval recording; ER = event recording; DUR = duration recording.

If one considers frequency of use to be an indicator of clinical utility, then event sampling appears to be, by far, the most useful sampling strategy in behavioral observation. This conclusion is consistent with a reasoned analysis of event sampling methods. In most cases, the client is brought into a clinical situation because some problem behavior or multiple behaviors are creating discomfort, social dysfunction, and/or harm (to self or others). Under these conditions, the clinician and client are most likely interested in gathering direct measures of the behavior frequency, intensity, and/or duration.

Data Collection and Reduction

Once the assessor has generated operational definitions of target and causal variables and determined a sampling strategy, who will conduct observations, and where observations will be conducted, decisions must be made about specific data-recording procedures. There are three classes of recording methods: written forms, audiovisual recordings, and computerized data-entry instruments. The most frequently used data-collection instrument involves a written form. On some occasions audiovisual recording devices will be used as well, but these recordings will ultimately need to be coded by observers who will most likely be using a written form to record their observations.

Event sampling (see Figure 12-2), event-within-interval sampling (see Figure 12-6), and real-time sampling procedures are used to yield a direct measure of the number of times (or frequency) that the target behavior was emitted by a client. These frequency counts are typically reduced by averaging them across a relevant time dimension (e.g., number of hits per hour or day) or causal dimension (e.g., number of hits in setting A, setting B, and so on).

Duration sampling also yields a direct measure of the time interval that occurs between the onset and termination of each bout of behavior. In this case, data are typically reduced by averaging the total amount of time that the behavior was observed by the number of target behavior bouts.

Partial interval sampling, whole interval sampling, and momentary-time sampling yield indirect estimates of behavior frequency. That is, rather than counting the occurrence of behavior, the assessor counts the number of intervals in which the behavior met some prespecified criterion (e.g., partial or whole interval criteria). As a result, the primary output of interval sampling systems is the number of intervals within which the behavior was observed. Often this number is divided by the total number of observation intervals to yield a proportion or percentage (i.e., # of intervals behavior observed/total number of observation intervals).

Evaluation of Observation Data

A primary goal of behavioral assessment is to generate a functional analysis. Hence, the more valuable data-analytic techniques will generate information about functional relations among target behaviors and hypothesized causal variables. As noted in Chapter 9, reliable covariation between a controlling event and some topographical aspect of a target behavior is an essential condition for inferring the presence of a causal relation. However, in order to differentiate causal from noncausal functional relations, the data-analytic technique should also help the assessor evaluate order effects—the extent to which variation in the hypothesized causal variable is associated with variation in the target behavior (Cook & Campbell, 1979; Saris & Stronkhorst, 1984).

Two predominant approaches to data evaluation—intuitive judgment and statistical testing—are available to the behavioral assessor. In the following paragraphs, each method will be described and evaluated more fully.

Graphing and Intuitive Evaluation

We summarized the data evaluation techniques used by the authors of studies summarized in Table 12-2. Out of the 19 studies that used observation methods, 74% used intuitive procedures (typically "visual inspection") to draw inferences from observational data. In most cases, the intuitive process involves generating a time-course plot of data and subjectively estimating whether there is covariation between the target behavior and the hypothesized causal variable.

Many authors have argued that intuitive data evaluation is an appropriate, if not preferred, method for evaluating behavioral observation data. The primary strengths associated with this method are that it requires a modest investment of time and effort on the part of the clinician, it is heuristic—it can promote hypothesis generation, and it is well suited for evaluating complex patterns of data.

An additional argument supporting intuitive evaluation is associated with clinical significance. Specifically, it has been argued that visual inspection is conservatively biased, and as a result, judgments of significant effects will only occur when the causal relation is of moderate to high magnitude. This latter supportive argument, however, has been challenged by Matyas and Greenwood (1990) who demonstrated that intuitive evaluation of data can sometimes lead to higher rates of Type I error when data are autocorrelated and/or when there are trends in single subject data.

A similar finding was reported by O'Brien (1995). In this simple demonstration of the fallibilities of covariation estimation, graduate students who had completed coursework in behavioral therapy were provided with a contrived set of self-monitoring data that presented data on three target behaviors: headache frequency, headache intensity, and headache duration. The data set also contained information from three potentially relevant causal variables: hours of sleep, marital argument frequency, and stress levels. The data were constructed so that only a single causal variable was strongly (i.e., r > .60) correlated with a single target behavior (remaining correlations between causal variables and target behaviors were of very low magnitude).

Students were instructed to (a) evaluate data as they typically would in a clinical setting, (b) estimate the magnitude of correlation between each causal variable and target behavior, and (c) select the most important causal variable for each target behavior. Results indicated that the students predominantly used intuitive evaluation procedures to estimate correlations. Additionally, the students substantially underestimated the magnitude of the strong correlations and overestimated the magnitude of weak correlations. In essence, they demonstrated a central tendency bias—guessing that two variables were moderately correlated. Finally, and most importantly, the students were able to correctly identify the most important causal variable for each target behavior only about 50% of the time. Taken together, these results suggested that intuitive data-analytic techniques were neither reliable nor valid.

The findings reviewed above are consistent with other research in human decision making where it has been reported that a fundamental limitation of intuitive evaluation is related to errors in covariation estimation (Arkes, 1981; Kleinmuntz, 1990; Matyas & Greenwood, 1990). As Arkes (1981) noted, many clinicians base covariation estimates on presupposition and/or cognitive biases rather than on objective interpretation of data patterns (see Chapman & Chapman, 1969 for an excellent illustration of the effect of the illusory correlation on clinical judgment). One reason for this phenomenon is that confirmatory information or hits (i.e., instances in which the causal variable and hypothesized effect co-occur) are overemphasized in intuitive decision making relative to other important information such as false positives, false negative, and true negatives.

In sum, intuitive data evaluation approaches are convenient and easily conducted. The validity of intuitive evaluation procedures, however, can be problematic. This is particularly true when the assessor attempts to intuitively estimate covariation between target behavior and causal variables. The problem of the invalidity of intuitive evaluation is compounded when one considers recommendations made throughout this book that multiple behaviors, multiple causes, and multiple interactions may need to be evaluated in a standard behavioral assessment situation.

Statistical Evaluation of Functional Relations

Conditional Probability Analyses

Conditional probability analyses are statistical techniques that are designed to evaluate the extent to which target behavior occurrence or nonoccurrence is conditional upon the occurrence and/or nonoccurrence of some other variable. Specifically, the assessor evaluates differences in the overall probability that the target behavior will occur (i.e., its unconditional probability) relative to the probability that the target behavior will occur given that some causal variable has occurred (i.e., its conditional probability). If there are substantial differences between the unconditional and conditional probabilities, the assessor concludes that the target behavior and causal variable are functionally related. The magnitude of this relation can also be tested using nonparametric statistical procedures such as chi-square analyses (Schlundt, 1985).

Consider for example, the hypothetical self-monitoring data presented in Table 12-3. To derive the conditional probability that the target behavior will occur, given that causal variable has occurred, the clinician would simply construct a 2×2 table as shown in Figure 12-8 and fill in the appropriate frequencies for each cell.

After determining the frequencies that fall into each cell, the clinician can determine the probability that the target behavior would occur regardless of causal variable occurrence. This quantity is the "base rate" or unconditional probability of target behavior occurrence. In this example, the unconditional probability of target behavior occurrence equals 8/21 or .38. Analogously, the unconditional probability of target behavior nonoccurrence is thus 13/21 or .62.

In order to gain an estimate of the association between the causal variable and the target behavior, the clinician would calculate conditional probabilities. The conditional probability is a ratio of target behavior occurrence divided by the number of times the causal variable occurred. In this case, the causal variable occurred a total of 11 times. Of these 11 occurrences, the problem behavior occurred twice. Thus, the conditional probability of target behavior occurrence given the occurrence of the causal variable is 2/11 or .18. Alternatively, the probability of target behavior occurrence given the nonoccurrence of the causal variable is 6/10 or .60.

By comparing the conditional probabilities against the unconditional probabilities, it can readily be seen that knowledge about causal variable occurrence improves one's ability to estimate the probability that the target behavior will occur. In this case, the causal variable is acting to suppress or reduce the likelihood that the problem behavior will occur.

Bayes theorem can also be applied to observational data. This approach is particularly helpful for data sets that contain missing data and multiple variables. In addition to using Bayesian formulas, the clinician can conduct many nonparametric statistical tests of observa-

Table 12-3

Conditional Probability Analysis of Hypothetical Observation Data
Collected in a Naturalistic Setting

Observation Number	Target Behavior Occurrence	Causal Variable Occurrence
1	0	1
2	1	0
3	0	1
4	0	0
5	0	0
6	1	0
7	1	0
8	0	0
9	0	1
10	1	0
11	0	0
12	0	1
13	0	1
14	1	0
15	1	1
16	0	1
17	0	1
18	1	1
19	0	1
20	1	0
21	0	1

Note: "1" indicates that the target behavior or causal variable occurred.

tional data (e.g., Chi-square, Cramer's V, Phi Coefficient) to determine the strength of association between variables and the likelihood that this pattern of results could have occurred by chance.

Conditional probability analyses, Bayes theorem, and the related nonparametric tests have several important strengths. First, the procedures require a relatively small number of data points (Schlundt, 1985). Second, the statistical procedures and concepts are straightforward and easily applied to clinical data. Third, virtually any PC-based statistical package can conduct most of the analyses. Fourth, the analyses can be used to evaluate data collected in analogue observation as well as naturalistic observation of unmanipulated target behavior-causal variable sequences. Finally, clients can be provided with a collaborative and complete analysis of observational data using procedures that are easy to explain and readily interpretable.

A main limitation associated with conditional probability analysis is that it can only be used to evaluate relations among a small set of variables. Further, because it is a nonparametric technique, it can only be used when the causal variables and target behaviors are measured with nominal or ordinal scales. Thus, ratio data such as frequency counts must be reduced into categories (e.g., high/low frequency) for evaluation. Finally, conditional probability analyses do not allow the assessor to evaluate and/or partition out the influence of serial dependency in data that may be autocorrelated.

T-tests, ANOVA, and Regression

When observation data are collected on two or more variables—most often the target behavior and a causal variable—conventional statistical tests of means and covariation can

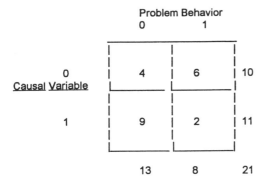

Unconditional Probabilities:

Overall probability of problem behavior occurrence = 8/21 = .38

Overall probability of problem behavior nonoccurrence = 13/21 = .62

Conditional Probabilities:

Probability of problem behavior occurrence given causal variable occurrence

= 2/11 = .18

Probability of problem behavior occurrence given causal variable nonoccurrence

= 6/10 = .60

Chi-Square (1) = 3.88, p < .05. Phi = .43, p < .05.

Figure 12-8. Contingency Table Summarizing Target Behavior-Causal Variable Interactions

sometimes be used. For example in an AB or ABAB design, the clinician can conduct an analysis of variance (ANOVA) to determine whether the mean level of target behavior occurrence differs as a function of causal variable occurrence and nonoccurrence (in this case the causal variable is systematically introduced and then removed). The clinician can also use regression techniques to evaluate whether the target behavior varies as a function of causal variable occurrence and nonoccurrence.

The primary advantage of using t-tests, ANOVA, and regression is that these procedures are well known to most clinicians who have received graduate training. The main disadvantage is that estimates of t and F are spuriously inflated when observational data are autocorrelated or serially dependent (Kazdin, 1998; Suen & Ary, 1989). This inflation of t and F is not trivial, for example Cook and Campbell (1979) noted that an autocorrelation of .7 can inflate a t value by as much as 265%. Thus, prior to using t-tests, ANOVA, or regression, the clinician must determine whether observational data are significantly autocorrelated.

Time-Series Analysis

Time series analyses involve taking repeated measures of the target behavior and one or more causal variables across time. An estimate of the relations among these variables is then calculated after the variance attributable to serial dependency is partitioned out (Barlow & Hersen, 1984; Hartmann et al., 1980; Wei, 1990). When assessment data are measured with nominal or ordinal scales, Markov modeling and lag sequential analysis can be used to evaluate functional relations (Gottman & Roy, 1990). With interval and ratio data, however, other time-series methodologies such as autoregressive integrated moving averages (ARIMA) modeling and spectral analysis can be used (Cook & Campbell, 1979; McCleary & Hay, 1980; Wei, 1990).

An example of the utility of time-series analyses is evident when data presented in Table 12-4 and Figure 12-9 are evaluated. These data represent two weeks (14 observations) of hypothetical baseline data and three weeks (21 observations) of hypothetical intervention data. In one series, data were very highly autocorrelated (i.e., the lag 1 autocorrelation was .90). In the other series, the exact same data were reorganized so that the autocorrelation was much less substantial (i.e., the lag 1 autocorrelation was .51). As is evident in Figure 12-9, the highly

Table 12-4

Hypothetical Data Representing High Autocorrelation and Moderate Autocorrelation During 14-Day Baseline and 21-Day Treatment Conditions

Observation Number	Phase	High Autocorrelation	Moderate Autocorrelation
1	1	1	7
2	1	3	13
3	1	4	10
4	1	2	1
5	1	5	4
6	1	7	14
7	1	6	3
8	1	8	9
9	1	9	8
10	1	10	12
11	1	12	5
12	1	11	11
13	1	13	2
14	1	14	6
15	2	16	31
16	2	15	30
17	2	17	23
18	2	19	35
19	2	18	17
20	2	20	28
21	2	23	19
22	2	22	32
23	2	21	16
24	2	24	33
25	2	27	15
26	2	26	18
27	2	25	20
28	2	29	29
29	2	28	21
30	2	30	25
31	2	32	28
32	2	31	24
33	2	33	34
34	2	34	26
35	2	35	22

Note: For Phase, 1 = baseline condition and 2 = treatment condition.

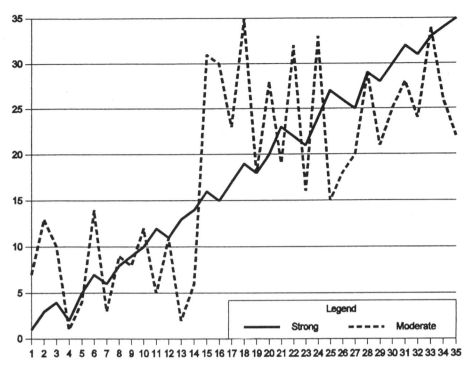

Figure 12-9. Line Graph of Highly Autocorrelated and Moderately Correlated Data

autocorrelated data do not suggest that there is a significant treatment effect. Instead, it appears that there is a linear progression of values across the baseline and intervention phases of the study. Alternatively, the moderately autocorrelated data appear to indicate that there is a substantial treatment effect.

Conventional statistical tests (t-tests, ANOVA, regression) of the highly autocorrelated and moderately autocorrelated data yielded equivalent results—both series of data were identified as exhibiting a very large and significant [t(34) = 9.23, p < .001] treatment effect. This equivalency of findings would be expected because the exact same numbers are contained in each data set and, as a result, the means and standard deviations are identical. In essence, the conventional statistical procedures yielded findings that are incompatible with apparent treatment effect differences between the two series of data.

An analysis of the data presented in Table 12-3 and Figure 12-9 using time-series methods yielded quite different findings. Using time-series ARIMA modeling (Cook and Campbell, 1979), it is clear that the highly autocorrelated series do not contain a significant treatment effect [t = 1.10, p = .28] while the moderately correlated series does [t = 3.41, p = .002].

It is beyond the scope of this book to provide detailed descriptions of the mathematical procedures that are used in time-series analysis. Books that do provide such information have been authored by Cook and Campbell (1979) and Wei (1990). Instead, our main goal is to briefly describe how time-series methods are applicable to the analysis of observational data.

Time-series methods can provide very accurate information about the strength and reliability of functional relations. They can also be used to examine the effects of controlling variables on target behaviors across different time lags. However, their applicability is limited because: (a) a minimum of approximately 50 points of measurement is required for estimation of functional relations (Gottman & Roy, 1990; Matyas & Greenwood, 1990), (b) the relations among only a few variables is typically feasible, and (c) the statistical procedures are not readily available on many statistical packages.

The first limitation can be reduced when the assessor designs an observational system that samples data at a rate that will yield a sufficient number of data points. The impact of the second limitation, that only a few interactions can be evaluated, will be diminished if the assessor carefully selects the most relevant target behaviors and causal variables using rational presuppositions and theory.

Psychometric Considerations

In Chapter 11, issues related to reliability and validity were extensively discussed. In this section, interobserver agreement, a particularly important psychometric characteristic of observational systems, will be reviewed.

A critical component for establishing the psychometric integrity of assessment data is reliability. In reference to behavioral observation, reliability most often refers to a statistic that reflects the extent to which observational data, collected with a specified sampling system, in a particular setting, is consistent among observers (Hops, Davis, & Longoria, 1995; also see Chapter 11 for a more extended discussion of reliability, stability, and consistency).

An evaluation of the consistency of a measurement system in behavioral observation is most often accomplished by evaluating the extent to which two or more observers agree that a target behavior and/or causal variable has occurred within the context of repeated measurements across sampling sessions (Suen & Ary, 1989). To generate a measure of interobserver agreement, two persons observe the same client, in the same setting, using the same sampling procedures, and identical operational definitions of target behaviors and/or causal variables. Arranging for two persons to collect client data under equivalent conditions is most often accomplished by having them conduct simultaneous "live" observations or conduct observations using a videotape that contains sequences of a client's behavior.

In Table 12-5 data are provided that illustrate how two observers may record occurrences and nonoccurrences of a target behavior across 15 observation sessions. A cursory examination of data in Table 12-5 indicates that Observer 1 recorded 3 occurrences of the target behavior while Observer 2 recorded 1 occurrence of target behavior. Additionally, Observer 1 recorded 12 nonoccurrences of target behavior while Observer 2 recorded 14 nonoccurrences. Observer 1 and Observer 2 agreed 11 out of 15 times. Is this an adequate level of agreement? Does it indicate that the observation system is consistent?

Data provided in Table 12-5 can be efficiently summarized in a 2 × 2 contingency table (see Figure 12-10). The value of Cell a is equal to the number of times the two observers agreed on target behavior occurrence. In this example, there were 0 occurrence agreements. The value of Cell b is equal to the number of times that Observer 2 recorded target behavior occurrence while Observer 1 recorded target behavior nonoccurrence. In this example, there was 1 disagreement of this type. The value of Cell c is equal to the number of times that Observer 2 recorded a nonoccurrence while Observer 1 recorded an occurrence. In this example, there were 3 disagreements of this type. Finally, the value in Cell d is equal to the number of times that Observer 1 and Observer 2 agreed on target behavior nonoccurrence. In this example, there were 11 agreements of this type.

Several additional features of Figure 12-10 should be mentioned at this point. The overall

Table 12-5
Hypothetical Observation Data Collected
by Two Observers of the Same Client

Observation Session	Observer 1	Observer 2	Agree/Disagree
1	0	0	a
2	0	0	a
3	0	1	d
4	1	0	d
5	0	0	a
6	0	0	a
7	0	0	a
8	0	0	a
9	0	0	a
10	1	0	d
11	1	0	d
12	0	0	a
13	0	0	a
14	0	0	a
15	0	0	a

Note: 1 indicates behavior was observed. 0 indicates behavior was not observed.

number of observations, labeled N, is equal to 15. Additionally, p1 is the proportion of the total N in which Observer 1 recorded target-behavior occurrence, while p2 is the proportion of the total N in which Observer 2 recorded target-behavior occurrence. Analogously, q1 is the proportion of the total N in which Observer 1 recorded target behavior nonoccurrence while q2 is the proportion of the total N in which Observer 2 recorded target behavior nonoccurrence.

While there are many different techniques that can be used to evaluate consistency among observers using data similar to those presented in Table 12-5 (see Suen & Ary, 1989 for a complete description of various options for measuring consistency and reliability), the most commonly used indicator is proportion agreement, which is often multiplied by 100 to yield the percentage of agreement.

The conceptual formula for calculating proportion agreement (po) is as follows: po = # agreements/# agreements + # disagreements. The computational formula, using Cell labels from Figure 12-10 is: po = (a + d)/(a + d) + (b + c). Returning to the data presented in Figure 12-10, we can readily calculate the proportion agreement:

$$po = (0 + 11)/(0 + 11) + (1 + 3)$$
$$po = 11/15$$
$$po = .73$$

At first glance, this might seem like an adequate level of agreement among observers. However, it has been noted by many authors that the proportion agreement index is significantly affected by chance agreement when the frequency of target behavior occurrence is low (e.g., less than 20% of observations) or high (greater than 80% of observations; Hops, Davis, & Longoria, 1995; Suen & Ary, 1989). Consequently, the proportion agreement index should never be used as the sole indicator of the reliability or consistency of an observation system.

Several additional agreement indicators will yield information that can supplement the proportion agreement index. The two most commonly computed and most relevant indicators are the proportion of occurrence agreements and proportion of nonoccurrence agreements. The

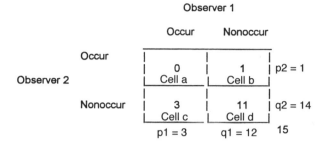

Observer 1

		Occur	Nonoccur	
Observer 2	Occur	0 Cell a	1 Cell b	p2 = 1
	Nonoccur	3 Cell c	11 Cell d	q2 = 14
		p1 = 3	q1 = 12	15

Agreement Indices for Data Presented Above

Statistic	Value
Proportion Agreement	.73
Occurrence Agreement	0
Nonoccurrence Agreement	.73
Chance Agreement	.76
Kappa	-.12

Figure 12-10. Data From Table 12-5 Entered into a 2×2 Contingency Table

conceptual formula for proportion of occurrence agreement is: poccurrence = # agreement on occurrences/# agreements on occurrences + # disagreements. The computational formula using Cell labels from Figure 12-10 is: poccurrence = (a)/(a) + (b + c). It can be seen that the numerator of this ratio is the number of times that the two observers agreed that the target behavior occurred (Cell a) while the denominator is composed of the number of times the observers agreed on target behavior occurrence (Cell a) plus the number of times they disagreed (Cells b and c). In essence, a ratio is being formed where the number of occurrence agreements is being divided by the number of times one or both judges recorded target behavior occurrence. Thus, Cell d, which contains information about agreements on target behavior nonoccurrence, is excluded from this computation.

Returning to the data presented in Figure 12-10, it is easily shown that the proportion of target behavior occurrence agreement is very poor:

poccurrence = (0)/(0) + (1 + 3)
poccurrence = 0/4
poccurrence = 0

Thus, while the overall proportion of agreement was high, these two observers did not agree about when the target behavior was exhibited by the client.

The conceptual formula for proportion of nonoccurrence agreement is: pnonoccurrence = # agreement on nonoccurrences/# agreements on nonoccurrences + # disagreements. The computational formula using Cell labels from Figure 12-10 is: pnonoccurrence = (d)/(d) + (b + c). It can be seen that this ratio is very similar to that used to calculate proportion of occurrence agreement. In this case, the numerator is the number of times that the two observer agreed about target behavior nonoccurrence while the denominator is comprised of the number of times that one or both judges recorded target behavior nonoccurrence. Thus, Cell a, agreements on target behavior occurrence is excluded from this computation.

Returning to the data presented in Figure 12-10, it can be shown that the proportion of target behavior occurrence agreement is relatively high.

$$\text{pnonoccurrence} = (d)/(d) + (b + c)$$
$$\text{pnonoccurrence} = (11)/(11) + (1 + 3)$$
$$\text{pnonoccurrence} = 11/15$$
$$\text{pnonoccurrence} = .73$$

By calculating proportion of occurrence and nonoccurrence agreement, the assessor is more able to form an opinion about the adequacy of the observational system. In this example, it is clear that the system does not yield consistent results; especially when target behavior occurrence is considered.

Although occurrence agreement and nonoccurrence agreement can be used to supplement the overall proportion of agreement index, they can also be adversely affected by chance agreement. An examination of the data in Figure 12-10 illustrates this point. Because the behavior occurred at a very low frequency (e.g., Observer 1 recorded three occurrences while Observer 2 recorded only one occurrence), there is an elevated probability that the proportion of nonoccurrence agreement is inflated by chance.

Consider, for example, a scenario where Observer 2 falls asleep during the observation session. He wakes up at the conclusion of the observation session and hurriedly records a 0 for all 15 observation points. If we recalculate the proportion of nonoccurrence agreement using these new data, it increases to .80! Thus, the increase is due to changes in the rates of nonoccurrences recorded by the observer as opposed to characteristics of the observational system.

Because of problems with chance agreement, it has been recommended that persons using observation systems calculate consistency indicators that correct for this error. The most commonly used indicator is Kappa (k), which is conceptually defined as the ratio of observed nonchance agreement divided by the highest value that nonchance agreement can attain in a given data-set. Like a correlation coefficient, Kappa can range from −1 (which indicates perfect disagreement) to +1 (which indicates perfect agreement) with 0 representing random agreement. Computationally, Kappa is calculated using the following formula:

$$k = po - pe/1 - pe$$

Where:

po = proportion of agreements (defined above),
pe = proportion of chance agreements (defined below),
po − pe = proportion of observed agreements minus proportion of chance agreements, and
1 − pe = highest possible value of nonchance agreement once chance agreement proportion is partitioned out.

As is evident above, in order to calculate Kappa, the assessor must determine the probability of chance agreements (pe). This is accomplished by multiplying the occurrence marginals (i.e., p1 and p2) and adding them to the nonoccurrence marginals (i.e., q1 and q2). Thus, the proportion of chance agreement is:

$$pe = p1p2 + q1q2$$

Where:

p1 = proportion of occurrences recorded by observer 1,
p2 = proportion of occurrences recorded by observer 2,
q1 = proportion of nonoccurrences recorded by observer 1, and
q2 = proportion of nonoccurrences recorded by observer 2.

For data presented in Figure 12-10,

p1 = 3/15 = .200,
p2 = 1/15 = .067,
q1 = 12/15 = .800, and
q2 = 14/15 = .933.

In turn,

pe = [(.200)(.067)] + [(.800)(.933)]
pe = [.013] + [.746]
pe = .759

Finally, we are in a position to calculate Kappa. Placing the appropriate numbers in the Kappa computational formula (k = po − pe/1 − pe), we arrive at the following:

Kappa = .73 − .759/1 − .759
Kappa = −.12

An interpretation of Kappa indicates that the two observers show very low agreement rates once chance agreement probabilities are partitioned out. In essence, the observational system, under these circumstances, would not be considered to be reliable or consistent.

The reliability and consistency of observational data are dependent upon the quality of the recording system. Specifically, reliable and consistent observational data can be collected when there are well-trained observers recording clearly specified target behaviors and causal variables in an appropriately defined setting. Alternatively, problems with reliability and consistency most commonly arise when (a) target behaviors and causal have not been adequately operationalized, (b) observers have not been adequately trained and monitored for continued accuracy, and (c) the observational setting does not permit accurate recording of target behavior occurrence.

An additional psychometric issue related to observation is reactivity. *Reactive effects* occur when the person or persons under scrutiny modify their behavior in the presence of observers. In some case, reactivity effects can lead to behavioral suppression (e.g., participants may suppress behaviors that they perceive to be socially undesirable) or behavioral intensification (e.g., socially desirable behaviors may occur at a higher rate of frequency, intensity, or duration). Reactive effects are sometimes indicated by transitional states and slope in obtained data. The degree of reactivity may be associated with the duration of observation, the amount of change in the natural environment associated with observation, the identity of the observers, instructions to subjects, the goals of assessment, and the methods of data recording. Reactivity effects associated with direct observation can be lessened when the salience and intrusiveness of an observational system are minimized (see reviews in Harris & Lahey, 1982; Haynes & Horn, 1982).

Summary

Behavioral observation emphasizes the quantification of minimally inferential variables. It is an assessment method that emerged out of, and is closely associated with, the empiricist tradition in behavior therapy. Behavioral observation is also one of the more frequently used methods of assessment in clinical and research contexts.

The primary goals of direct observation are to provide precise, quantifiable, information about behavior, controlling factors, and the relations among them. Direct observation systems can use several methods for sampling behavior in settings that range from naturalistic settings to analogue settings. Different types of human observers or technological devices can record the occurrence of target behaviors and controlling factors.

The reliability and validity of direct observation varies with the integrity of the methods used to collect data. Enhanced levels of reliability and validity are expected when carefully defined behaviors and controlling factors are recorded by properly trained observers or correctly calibrated technical devices in settings that promote target behavior occurrence and unobstructed observation. Additionally, the use of quantitative data-analytic procedures should be used to enhance intuitive evaluation of data.

Suggested Readings

Barrios, B. A. (1993). Direct observation. In T. H. Ollendick & M. Hersen (Eds.), *Handbook of child and adolescent assessment* (pp. 140–164). Boston: Allyn & Bacon.

Foster, S. L., Bell-Dolan, D. J., & Burge, D. A. (1988). Behavioral observation. In A. S. Bellack & M. Hersen (Eds.), *Behavioral assessment: A practical handbook* (3rd ed., pp. 119–160). Elmsford, NY: Pergamon.

Hartmann, D. P., & Wood, D. D. (1990). Observational methods. In A. S. Bellack, M. Hersen, A. E. Kazdin (Eds.), *International handbook of behavior modification and therapy* (2nd ed., pp. 107–138). New York: Plenum.

Paul, G. L. (1986). *The time sample behavioral checklist: Observational assessment instrumentation for service and research.* Champaign IL: Research Press.

Suen, H. K., & Ary, D. (1989). *Analyzing quantitative behavioral data.* Hillsdale, NJ: Lawrence Erlbaum Associates.

Tryon, W. W. (1998). Behavioral observation. In A. S. Bellack & M. Hersen (Eds.), *Behavioral assessment—A practical handbook* (4th ed., pp. 79–103). Boston: Allyn & Bacon.

13

Clinical Case Formulation

Introduction

Intervention paradigms differ in the degree to which their strategies are individualized across clients. In some intervention paradigms, the methods of intervention are similar for all clients with the same behavior problem or are similar for all behavior problems. This would be illustrated by a treatment program that involved exposure and desensitization treatment protocols with all children with anxiety disorders (see discussions in March, 1995) or adults with a panic disorder (Craske, Rapee, & Barlow, 1992).

Treatments can be similar or individualized in several ways. As noted above, a general treatment program can be similar, standardized,[1] or individualized for clients with a particular problem or diagnostic label. Additionally, the components of a specific treatment can be standardized or individualized. This would be illustrated by a training program for children exhibiting autistic behaviors in which different reinforcers and schedules of reinforcement were used for different children (see discussion in Schreibman, Charlop, & Kurtz, 1992).

Behavioral intervention programs are sometimes standardized but often individualized (e.g., Bellack & Hersen, 1993; Turner, Calhoun, & Adams, 1992). The use in behavior therapy of individualized intervention reflects several characteristics and assumptions of the behavioral paradigm, particularly behavioral models of causality. This chapter reviews assumptions underlying the close assessment-intervention relationship in behavior therapy. We review several models of clinical case formulation and discuss the functional analysis.

We discuss behavioral clinical case formulation as it affects both the selection of treatment program components and the specific application of those components. We suggest that, for many clients, a pretreatment assessment of a client's multiple problems and causal variables can aid decisions about which treatment foci are likely to be the most effective and how treatment components should best be designed.

This chapter emphasizes several concepts:

1. Treatments are likely to be most effective when individualized and designed from information about the causal variables related to the behavior problem and other characteristics of the client.
2. The emphasis on individualized interventions is a result of several assumptions and characteristics of the behavioral paradigm: there are multiple methods of intervention available to the therapist with limited focus and effects for different treatment methods; clients have multiple behavior problems with multiple causal variables; classification of a client's behavior problems is insufficient to select treatment foci; and many variables can moderate or mediate intervention effects.
3. The clinical case formulation links preintervention behavioral assessment measures, clinical judgments, and the design of individualized intervention programs.
4. Nezu and Nezu's "problem solving" approach to clinical decision making and clinical case formulation involves the identification and analysis of the client's problems, intervention possibilities and goals, a general systems approach to assessment and treatment, selection of the best intervention strategy, and a Clinical Pathogenesis Map to guide and illustrate treatment decisions.
5. Person's Cognitive Behavioral Case Formulation includes four components: behavior problems list, core beliefs list, activating events and situations, and working hypotheses.

---

[1]A "standardized" treatment usually involves a specifically delineated procedure, usually with the aid of a treatment manual, within and across sessions.

6. Linehan's Dialectical Behavior Therapy, a contextual approach, integrates a stage theory of intervention, a biosocial theory of the original and maintaining causes of borderline personality disorder (BPD), learning principles, and aspects of the client's behavior problems that undermine intervention.
7. Haynes and O'Brien's functional analytic approach to case formulation emphasizes the identification of important, controllable, causal, and noncausal functional relations applicable to specified behaviors for an individual.
8. The functional analysis emphasizes idiographic functional relations relevant to the client's behavior problems and important and controllable causal variables.
9. Case formulations are dynamic, subjectively estimated, and have limited domains of validity.
10. Research on the clinical utility of clinical case formulations is sparse and mixed, but clinical case formulations are most likely to be useful when the clinical case is complex, there is a valid intervention strategy to modify the causal variables identified in the functional analysis, or where a standardized intervention program is not maximally effective or has failed.
11. A Functional Analytic Clinical Case Model is a vector-graphic diagram of a functional analysis.

Preintervention Assessment and the Design of Individualized Intervention Programs

As we discussed in Chapter 10, standardized interventions may be particularly effective when there is a close relationship between causal variables for a behavior problem and the causal variables affected by the intervention. Infrequently, a behavior problem may be a result of a single causal variable or common causal mechanism that is addressed by a treatment. More commonly, a behavior problem results from different permutations of multiple causal variables, and an intervention program is effective across these different causal variables. Examples of the latter case would be treatment programs involving a combination of exposure, self-instruction training, shaping, and reinforcement approaches to anxiety and mood disorders. Some intervention strategies are implemented from a constructional, goal-oriented approach and focus less on causal variables underlying the targeted deficit and more on positive goal attainment. This approach is exemplified by reinforcement-based learning programs for the acquisition of speech and self-help skills for persons with developmental or neurological deficits.

Although research on this complex issue is at an early stage (see discussions in Eels, 1997; Haynes, Leisen & Blaine, 1997), treatments are likely to be most effective when validated components are selected for use with clients on the basis of careful assessment of causal variables and behavioral characteristics of the client. Standardized treatment programs will be effective to the degree that their components address the particular causal variables and behavior problems most relevant for a client, but they will not be optimally effective. For example, a standardized treatment program for mood disorders that includes multiple validated components would be effective, on average, for persons with a mood disorder. However, it would be less effective, cost-effective, and efficient, on average, than a program that is modified to proportionately address the specific problem and causal factors for the individual client.

Several characteristics of the behavioral assessment and treatment paradigms, introduced in previous chapters, account for the emphasis on individualized behavioral intervention programs:

- The behavioral intervention paradigm includes many intervention methods. For example, behavioral intervention with clients with severe social anxiety may include different permutations of graded exposure to feared social situations in the natural environment, education about how anxiety responses are learned, role playing, imaginal desensitization, flooding, interoceptive reconditioning, medication, rational discourse about core beliefs, and self-monitoring of automatic thoughts (e.g., McNeil, Ries, & Turk, 1995).
- The same behavior problem can be a result of different permutations of causal variables across clients. Because each intervention method affects a limited array of causal variables for a client's behavior problems, interventions are likely to differ across clients.
- Clients often have multiple behavior problems, and their functional interrelations can affect decisions about the most effective intervention strategy.
- Each behavioral intervention strategy targets a limited array of potential causal variables and a limited array of behavior problems. It is likely that a specific intervention will have a greater impact on some causal variables and behavior problems than on others (see discussions in Newman et al., 1994).
- The components of behavior problems and characteristics of a behavior disorder can differ across clients, and the identification or classification of a client's behavior problems are insufficient to determine treatment foci.
- Variables that moderate or mediate intervention effects can differ across clients. Clients can differ in cognitive abilities, motivation to change, reinforcement associated with the maintenance of a behavior problem, support for change by family members, and concurrent problems and stressors.

Our main point here is that assumptions of the behavioral assessment paradigm about the nature and causes of behavior problems and the multimethod nature of behavioral interventions means that preintervention assessment is a crucial component in behavioral intervention. Even when standardized interventions are used, preintervention assessment is necessary to estimate which standardized intervention and which intervention components are likely to be the most effective for a client.

To design the best intervention plan for a client, the clinician must estimate the characteristics and dimensions of a behavior problem, whether other behavior problems are occurring currently and the relations among those behavior problems, the operation of variables likely to moderate intervention outcome, and the operation and relations among these multiple causal variables. These are difficult decisions, based on complex data sets, fraught with many sources of potential error. The integration of assessment data for the purpose of designing an intervention program is best approached through systematic clinical case formulation strategies.

Clinical Case Formulation

An individualized intervention program can be difficult to design because it is based on an integration of many clinical judgments. Each judgment is affected by multiple sources of data, is often made in the absence of sufficient or valid data or in the presence of conflicting data, and is subject to many sources of error and bias (see discussions in Chapter 3; Garb, 1998; Nezu & Nezu, 1989; Persons, 1991; Turk & Salovey, 1988).

The clinical case formulation links the numerous preintervention clinical judgments to the design of individualized intervention programs. Clinical case formulations are an integrated array of intervention-relevant clinical judgments about a client's behavior problems and important functional relations. Clinical case formulations include both strategies and conceptual models to help the clinician integrate preintervention assessment data, data from nomothetic research, and the clinician's hypotheses about potentially relevant client characteristics and causal variables. Clinical case formulation strategies inform the clinician about the information that should be acquired to make valid intervention decisions and help reduce the influences of judgment biases and errors. It is not surprising that many clinical scholars (see review in Haynes & O'Brien, 1990) have suggested that an invalid functional analysis may be a frequent cause of intervention failure.

Models for behavioral clinical case formulation have been proposed by Haynes and O'Brien (1990), Linehan (1993), Nezu and Nezu (1989), and Persons (1989). Many models of clinical case formulation were presented in greater detail in an edited book on clinical case formulation by Eels (1997). In this section we present an overview of the models articulated by Nezu and Nezu, Persons, and Linehan. In the subsequent section we describe the functional analysis and functional analytic clinical case models of Haynes and O'Brien.

A Problem-Solving Approach to Case Formulation

Nezu and Nezu (Nezu & Nezu, 1989; Nezu, Nezu, Friedman, & Haynes, 1997) have outlined a "problem-solving" approach to clinical decision-making and clinical case formulation. Nezu and Nezu suggested that during initial psychological assessment, the clinician is faced with a supraordinate "problem"—what intervention strategy is likely to be the most effective for this client? Nezu and Nezu noted the complexity of the problems facing the clinician—each client enters the assessment situation with a unique learning history, pattern of behavior problems, biological makeup, and set of causal factors.

The problem-solving process involves two components. First is problem orientation, which involves the clinician's beliefs, values, and expectations concerning a client's behavior problems, which guides the clinician's problem-solution strategies. These form the psychological assessment paradigm within which the clinician operates.

Second, is the clinician's problem-solving skills, which are the behaviors involved in solving the problems presented by a client. Problem-solving skills include problem definition and formulation, generating possible solutions to problems, making decisions about possible solutions, and implementing the selected solutions.

Nezu and Nezu suggested that there are three sequential judgments, or three specific problems, to be solved in order. Each contributes to the supraordinate judgment of selecting the best intervention strategy for a client:

(1) *The identification of the client's problems and determining if intervention is possible.* The assessor must translate the client's complaints into clinically useful, more specific operationalized problems and intervention goals. Intervention goals can be immediate and intermediate (i.e., instrumental) or ultimate. This first step begins with the process of gathering information relevant to the client's concerns, using a "funnel approach"—beginning with a broadly focused assessment across many domains of the client's life and gradually narrowing down the focus to more specific factors—guided by the SORKC (S, antecedent events; O, biological status; R, behaviors; K, schedules of reinforcement; c, response consequences) model (Ciminero, 1986).

(2) *Analysis of the client's problems and determining intervention goals.* Consistent with the functional analysis, discussed later in this chapter, the problem-formulation step leads to the

identification of instrumental outcomes for the client. These outcomes often operate as causal variables for the client's behavior problems and become the immediate targets of behavioral intervention.

Nezu and Nezu presume that there are multiple possible causal variables for a behavior problem, that the patterns of causation may differ across clients with the same disorder, and that there are reciprocal influences among multiple response modes (which they label a **general systems approach**). Thus, a major problem to be solved in the case formulation process is the identification of the factors that serve to maintain the client's behavior problems and affect the resolution of the problems.

(3) *Determination of the best intervention strategy.* This decision is guided by the outcome of the two previous steps. Decisions about the best intervention strategy are also informed by research on the effects, cost-effectiveness, moderator variables, and incremental validity and utility of potential intervention strategies.

Nezu and Nezu use a Clinical Pathogenesis Map (CPM) (Figure 13-1) to guide and illustrate the judgments necessary in clinical case formulation process and problem solving. The CPM is similar to the Functional Analytic Clinical Case Models presented later in the chapter in that they are idiographic vector diagrams that illustrate the functional relations relevant to a client's behavior problems. CPMs are illustrated in Nezu et al. (1997) and Nezu and Nezu (1989).

Successful resolution of the problem of selecting the optimal treatment strategy is the formation of a Goal Attainment Map, which identifies optimal strategies for each clinical goal. Clinical goals are identified by selecting the targets from the CPM that have the greatest likelihood of improving upon the ultimate goals of treatment.

Cognitive Behavioral Case Formulation

Persons (1989; Persons & Tompkins, 1997) presented a rationale and strategy for cognitive behavioral (CB) case formulation. Like other models of behavioral case formulation, CB is designed to facilitate decisions about the best intervention strategy for a client. To that end, CB Case Formulation incorporates assessment of the topographical (structural) features of a client's behavior problems, the assessment of causal mechanisms, and the identification of functional relations. The CB Case Formulation is designed to help the clinician develop working hypotheses about the factors that serve to maintain a problem behavior.

Cognitive Behavioral Case Formulation is congruent with cognitive theories of behavior problems, which emphasize the causal importance for behavior problems of core beliefs and the life events that activate the core beliefs. CB Case Formulation can be used to help conceptualize a client's behavior problems and also to help conceptualize individual problems or events (such as a specific self-injurious response).

CB Case Formulation includes four components which are central to the clinical case formulation:

1. *Behavior problems list.* This is an exhaustive, highly specific list of the client's behavior problems.
2. *Core beliefs list.* The client's specific beliefs about himself or herself or the world that may affect the client's behavior problems. These are the primary causal variables in CB Case Formulation. They can be suggested by a diagnosis and estimated on the basis of research. A common method of identify core beliefs is through a "Thought Record," a self-monitoring method in which a client records the situation and the behaviors, emotions, thoughts, and responses to the situation.

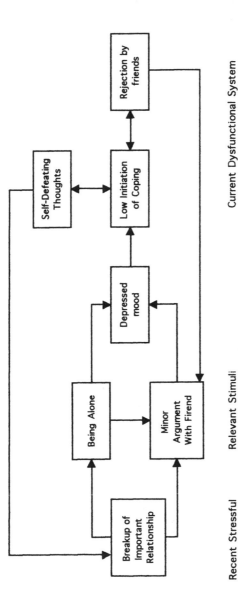

Recent Stressful   Relevant Stimuli   Current Dysfunctional System
Events

Figure 13-1. A simplified example of a Clinical Pathogenesis Map for a client whose main problem was depressed mood. An elaborated version of the model would include developmental history (e.g., poor problem-solving skills, irrational cognitions), additional relevant stimuli, and additional elements in the dysfunctional system.

3. *Activating events and situations.* These are the external events that activate core beliefs, which lead to the behavior problems.
4. *Working hypotheses.* This is a model of the interrelations between the client's problems, core beliefs, and activating events.

CB Case Formulation involves three other components: (1) the origins of core beliefs (The early learning history that explains the core beliefs), (2) the intervention plan, and (3) predicted intervention obstacles.

The product of these seven components is a written case formulation, designed to guide intervention decisions and intervention strategies. (An example of a CB Case Formulation is provided in Eels, 1997, pp. 330–331).

Dialectical Behavior Therapy Clinical Case Formulation

Linehan (Koerner & Linehan, 1997; Linehan, 1993) has outlined a model for the case formulation and intervention, primarily focusing on borderline personality disorder (BPD). Her approach, which she terms Dialectical Behavior Therapy (DBT), integrates a stage theory of intervention, a biosocial theory of the original and maintaining causes of BPD, learning principles, aspects of the client's behavior problems that undermine intervention, and a dialectic orientation to change.

It is a contextual, extended systems approach to clinical case formulation. DBT Case Formulation emphasizes the importance of the client's behavior problems in the context of the client's community. The case formulation also includes interactions with the therapist, and the variables affecting the therapist (Koerner & Linehan, 1997), and it presumes that the interactions among multiple factors affecting the client are dynamic.

Several aspects of the DBT model highlight the importance of preintervention assessment and clinical case formulation for intervention design.

1. Linehan noted that BPD can result from different permutations of causal factors. The DBT model stresses the importance of biological vulnerability and high sensitivity to emotional stimuli and high reactivity and slow recovery in response to emotional stimuli. In an interactive causal model, these responses to emotional stimuli are moderated by the characteristics of the client's social environment. An "invalidating" social environment (e.g., environments that teach the individual that their emotional responses are pathological or incorrect) can trigger or exacerbate dysfunctional emotional reactions.
2. Intervention strategies are influenced by the identification of functional relations, particularly the antecedents and consequent events (the behavioral chains) that maintain problem behaviors. The therapist and client identify each environmental event, thought, behavior, emotional reaction, and response by others that is associated with each problem behavior. This analysis of causal chains allows the therapist to identify multiple places where alternative responses by the client might be helpful.
3. The client's capabilities are likely to vary across different settings and contexts. For example, emotional responses to environmental events may be stronger in the context of sleep deprivation or as a function of recent life stressors.
4. There are reciprocal influences between the client's responses and environmental events. The client plays an active role in shaping his or her contexts and the responses of other persons.
5. Insufficient skills in dealing with environmental challenges may be a function of:

(a) lack of necessary skills, (b) a history of reinforcement for dysfunctional behavior, (c) disruption of skilled responses by heightened emotional responses, and (d) inhibition by faulty beliefs. Clients differ in the reasons that they do not deal with environmental events in a more effective manner.

6. The behavior problems of persons with BPD can interact in complex ways. These interactions have an important effect on decisions about the best strategy and focus of therapy. For example, inhibited grieving, avoidance of painful thoughts, negative self-statements, the inability to control intense emotional reactions, and overly active and passive responses to life events may affect life-threatening behaviors (e.g., parasuicidal behaviors) and affect the success of intervention focused on these behaviors.

7. DBT emphasizes task analyses relevant to the client's problems. Basing judgments on the identification of causal chains for dysfunctional behaviors, the therapist and client construct situation-specific step-by-step sequence of behaviors necessary to acquire desired behavioral responses to environmental challenges.

8. DBT Case Formulation involves a written summary. As with Functional Analytic Clinical Models and Clinical Pathogenesis Maps, the recommended format is a flow chart (see example in Koerner & Linehan, 1997, p. 363) that highlights antecedents and precipitating events, specific thoughts, causal mechanisms and "links," primary target behaviors, and consequent events.

Presuming that a causal model of BPD is valid and that effective intervention strategies are available to address the components of the model, Linehan suggested that a standardized intervention program that addressed all components of the model would result in clinically meaningful benefits for all clients (acknowledging that many other factors contribute to intervention outcome). However, a standardized intervention program would not be as effective or cost-efficient as an individually tailored intervention program that covaried intervention components to match the components that are most relevant to a particular client. A standardized program would have a disproportionate focus on unimportant components and an insufficient focus on important components for every client.

Common Features

The models presented by Nezu and Nezu, Persons, and Linehan use different terms and focus on different aspects of clinical case formulation. However, they are congruent in their underlying strategies and rationales. For example, the identification of core beliefs (Persons) and the identification of causal chains (Linehan) could be considered as problems to be solved within the model by Nezu and Nezu. The models by Nezu and Nezu and Linehan both emphasize the reciprocal causal relations among behavioral, cognitive, and emotional response modes. The emotional stimuli of Linehan's model can be considered as activating events in Persons's model.

The three models include several other common assumptions and elements: (a) the importance of preintervention assessment for clinical case formulation and individualized treatment, (b) the central role of clinical case formulation for determining the best intervention strategy, (c) the need for careful specification of a client's behavior problems, (d) the presumption that there are multiple causal factors for a behavior problem, which may differ across clients and across time, (e) the clinician's orientation and judgment can affect clinical case formulation and intervention decisions, (f) the importance of a written or visual display of the clinical case formulation, and (g) the fact that all models are amenable to a constructional approach that emphasizes positive treatment goals.

The Functional Analysis

The components of models by Nezu and Nezu, Persons, and Linehan are similar to those of the functional analysis. In addition to the components listed above, the functional analysis includes a more specific description and weighting of behavior problems, causal variables, and functional relations. In this section, we discuss the components, rationale, empirical basis, and methods for development of the functional analysis. In the subsequent section we present Functional Analytic Causal Models as a method of illustrating the functional analysis. Our discussion summarizes material presented in Haynes (1997), Haynes, Leisen, and Blaine, (1998), Haynes and O'Brien (1990), Haynes et al. (1993), and O'Brien and Haynes (1995b).

Definition

As with the models presented by Nezu and Nezu, Persons, and Linehan, the functional analysis is designed to organize and present the component judgments in clinical case formulation. The ultimate goal of the functional analysis is to guide assessment and intervention decisions for a client.

The functional analysis is "the identification of important, controllable, causal and noncausal functional relations applicable to specified behaviors for an individual" (Haynes & O'Brien, 1990). Like other models for clinical case formulation, the functional analysis is a working model of a client's problem behaviors, intervention goals, the variables that maintain and moderate the client's behavior problems, and the functional relations among those variables (see Box 13-1).

There are several aspects of the definition of the functional analysis:

- The functional analysis emphasizes *functional relations* relevant to the client's behavior problems.
- Functional relations in a functional analysis can be causal or noncausal, but *causal relations* are emphasized because they are especially relevant for intervention design.
- The functional analysis emphasizes *important* causal relations. Only some variables that have a causal relation with a particular target behavior are important in terms of their magnitude of effect or magnitude of shared variance. In the functional analysis, we are interested in those causal relations that account for the greatest proportion of variance in behavior problems, because they are the variables whose modification is estimated to have the greatest benefits for the client.
- *Controllable* variables are emphasized because of their relevance to the design of intervention programs. There are many examples of important causal variables that are amenable to modification (e.g., stroke, developmental disabilities, or severe life trauma). As we discussed in Chapter 9, historical causal events are often confused with their controllable sequelae.

Several classes of variables are important, in that they can account for a significant proportion of variance in behavior problems (across persons or across time with a person) but are not modifiable in the intervention process. Examples of unmodifiable causal variables include: (a) historical life events (e.g., a traumatic life experience), (b) biological attributes (e.g., a genetic predisposition for a disorder, effects of aging), (c) medical status (e.g., head trauma, cancer) and sociodemographic characteristics (e.g., economic status, age), (d) an uncontrollable environment (e.g., an aversive job setting from which the client cannot easily escape), and (e) epidemiological factors (e.g., economic status, racism).

Consistent with the tenet of the behavioral assessment paradigm that there are important between-person differences in the causes of behavior, functional analyses are *idiographic*. There are likely to be important differences in the functional analyses of clients with the same behavior problem. The functional analysis is in contrast with nomothetic models of behavior disorders, associated with structural equations modeling (see Lochlin, 1998), that are based on patterns of shared variance estimated from data on many persons.

Nomothetic models can indicate an array of possible causal variables for a particular behavior problem, which may or may not be relevant for a particular client. Nomothetic models can help the assessor focus assessment efforts on variables that are most likely to contribute to a valid functional analysis.

The definition of the functional analysis does not restrict it to a particular *class of variables* or a particular *method of assessment*. Functional relations can be identified through several methods and can include many classes of variables that have historically been de-emphasized in applied behavior analysis (e.g., physiological, cognitive, personality variables).

Components

There are 11 components of the functional analysis. All components contribute to the main goal of the functional analysis—to help the clinician decide on which causal variables to focus the intervention efforts. This goal is approached by estimating the variance in the client's behavior problems or intervention goal attainment associated with each causal variable in the functional analysis: the expected relative magnitude of effect of focusing treatment on

---

Box 13-1
Alternative Definitions

As noted in Haynes and O'Brien (1990), the term "functional analysis" has been defined differently across disciplines and across scholars in behavior therapy. The definitions differ in the degree to which they are congruent with the concepts of functional analysis outlined on pages 276–278. The degree to which they are tied to a particular method of assessment, and the degree to which functional variables are limited to a contiguous antecedent and consequent environmental events and whether it is defined as a process or as a product.

Some authors have recommend the use of "functional assessment" as an alternative label for a multimethod analysis of functional relations for a client. However, "functional assessment" has been used in rehabilitation psychology, neuropsychology, and other disciplines to mean "an assessment of a client's functional abilities," such as memory, hand-eye coordination, speech, and executive function abilities, and is less precise than functional analysis. (Martin and Pear [1996] label the derivation of causal hypotheses from observations in the natural environment or other "indirect" methods of assessment as "descriptive analysis.")

Some authors in applied and experimental behavior analysis have defined "functional analysis" as the estimation of functional relations through systematic manipulation (experimentation), or as the analysis of the functional relations of particular behavior problems with discrete antecedent and consequent environmental events. This restriction on the methods and type of functional variables in the functional analysis increases the precision of the definition and is based on a long history of behavior analysis. However, this more restricted definition unnecessarily limits the role of other important methods (e.g., time-series regression analyses) and other important variables (e.g., physiological and cognitive events) in the functional analysis.

particular causal variables. In Functional Analytic Clinical Case Models this estimation is aided by assigning each component a numerical value.

1. *The client's behavior problems and/or intervention goals.* The primary focus of the functional analysis is the major behavior problems or intervention goals of the client. The functional analysis may include multiple problems and goals and may include different response modes and dimensions.

2. *The relative importance of behavior problems and goals.* Most clients have multiple behavior problems, which differ in importance (see Chapter 8).

3. *The relations among a client's behavior problems.* A client's multiple behavior problems can have no functional relations, noncausal relations, or unidirectional causal or reciprocal causal relations. Reciprocal causal relations are particularly important for intervention decisions. Intervention in a reciprocal causal relation reverberates and has an enhanced magnitude of effect.

4. *The effects of a client's behavior problems.* Many behavior problems have important sequelae—effects on occupational, social, legal, medical, or family areas of the client's life. The effects of behavior problems are important components of a functional analysis because they influence the estimated magnitude of effect of a particular intervention focus. For example, a child's physical aggression can harm peers and siblings, cause marital distress between his or her parents, and lead to dismissal from school. When estimating whether to focus an intervention program on the child's aggressive behaviors, as opposed to his or her hyperactive or oppositional behaviors, one of many considerations is the system's level effects, reflected by the effect of aggression on other arenas.

5. *The identification of important social/environmental and contemporaneous causal variables for a client's behavior problems.* Causal variables can include all classes that were discussed in Chapter 10. However, the functional analysis emphasizes contiguous antecedent behaviors, environmental events, situational events, response contingencies, and cognitive antecedent and consequent variables because these have been shown to function as important triggering or maintaining variables for many behavior problems.

6. *The modifiability (clinical utility) of causal variables.* As we noted, causal variables differ in the degree to which they are clinically useful and the degree to which they are amenable to modification in an intervention program.

7. *The relation between causal variables and behavior problems.* Causal relations differ in their strength (the magnitude of causal effect) and whether the causal relation is unidirectional or bidirectional, and linear or nonlinear.

8. *The relation among causal variables.* Causal variables can affect one another in a unidirectional or bidirectional fashion.

9. *Chains of causal variables.* Behavior problems are often the end point of (or imbedded in) chains of causal variables and other behavior problems. Chains can include environmental events and client behaviors. Chains are important elements of the functional analysis because they can point to several possible intervention points.

10. *The operation of causal mechanisms and mediating variables.* As we discussed in Chapter 10, mediating variables explain "how" or "through what means" a causal variable affects a behavior problem. Mediating variables are important because interventions often focus on their modification. Mediating variables are particularly important when unmodifiable variables have important causal effects.

11. *The operation of moderating variables*. Moderating variables affect the strength of relation between two other variables. As with mediating variables, moderating variables are particularly important when the important causal variables are unmodifiable.

Additional Characteristics

Because the functional analysis emphasizes the form, direction, and magnitude of functional relations relevant to clients' behavior problems, it is congruent with many characteristics of idiographic functional and causal relations and models described in Chapter 10:

1. *Different types of functional relation* are included in a functional analysis. Functional relations can be causal or noncausal, important or unimportant, unidirectional or bidirectional, and controllable or uncontrollable. A causal variable in a functional analysis can also be necessary, sufficient, necessary and sufficient, or neither necessary nor sufficient to account for variance in the behavior problem.

2. Because there are always unmeasured variables that are functionally related to a behavior problem and always errors in estimating functional relations, a functional analysis is a tentative, temporary, *"best estimate."* A functional analysis should be considered as *hypothesized, probabilistic, subjectively estimated*, and *incomplete* clinical case formulation. Although the validity of a functional analysis can be increased by basing it on valid assessment data, it unavoidably incorporates clinical judgmental errors.

   The technology of behavioral assessment is nascent. The technologies for estimating causal relations are particularly weak—few of our assessment methods satisfy all the requirements for identifying a causal relation as discussed in Chapter 10. Additionally, the variables and relations in the functional analysis will be affected by which assessment instruments are used.

3. Functional relations and the functional analysis are *nonexclusionary*: A valid functional analysis does not preclude the existence of other valid and important functional relations for a client's behaviors problems. For example, a functional analysis that emphasizes a strong functional relation between depressed mood and automatic negative thoughts does not preclude the possibility that there is also a strong functional relation between depressed mood and the valence or frequency of social interactions or with neurotransmitter synthesis.

4. Congruent with the dynamic nature of client behavior problems, causal variables, and functional relations, the functional analysis is likely to be *dynamic*. The dynamic nature of the functional analysis is a result of real changes in the client's behavior and functional relations and from new information that changes the assessors judgments about problems and functionally related variables.

5. A functional analysis has *limited domains of validity*: The validity of a functional analyses is *conditional*. The validity of the functional analysis may be limited in many domains, including (a) setting (e.g., the functional analysis of aggressive behaviors by a child may be valid only in the home), (b) state of the client (e.g., a child's medication level), (c) response modalities of the behavior problem (e.g., a functional analysis may be valid for depressed thoughts but not for depressed overt behavior), (d) dimensions of behavior problems (e.g., for the magnitude but not for the onset on a panic episode), and (e) developmental stages (e.g., the causes of aggression may be different for a young child than for an adolescent).

6. Functional analyses can differ in their *level of specificity*. As we discussed in Chapter 7, higher and lower level variables can be valid in a functional analysis, depending on how the functional analysis will be used. However, functional analyses often err by including excessively higher-level variables, which do not facilitate intervention decisions. Variables such as "depression," "anxiety," "stress," "self-esteem," and "marital distress" are not sufficiently specific to point to specific intervention strategies.

7. Each component of the functional analysis integrates *nomothetic and idiographic empirical research findings* with the results of quantitative and qualitative assessment of the client. Empirically derived, nomothetic causal models for a behavior problem can point to possible causal relations for an individual client's behavior problem and guide initial assessment foci with that client. The validity of a functional analysis is probably affected by the assessor's degree of familiarity with empirical research on the targeted behavior problems and functionally related variables.

8. A functional analysis can include *extended social systems*. Chains of causal variables related to a client's behavior problem often include the behavior of others, who are, in turn, affected by the behavior of others and by other variables in their lives. Consequently, important sources of variance in a client's behavior problems can lie in variables far removed, geographically and temporally. The inclusion of social systems variables is particularly relevant in the functional analysis of children's and adolescents' behavior problems. A child's behavior is often affected by the behavior of parents, siblings, teachers, and peers, all of whom are influenced by other events and persons in their social system.

9. As suggested by the importance of social systems variables, a functional analysis can also include *noncontiguous variables*—causal events that are temporally distant from the target behaviors, such as childhood sex abuse and learning history. Although noncontiguous causal variables are often clinically useful, their mechanism of action (e.g., specific social skills deficits of the abused child, attention deficits by a stressed parent) is more often the target of intervention and must be carefully specified.

10. The functional analysis is congruent with and amenable to a *goal-oriented, constructional approach* to assessment. We have mostly focused on the identification and modification of causal variables for a behavior problem. However, the goal of intervention is often to strengthen behaviors that are desirable alternatives to undesirable behaviors or behavioral deficits. The functional analysis is also central to a constructional, goal-oriented approach to intervention. Positive goal-oriented intervention strategies are still affected by estimates of shared variance and magnitude of effect—estimates about which variables (e.g., instructions, exercises, thoughts, response contingencies) can be manipulated to affect the desired intervention outcome.

11. The functional analysis can include *functional response classes*. As we noted in Chapter 8, behaviors that are dissimilar in form can be similar in function and exhibit similar functional relations with other variables.

Methods of Derivation

Methods of estimating functional and causal relations were presented in Chapter 10. These included: (a) nomothetic research, (b) causal markers, (c) analogue assessment (manipulation designs), (d) time-series regression analyses, and (e) client estimates of causal relations. Additionally, in Chapter 8, we discussed several methods of estimating the relative importance of behavior problems. These included judgments about the rate and magnitude of a behavior problem, judgments about the probability that the behavior problem will lead to harm, judgments about the degree of impact on the client's quality of life, the degree to which a behavior problem functions as a cause of other behavior problems.

As we suggested earlier in this chapter, a valid functional analysis can be difficult to develop. Component judgments must sometimes be based on insufficient data, and data from different assessment methods or different informants may conflict (see Box 13-2).

Schill, Kratochwill, and Gardner (1996) discussed methods of conducting a functional analysis with children with behavior problems. They recommended a sequence of descriptive and experimental procedures, beginning with more easily implemented methods (which they term "descriptive functional analysis"), such as self- and participant report measures, interviews, questionnaires, and rating scales. These descriptive methods would be followed by observations in the natural environment and controlled manipulations in analogue clinic settings (which they refer to as "analogue experimental assessment"). They suggested that the descriptive procedures could help the assessor generate causal hypotheses, which could be evaluated in controlled analogue assessment. They also noted that parents and teachers can be valuable sources of hypotheses about functional relations and can be involved in experimental assessment protocols.

Groden (1989) discussed and illustrated a "guide for conducting a comprehensive behavioral analysis of a target behavior." This is a structured format for conducting a behavior analytic functional analysis that can be used to guide treatment. This "behavior analysis" emphasizes important antecedent events, consequent events, and covert antecedents such as thoughts, distant functionally related antecedent events, and the contexts for behavior.

Issues of Validity and the Utility of the Functional Analysis

Although the functional analysis, and other models for behavioral case formulation, has a compelling rationale, its validity and utility have not been extensively evaluated. Given that an ultimate goal of the functional analysis is to increase intervention effectiveness, the ultimate criterion is incremental intervention validity (Hayes, Nelson, & Jarret, 1987; Kratochwill & Plunge, 1992; Silva, 1993). The functional analysis has incremental intervention validity to the

---

Box 13-2
Drawing Inferences When There Are Discrepancies Between Informants

Kamphaus and Frick (1996) discussed methods of integrating data from multiple informants in child and adolescent assessment. When using multiple informants who are providing discrepant data, they suggested that the assessor: (a) consider the degree to which data from different informants reflect real difference in the child's behavior across settings, (b) consider the degree to which informants are providing data at different levels of specificity, and (c) consider the degree to which data from different informants are derived from different assessment instruments. Additionally, information from one informant may be weighted more heavily, on the basis of frequency of contact or other indications of validity of the data (e.g., cognitive competency, motivation, and bias of the informant). Finally, the authors suggested that convergent findings, looking for agreement among multiple sources, are particularly meaningful when using multiple informants and that the causes of discrepancies should be investigated.

degree that intervention based on it is more effective than intervention not based on it. Judgments about the intervention validity of the functional analysis are also affected by the degree of content and criterion validity of the model and characteristics of the available interventions.

The validity of the functional analysis depends on the validity of the component judgments and the validity of the assessment data upon which they are based. Although the functional analysis can reflect judgments derived from nomothetic research, it mostly reflects quantitative and qualitative assessment information on the client derived in the assessment process.

Content Validity

The content validity of a functional analysis is the degree to which it reflects the client's behavior problems and the important causal variables relevant to the client's behavior problems. Are the behavior problems and causal variables in the functional analysis relevant and representative of those operating for the client?

Perhaps the most common errors in the functional analysis are errors in content validity. These include the failure to identify important causal variables or behavior problems, the inclusion of irrelevant problems or causal variables, and the inclusion of causal variables and behavior problems that are insufficiently specific to guide intervention decisions. All three errors can seriously undermine the clinical utility of the functional analysis. In the case of each error, the intervention strategy designed on the basis of the functional analysis would not be focused on the variables with the greatest magnitude of shared variance with the behavior problem.

Content validity of a functional analysis can be enhanced by following the principles of assessment intrinsic to the behavioral assessment paradigm. The functional analysis should be based on multiple sources of information, information about the client in the natural environment, an initial broadly focused assessment strategy, and a thorough knowledge of the relevant empirical literature.

Criterion-Related Validity and Accuracy

Criterion-related validity and accuracy of the functional analysis refer to the degree to which the specific judgments included in a functional analysis (see "Components" in this chapter) represent the "true" state of affairs for the client. With criterion-related validity, we ask questions such as: Does the functional analysis accurately rank order the importance of the client's behavior problems? Does the functional analysis accurately estimate the strength of functional relations relevant to the client's behavior problems and goals?

As we discussed in Chapter 10, validity is best estimated from the magnitude of congruence among multiple indices. For example, an assessor may estimate, on the basis of an interview, that a client's episodes of depressed mood are strongly related to marital conflicts, and that subsequent thoughts about a hopeless and uncontrollable future serve to maintain the depressed mood. The validity of these judgments can be estimated by examining the degree to which data from self-monitoring, questionnaires, or analogue assessment of marital conflict confirms these hypothesized relations.

Applications and Restrictions on Clinical Applicability of the Functional Analysis

The functional analysis is applicable to all behavior problems that are affected by controllable variables. As we noted earlier, the underlying concepts or methods of the functional analysis are not limited to a particular type of functional variable or a particular mode of behavior problem.

Several papers (e.g., Haynes and O'Brien, 1990; Lennox, Miltenberger, Spengler, & Efanian, 1988; Singh, Deitz, Epstein, & Singh, 1991) have examined the frequency with which behavioral intervention decisions are based on preintervention data on behavior problems or functional relations. All studies lead to similar inferences: Intervention decisions were most often based on nomothetic causal models of the behavior problems and infrequently based on a functional analysis of behavior problems and functional relations. Furthermore, despite frequent emphasis in the literature on the importance of the functional analysis and clinical case formulations, there is no evidence that the use of the functional analysis is increasing over time. For example, in a review of 259 single-subject assessment and intervention studies on behavior problems, published from 1985 through 1993 in major behavioral journals (*Behavioral Assessment*, *Behavior Modification*, *Behavior Research and Therapy*, *Behavior Therapy*, *Journal of Applied Behavior Analysis*), O'Brien and Haynes (1997) found that only 20% used a preintervention functional analyses to guide intervention design.

Can interventions that are instituted without a functional analysis harm clients? Adverse effects are most likely when interventions can be aversive for the client, such as in the use of restraint, imaginal flooding, or punishment. It may be particularly important to precede use of aversive procedure with a careful functional analysis that supports the importance of such decelerative procedures.

Often, there are few adverse consequences associated with an intervention that are not based on a functional analysis. In these cases the main benefit of the functional analysis may be increased intervention efficiency or cost-effectiveness. For example, the use of muscle relaxation techniques in treatment of a client with tension headaches when those headaches are not a function of increased muscle tension may not be the most effective intervention but is unlikely to harm the client (acknowledging that a delay of positive intervention effects could be considered "harmful"). However, even in cases of "no harm," the magnitude or speed of behavior change is an important consideration in judging the intervention utility of the functional analysis.

We strongly endorse the potential utility of the functional analysis in clinical assessment—a validly constructed functional analysis can serve as a guide to intervention strategies, help the clinician clarify his or her judgments about the client, and help the clinician communicate these judgments to others. Nevertheless, all clinical case formulations are likely to be more useful in some conditions than in others. Given that the functional analysis takes time to construct and that it should be based on valid multisource preintervention assessment, it is likely to be cost-effective when:

- The clinical case is complex. It may be more useful with clients who have multiple behavior problems and the behavior problems are affected by multiple and complexly interacting causal variables.
- Causal variables differ across persons with the same behavior problem. In these cases, which seem to include most behavior problems encountered in behavior therapy, a diagnosis or problem behavior identification is not sufficient to identify causal factors and, consequently, is insufficient to plan intervention strategies.
- Valid methods are available for the measurement of a particular behavior problem and causal variables and other moderators of intervention outcome.
- There is a valid intervention strategy to modify the causal variables identified in the functional analysis.

- A standardized intervention program does not effectively and efficiently address all of the causal variables for a particular behavior problem.
- A standardized intervention program not based on a functional analysis has failed for a particular client.
- Variables that have been identified in nomothetic research are important as moderators of intervention outcome.

Several factors may explain why the functional analysis appears to be infrequently used in behavior therapy. First, financial incentives may sometimes be involved. Although financial contingencies are changing with an increasing focus on accountability and the mandate to document intervention decisions (Hayes, Follette, Dawes, & Grady, 1995), the time required to construct clinical case formulations is often not reimbursed by third-party payers and detracts from time devoted to reimbursed intervention. Cost-effectiveness issues are important—the time required to construct the functional analysis must be associated with enhanced intervention effectiveness or efficiency. Functional analyses will be reimbursed if it can be shown that the time devoted to their construction is warranted by increased effectiveness and efficiency.

Second, the complex functional relations in a functional analysis are difficult to organize in a clinically useful manner. It is insufficient to collect data on multiple variables and relations from multiple sources. Those data must be organized in a manner that facilitates intervention decisions and other clinical judgments. The Functional Analytic Clinical Case Model is one strategy of organizing the results of behavioral assessment and describing a functional analysis. The visual models presented by Nezu and Nezu and Linehan are other ways.

Treatment Validity

As we noted, the main measure of utility and validity of the functional analysis is the degree to which intervention based on a functional analysis is more effective than treatment not based on a functional analysis. Haynes, Leisen, and Blaine (1997) reviewed 20 studies on the relationship between components of the functional analysis and intervention outcome.[2] For example, Chorpita and associates (1996) used parent and child interviews to identify the maintaining variables for school refusal. The authors found that interventions specific for each of the maintaining variables identified in the assessment resulted in reduced school refusal. Iwata and associates (1994) used systematic observation during clinic analogue situations to identify the factors maintaining self-injurious behaviors. They found that 80% of treatments based on the results of the functional analysis were successful; treatments not based on the functional analysis had minimal success.

Other authors designed and evaluated treatments that matched the results of a pretreatment functional analysis. Supportive studies include: Chapman, Fisher, Piazza, and Kurtz (1993), for drug overdose with an individual with autistic behaviors; Kearney and Silverman (1990) for school refusal by children and adolescents; Kennedy and Souza (1995), for eye poking. The results of these studies are moderately supportive of the treatment utility of the functional analysis. However some negative results have been obtained (e.g., Schulte et al., 1992), and methodological limitations limit the inferences that can be drawn from these studies. Few studies compared the outcome of treatments based versus those not based on the functional analysis. Furthermore, all studies involved only a few components of the functional

[2]Studies were drawn from a survey of behavioral intervention and assessment journals and were selected for inclusion if they tailored intervention to the results of a preintervention behavioral assessment. Few of these are methodologically sound. Often there are no appropriate control groups, some are single uncontrolled cases, some did not match interventions to identified functional relations, and some use unvalidated interventions.

analysis, such as a small set of functional relations or treatment effects across different behavior problems. The value of a complete functional analysis has not been investigated. In sum, the functional analysis has a strong conceptual basis. It has promising but undemonstrated treatment validity.

Functional Analytic Clinical Case Models

Introduction and Illustration

A Functional Analytic Clinical Case Model (FACCM) is a vector-graphic diagram of a functional analysis (Haynes, 1994; Haynes, Leisen, & Blaine, 1997). The FACCM includes behavior problems, the importance and relations among behavior problems, the strength and direction of causal and noncausal functional relations, and the modifiability of causal variables. The FACCM illustrates and quantifies all elements of the functional analysis.[3]

Figure 13-2 illustrates two FACCMs. These were based on data from interviews and questionnaires, self- and participant monitoring (by staff and the mother), and behavioral observations (in the institution classroom and in the clinic). The first is of an eight-year-old institutionalized boy with pervasive developmental disabilities. The immediate concerns of staff were that he was hitting his head and ears with his fists and thrusting his head back against chairs and walls. Because of his self-injurious behaviors, his hands were often gloved and a foam brace was often placed around his neck, both of which restricted his movement and ability to interact with his environment. The FACCM was also congruent with findings in the literature on functional relations with severe behavior problems (e.g., Iwata et al., 1994).

The second FACCM is of a 36-year-old woman who had recently left her friends and family in her hometown to be with her husband in a different state, who died suddenly, six months prior to the assessment, of a heart attack. At the time of his death she had been taking courses at a community college and working part time as a medical technician. After his death, she lived alone with her eight-year-old daughter and became increasingly seclusive, dropped out of school and quit her job, had difficulty engaging in daily activities (e.g., cleaning, care of her daughter), and had intermittent panic episodes when outside of the home. Her daughter began taking more responsibility for household tasks, such as shopping and housework, and during observations the daughter was highly solicitous, reflective, and reassuring whenever the mother expressed any self-doubts or feelings of negative mood.

The information contained in the FACCMs is explained in Figure 13-3. Other examples of FACCMs can be found in O'Brien and Haynes, 1995a; Haynes, Leisen, and Blaine, 1997; Floyd, Haynes, and Kelly, 1997; and Nezu, Nezu, Friedman, and Haynes, 1997. The FACCM can be useful in several ways. First, the FACCM organizes the assessor's clinical judgments relating to a client's behavior problems and their causes. Second, the FACCM encourages a sequential, systematic, and specific approach to clinical case formulation and decision making by decomposing the functional analysis into its component clinical judgments. This approach may be particularly helpful to new clinicians. Third, the FACCM can help guide assessment efforts by indicating variables and relations in need of additional assessment. Fourth, the FACCM facilitates clinical case presentations to other professionals. It presents the clinician's hypoth-

---

[3]Some elements of FACCMs are borrowed from structural equations modeling (Loehlin, 1998) and vector geometry. However, FACCMs are not nomothetic models and do not adhere to constraints associated with traditional path models. Crewe and Dijkers (1995) noted that variables in a functional analysis correspond to latent variables, and that a full structural model would have multiple observed variables for each latent variable.

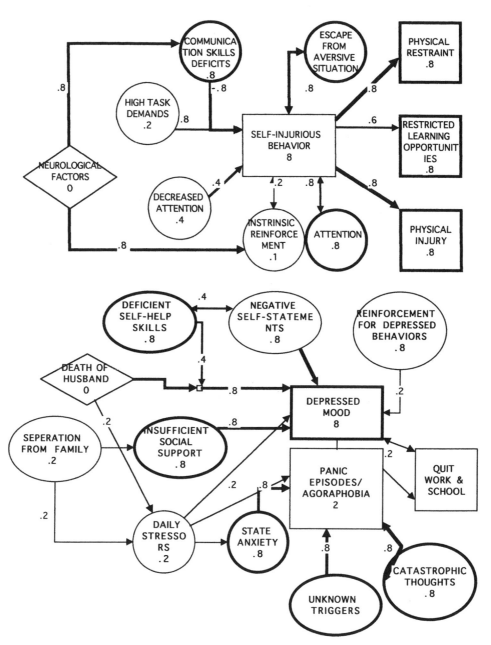

Figure 13-2. A Functional Analytic Clinical Case Model of a boy with self-injurious behaviors and a woman with panic episodes.

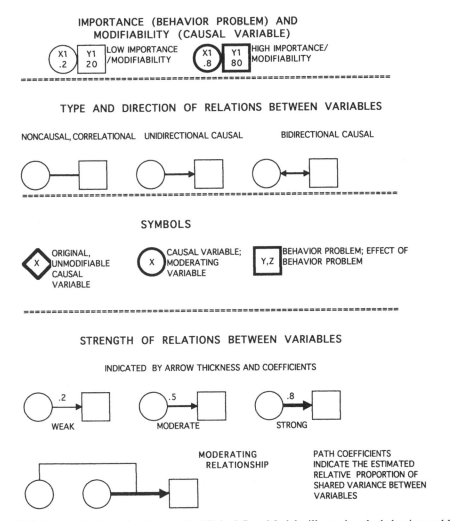

ILLUSTRATING A FUNCTIONAL ANALYSIS WITH A
FUNCTIONAL ANALYTIC CLINICAL CASE MODEL

IMPORTANCE (BEHAVIOR PROBLEM) AND
MODIFIABILITY (CAUSAL VARIABLE)

TYPE AND DIRECTION OF RELATIONS BETWEEN VARIABLES

NONCAUSAL, CORRELATIONAL   UNIDIRECTIONAL CAUSAL   BIDIRECTIONAL CAUSAL

SYMBOLS

STRENGTH OF RELATIONS BETWEEN VARIABLES

INDICATED BY ARROW THICKNESS AND COEFFICIENTS

Figure 13-3. Legend for Functional Analytic Clinical Case Models, illustrating the behavior problems, causal variables, and functional relations.

eses about a client in a manner that allows professionals from other disciplines and non-behavioral clinicians to understand the clinical case formulation and the basis of treatment decisions.[4] Fifth, because the FACCM quantifies clinical judgments, it encourages research on the clinical judgment process. Sixth, a FACCM can be used to illustrate variables and relations that affect treatment goals, as part of a constructional approach to assessment and treatment. Lastly, and most importantly, the FACCM guides decisions about which variables should be

[4]We have found that removing the numbers in the FACCM and using line widths and arrows increases the acceptance of FACCMs by professionals who are not quantitatively oriented.

selected as treatment targets for an individual client. By using numerical estimates of many judgments, the assessor can estimate the relative magnitude of effect that would be associated with treatment focused on each causal variable.

Estimating the Magnitude of Treatment Foci: The Elements of a FACCM

An important goal of an FACCM is to quantify elements of the functional analysis to help estimate the relative magnitude of treatment effects that would be associated with the modification of each causal variable associated with the client's behavior problems. As illustrated by the previous figures, FACCMs quantify judgments about the type and direction of all elements of the functional analysis.

Type and Direction of Functional Relations

A client's multiple behavior problems and related variables can have no functional relations, noncausal functional relations, or unidirectional causal or reciprocal causal relations. Reciprocal causal relations are particularly important for intervention decisions and are illustrated by several arrows in Figure 13-2a and 13-2b.

The Strength of Functional Relations: Path Coefficients

Path coefficients are the estimated degree of correlation $(0 > 1)$ between two variables across time for a client. For causal paths, FACCM path coefficients represent the estimated magnitude of causal relation—the degree to which change in the causal variable will result in change in the behavior problem (or goal attainment). Changes in a behavior problem are presumed to result in no change in a correlated, noncausal behavior problem unless treatment affects causal variables for both behavior problems.

Causal Variable Modifiability Coefficients

As we noted earlier, some causal variables have an important effect but are not modifiable (e.g., historical, genetically based, those that depend on help from uncooperative staff or family). The modifiability of a causal variable affects the clinicians decision about whether treatment should focus on that variable. The estimated modifiability of a causal variable is represented in FACCMs by a coefficient $(0 > 1)$. "0" indicates a causal variable that cannot be modified and "1" indicates a causal variable that is totally modifiable.

Causal Chains

We also noted that unmodifiable variables often have modifiable sequelae, which mediate the effects of the original causal variable. These are illustrated by chains of causal variables leading to a behavior problem.

The Importance of Behavior Problems

Decisions regarding the best initial treatment focus for clients with multiple behavior problems are also affected by the clinician's estimates of the relative importance of the behavior problems for each client and are indicated by values associated with problem behaviors. The scale used to depict relative importance of behavior problems is unimportant because FACCMs are idiographic. The only purpose of the numerical values is to place behavior problems on some ordinal scale of importance, for a particular client. Decisions about treatment focus will not differ as a function of whether two behavior problems are rated .8 and .4 or they are rated .4 and .2. In each case the first problem has been rated as twice as important as the second. Consequently, the relative magnitude of effect estimates are influenced only by the relative indices of importance of the behavior problems.

Behavior Problem Sequelae and Interrelations

Behavior problems can have effects and functional interrelations that influence the estimated magnitude of effect of a causal variable. As we noted in our discussion of reciprocal causation, a behavior problem may be an early or intermediate element in a chain of behavior problems and may function as a causal variable for other behavior problems. Excessive alcohol intake may lead to marital conflicts, domestic violence, and disrupted sleep. The contribution of behavior problem interrelations and sequelae to the magnitude of effect of an intervention is estimated using variable weights and path coefficients, as outlined above. Because sequelae are additive effects, they are treated as separate paths and their effects are added to the effects of preceding paths, as indicated in Figures 13-4 to 13-6.

FACCM and Treatment Decisions: Estimating the Magnitude of Effect

FACCMs help the clinician make decisions about the focus of intervention programs by estimating the relative magnitude of effect that would be expected from intervening with any

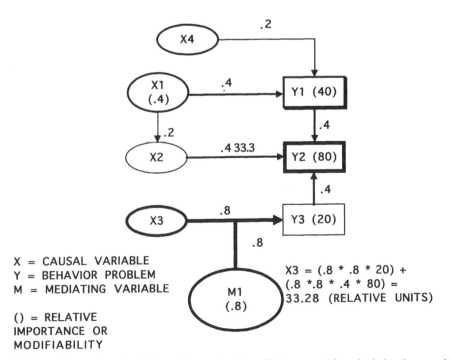

Figure 13-4. An illustration of variable weights and path coefficients, used for calculating the magnitudes of effect in Functional Analytic Clinical Case Models.

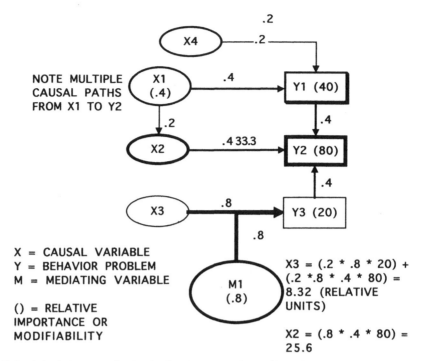

Figure 13-5. Calculating Magnitude of Effect in an FACCM: Effect of Changing Clinical Utility of X3 (from Figure 13-4).

causal variable hypothesized to affect the client's behavior problems or goals. The concept of magnitude of effect is invoked to help the behavior therapist estimate the relative benefits (and disadvantages) to a client of modifying any causal variable in an FACCM. The magnitude of effect is a quantitative estimate of the aggregated effects, weighted for importance, expected to result from the modification of a causal variable.

Acknowledging that there are other important considerations that affect intervention decisions (see Chapter 3), intervention efforts should be focused on those variables that have the greatest benefit for the client—those causal variables whose modification will result in the greatest reduction in the client's behavior problems or in the closest approximation to the client's treatment goals.

The estimated magnitude of treatment effects is derived from a multiplicative function that includes the strength of functional relations, the direction of causal relations, the modifiability of causal variables, all causal paths, the operation of moderating variables, and the relative importance of behavior problems. Essentially, the estimated magnitude of effect for a causal variable is derived by calculating the sum of all path coefficients between a causal variable and the client's behavior problems.

Figures 13-4 through 13-6 illustrate calculations of the relative magnitude of effect for a causal variable. They also illustrate the impact on the estimated magnitude of effect of changing judgments regarding the modifiability of a causal variable and of the importance of behavior problems. As these diagrams illustrate, small to moderate changes in a clinician's judgments about the elements in the functional analysis can have an important effect on treatment decisions.

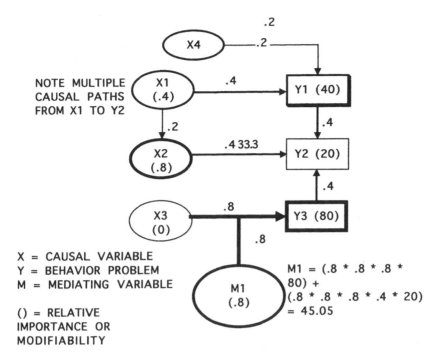

Figure 13-6. Calculating Magnitude of Effect in an FACCM #3 Changing Clinical Utility and Importance (from Figures 13-4 and 5).

As Figures 13-4 through 13-6 illustrate, the estimated magnitude of effect of the causal variable in an FACCM is a multiplicative function of all path and variable coefficients leading from the causal variable to the behavior problem. The sum of coefficients of paths emanating from a variable is an estimate of the treatment-related importance of that variable to contiguous downstream variables. In the case of multiple routes between a causal variable and a behavior problem, the magnitude of effect of a causal variable is the sum of the products of the coefficients of all routes between the causal variable and connected behavior problems. The magnitude of effect associated with a causal variable is useful only when contrasted with the estimated magnitudes of effects associated with other causal variables for the same client.

It may be helpful to reiterate the importance of "context" for interpreting the estimated magnitude of effect. The units of effect do not necessarily correspond to units of change in a dimension of a behavior problem. The behavior problem weights are subjectively scaled "importance" ratings. They could, but do not necessarily, correspond to behavior problem dimensions such as magnitude, duration, or rate.

Limitations of FACCMs

Functional Analytic Clinical Case Models have all the limitations ascribed to the functional analysis. They have a limited domain, their validity is limited by the validity of the measures used to guide the component judgments, they are only best estimates at a particular time, and they are unstable. FACCMs are limited in additional ways. First, the numerical values in an FACCM appear *pseudoprecise*, that is, they can imply an unwarranted level of measurement precision. The numerical values in an FACCM are derived from imperfect measures and they incorporate judgment errors. FACCMs are always "hypothesized" and subjectively constructed. Although hopefully based on systematically collected multimethod, multisource, time-series assessment data, FACCMs are often constructed from insufficient and conflicting assessment data. Consequently, FACCMs, and treatment decisions based on them, should be advanced prudently and tentatively.

Second, FACCMs take time to construct[5] and the cost-effectiveness limitations noted for the functional analysis are amplified for the FACCM. The utility of the FACCM is likely to covary with the complexity of the clinical case, the purpose of the clinical case formulation, the impact of treatment decisions, and the estimated effect of a standardized treatment program that can be implemented independent of a functional analysis. FACCMs are likely to be most useful in professional presentations, in training students in clinical assessment and case formulation, in making treatment decisions with client who have multiple behavior problems and multiple sources of causation, and in cases of failing treatments.

Third, an FACCM may be valid only within a limited domain. The FACCM may be valid for a limited time, for some situations and contexts but not others, and for only some client "states" (e.g., alcohol intoxication, medication).

Summary

Intervention paradigms differ in the degree to which intervention strategies are standardized or individualized across client. Behavioral interventions are sometimes standardized but are often individualized.

Individualized interventions reflect several characteristics and underlying assumptions of behavioral assessment and intervention paradigms: (a) the behavioral intervention paradigm includes many intervention methods, (b) client often have multiple behavior problems, (c) a behavioral intervention strategy usually targets only a limited array of causal variables and behavior problems, (d) the characteristics of a behavior problem and disorder can differ across clients, (e) variables that moderate intervention effects can differ across clients, and (f) the same behavior problem can be a result of different permutations of causes across clients.

Preintervention clinical assessment is an important component of the intervention process and is linked to the design of individualized intervention programs through the clinical case formulation—an integrated array of intervention-relevant clinical judgments about a client. Models for behavioral clinical case formulation have been proposed by Haynes and O'Brien (1990), Linehan (1993), Nezu and Nezu (1989), and Persons (1989).

Nezu and Nezu (1989) have developed a "problem-solving" approach to clinical case formulation, which focuses on "problems" faced by clinicians, such as selecting the best intervention strategy. Problems to be solved by the clinician include the identification of the client's problems and determining if intervention is possible, analysis of the client's problems and determining intervention goals, and determination of the best intervention strategy. Nezu and Nezu also suggest that a Clinical Pathogenesis Map (CPM) can guide and illustrate these judgments.

Persons and Tompkins (1997) have developed a cognitive behavioral (CB) Case Formulation model that integrates topographical features of a client's behavior problems and functional

[5]Haynes, Richard, O'Brien, and Grant (1999) have developed an interactive computer program to help construct an FACCM and calculate magnitudes of effects. Information about this program is available from the first author.

relations. CB Case Formulation is particularly congruent with cognitive theories of behavior problems and includes four components: (1) a behavior problems list, (2) a core beliefs list, (3) activating events and situations, and (4) working hypotheses.

Linehan (1993) presented a contextual and systems-oriented model for the case formulation focused on the intervention of a client with borderline personality disorders. Her model integrates a biosocial causal model of the original and maintaining causes of BPD, learning principles, and a stage theory of intervention (which she termed Dialectical Behavior Therapy).

These models are congruent in that they emphasize the importance of preintervention assessment, clinical case formulation, specification of a client's behavior problems, multiple and idiosyncratic causal factors for a behavior problem, the impact of the clinician's orientation and judgment, and the utility of a written or visual display of the clinical case formulation.

The functional analysis (Haynes & O'Brien, 1990) is "the identification of important, controllable, causal and noncausal functional relations applicable to specified behaviors for an individual." The functional analysis emphasizes important, controllable, causal relations relevant to a client's behavior problems. It is a clinical case formulation that may be informed by multiple methods of assessment.

There are several components of the functional analysis. They include (a) the client's behavior problems and/or intervention goals and their relative importance, sequelae, and interrelations, (b) the importance, modifiability, and interrelations among contiguous social/environmental antecedent and consequent causal variables, and (c) the operation of moderator and mediator variables.

The functional analysis includes different types of functional relations and is a "best estimate" derived from multiple clinical judgments by the assessor. A valid functional analysis does not preclude the possibility of other valid functional analyses. It is also unstable over time, can be at different levels of specificity, and has domains of validity. A functional analysis is an integration of nomothetic and idiographic data and can include extended social systems. It is congruent with and amenable to a goal-oriented, constructional approach to assessment.

The content and criterion validity of a functional analysis refers to the degree to which it reflects and accurately represents the important causal variables relevant to the client's behavior problems. Insufficient content validity is a major threat to intervention utility.

Although the functional analysis is applicable to all behavior problems that are affected by controllable variables, it is infrequently used to guide behavioral intervention strategies. This points to the difficulties in developing a functional analysis and the conditional nature of its utility. Clinical case formulations may be most useful in situations involving a complex clinical case, where causal variables differ across persons with the same disorder, where valid assessment methods are available, where there is a valid intervention strategy that can be implemented, and where a standardized intervention program was not effective or a valid program has failed. Additional research is needed on types and patterns of behavior problems, client characteristics, causal variables, and assessment methods that affect the utility and validity of the functional analysis.

Intervention validity, the degree to which intervention based on a functional analysis is more effective than treatment not based on a functional analysis, is the main index of validity. The results of these studies are moderately supportive of the treatment utility of the functional analysis. However some negative results have been obtained (e.g., Schulte et al., 1992).

In sum, in many clinical assessment contexts, the clinical case formulation is an important component of the assessment-treatment process. Although still in development, in terms of concepts and methods, clinical case formulations will grow over time.

Clinical judgments are often influenced by the clinicians biases, but these biases may be reduced with FACCMs. An FACCM is a vector diagram of a functional analysis of an individual client. FACCMs help determine the focus of intervention programs by indicating the estimated relative magnitude of effect expected from intervening with various hypothesized causal variables operating on the client's behavior problems or goals. The magnitude of effect of a particular treatment focus can be estimated by using path coefficients.

FACCMs have several limitations. They are unstable, hypothesized, and may be limited to particular situations. However, the validity and clinical utility of FACCMs can be enhanced with multimethod, multisource, multimodal time-series assessment and by attending to the level of variables and the comprehensiveness of the model.

Suggested Readings

Clinical Case Formulation in Behavior Therapy

Koerner, K., & Linehan, M. M. (1997). Case formulation in dialectical behavior therapy. In T. D. Eells (Ed.), *Handbook of psychotherapy case formulation* (pp. 340–367). New York: Guilford.

Nezu, A. M., Nezu, C. M., Friedman, S. H., & Haynes, S. N. (1997). Case formulation in behavior therapy: Problem-solving and functional analytic strategies. In: T. D. Eells (Ed.), *Handbook of psychotherapy case formulation* (pp. 368–401). New York: Guilford.

Persons, J. B., & Tompkins, M. A. (1997). Cognitive-behavioral case formulation. In T. D. Eells (Ed.), *Handbook of psychotherapy case formulation* (pp. 314– 339). New York: Guilford.

Functional Analysis Concepts

Alessi, G. (1988). Direct observation methods for emotional/behavior problems. In E. S. Shapiro & T. R. Kratochwill (Eds.), *Behavioral assessment in schools, Conceptual foundations and practical applications* (pp. 14–75). New York: Guilford.

Haynes, S. N. (1998). The assessment-treatment relationship and functional analysis in behavior therapy. *European Journal of Psychological Assessment, 14*(1), 26–34.

Haynes, S. N., Leisen, M. B., & Blaine, D. D. (1997). Functional analytic clinical case models and clinical decision-making. *Psychological Assessment, 9,* 334–348.

Haynes, S. N. & O'Brien, W. O. (1990). The functional analysis in behavior therapy. *Clinical Psychology Review, 10,* 649–668.

O'Brien, W. H. & Haynes, S. N. (1995). A functional analytic approach to the conceptualization, assessment and treatment of a child with frequent migraine headaches. *In Session, 1,* 65–80.

Methods of Deriving a Functional Analysis

Journal of Applied Behavior Analysis, 27, 1994, p. 211 (presentations of functional analysis of severe behaviors of children with developmental disabilities using mostly ABA experimental manipulation designed and carried out in clinic situations).

Schill, M. T., Kratochwill, T. R., & Gardner, W. I. (1996). Conducting a functional analysis of behavior. In M. J. Breen & C. R. Fiedler (Eds.), *Behavioral approach to assessment of youth with emotional/behavioral disorders—A handbook for school-based practitioners* (pp. 83–180). Austin, TX: PRO-ED.

Glossary

Listed below are definitions for terms and phrases used in psychological assessment. Often, a term has been used in different ways. When multiple definitions are provided, the first one most closely approximates the definition used in this book. Citations are provided where definitions were strongly influenced by other sources or where terms are discussed in greater detail.

Acceleration   The rate of change of speed; for example, it can be measured in units of x axis, per unit of y axis, per units of y axis, or (x/y^2).

Accuracy   (1) The extent to which obtained measures approximate the "true" state of nature (Foster & Cone, 1995; Johnston & Pennypacker, 1993; Silva, 1993). (2) Correctness. Precision. Exactness (James & James, 1992). (3) The degree to which obtained data are correct measures of targeted phenomena. (4) The degree to which the measurement represents the objectively defined topographic characteristics of the measured event (Cone, 1988). Used most often but not exclusively with behavioral observation.

Actimeter   An instrument used to measure movement.

Acquiescence   A *response set*. The degree to which measures derived from an assessment instrument reflect the respondents tendency to answer "yes" or "true" to instrument items (Anastasi & Urbina, 1997).

Adaptive testing   A procedure in which the set or sequence of items on an assessment instrument are administered to an individual as a function of the individual's status on the trait being measured. Can be fixed length adaptive testing, clinical decision adaptive testing, or countdown method. Done to decrease administration time with long assessment instruments.

Aggregated measure   A measure composed of multiple elements joined in an additive or multiplicative process. Also termed a *composite measure*.

Agreement   (1) The degree of correspondence between the output of two or more assessment instruments. (2) The degree of overlap between two more independently obtained measures.

Analogue assessment   (1) A procedure in which the subject is systematically exposed to one or more hypothesized causal variables while measures of dependent variables (usually the target behavior) are obtained. (2) Assessment under conditions different from the situation to which one wishes to generalize (Kazdin, 1998).

Analogue assessment, behavior   Direct measurement of behavior in situations different from the participant's natural environment (e.g., role-play assessment of social skills; observation of parent–child interactions in clinic play room) and in which the behavior measured is assumed to be analogous to the primary behavior of interest (e.g., measuring bar-press of a client to estimate how he or she would respond to various classes of reinforcers).

Antecedent event   A stimulus or event that occurs immediately before a response or another event.

Assessment instrument   A specific procedure for deriving data on the behavior of a person or persons on a specific assessment occasion (e.g., a specific self-report depression questionnaire; a specific marital interacting observation and coding system).

Assessment method   A class of procedures for deriving data on the behavior of a person or persons (e.g., self-report questionnaires, behavioral observations in the natural environment, interviews).

Assessment strategy   The overall plan of action for deriving assessment data. It involves a particular set of assessment instruments, instructions to client, and time-sampling parameters.

Attenuation   A reduction in estimates of covariance, usually a result of measurement error.

Autocorrelation (serial correlation; serial dependency)   The extent to which values in one part of a time-series predict values in subsequent parts of the time-series. It occurs when residual error terms from measures of a variable taken at different times are correlated (Vogt, 1993).

Baseline condition   (1) A phase of data acquisition prior to intervention. (2) A condition or phase of an experiment in which the independent variable is not present (Johnston & Pennypacker, 1993).

Base rate   The unconditional probability of an event or category for a specified time, condition, or place (e.g., rate of persons coming to a mental health center from a specific ethnic group or who report family violence; rate of a client's panic episodes prior to treatment).

Behavior   Most often used to refer to a class of responses (e.g., hitting, interrupting); often used synonymously with response class (Johnston & Pennypacker, 1993).

Behavior avoidance test (BAT)   An assessment method in which a person is requested to approach a feared object, or emit a feared behavior. Obtained measures during the BAT often involve physical proximity to the feared object, "anxiety" behaviors, thoughts, psychophysiological responses, and subjective distress.

Behavior disorder/behavior problem   Generic terms of convenience used to refer to a target of clinical intervention. The use of these terms does not imply that the disorder/problem is an empirically validated construct or that it is composed of a reliably covarying set of behaviors, such as is implied in DSM-IV. It also does not imply that there is an "underlying" cause to a group of "symptoms." Thus, "behavior disorders" or "behavior problems" may be used, interchangeably, at a variety of levels to refer to self-stimulatory behaviors, self-reported depressed affect, amount of exercise, negative self-statements, excessive caloric intake. Sometimes referred to as "maladaptive behavior."

Behavior therapy   A term referring to multiple intervention strategies and models such as contingency management, systematic cognitive therapies, behavioral marital and family therapy, and desensitization. Behavior therapies are often closely tied to principles derived from basic areas of psychology research, such as cognitive psychology, social psychology, psychobiology, and especially learning.

Behavioral chaining   A series of behavior-environment events in which each event serves as a discriminative stimulus for the following event (Donahoe & Palmer, 1994).

Behavioral scientist-practitioner   A generic term used to refer to a clinician or behavioral scientist who is assessing, treating, or conducting research on behavior disorders. This term implies an integration of empirical methods with clinical assessment and treatment.

Believability   The extent to which judges believe that the data from an assessment instrument represent the phenomena they are intended to represent and therefore warrant interpretation (Johnston & Pennypacker, 1993).

Beta   The probability of erroneously accepting a null hypothesis (Type II error).

Bias, clinical judgment   A systematic, nonrandom error in clinical judgment. Sources of bias may be age, sex, ethnicity of the client, or a priori ideas of the clinician.

Bias, measure or assessment instrument   A statistical characteristics of the test score derived from an assessment instrument or inferences based on the test score. When a score or inferences derived from an assessment instrument errors in a systematic manner (Murphy & Davidshofer, 1994).

Bias, measurement   When an assessment instrument errors systematically in measuring a variable or construct (Murphy & Davidshofer, 1994) (see *Bias, measure or assessment instrument*).

Bias, prediction   Systematic errors in predicting a criterion (Murphy & Davidshofer, 1994) (see *Bias, measure or assessment instrument*).

Calibration   A method of establishing the scales of an assessment instrument by comparing obtained scores with the scores obtained from a "gold standard" instrument.

Catalytic variable   A variable that is necessary for the causal relation between two other variables. It "enables" such a relation.

Categorical variable   A variable (nominal) that distinguishes among subjects by placing them into categories (Vogt, 1993).

Causal discontinuity   Variation in the strength or form of a causal relation between two variables. The variation may be a function of time, the magnitude (or other dimension) of the variables, or developmental epochs of the person (Haynes, 1992).

Causal indicators   When an aggregated score of an assessment instrument is presumed to be a function of the variables of which it is composed (Bollen & Lennox, 1991).

Causal latency   The time between a causal event (or a change in a causal variable) and its effect. Effect can be defined as the initial effect, maximum effect, or some other criteria.

Causal marker   A variable that covaries with the strength of causal relation between two other variables (e.g., when response to a laboratory stressor is highly corrolated with responses to a stressor that occurs in the natural environment).

Causal mechanism   The means through which a causal effect is produced. It answers the questions of "How or why does X cause Y."

Causal model (of behavior disorders)   A qualitative and/or quantitative description of the variables hypothesized to be associated with variance in a behavior disorder. It emphasizes important, controllable causal variables and depicts the form, strength, and direction of causal and noncausal (correlational) relations (Haynes, 1992).

Causal relation   Two variables have a causal relation when they have a functional relation, when the hypothesized causal variable reliably precedes the effect, when there is a logical mechanism for the hypothesized causal relation, and when alternative explanations for the observed covariance can reasonably be excluded.

Causal variable   A variable that controls a proportion of the variance in another variable; causal variables precede and are correlated with their effects, have a logical connection with their effects, and the association between the causal variable and the effect cannot be wholly attributed to a common effect of another variable (Haynes, 1992).

Causal vector diagrams   Illustrate the strength and direction of functional and causal relations among a set of variables.

Ceiling effect   Low magnitudes of variability or shared variance because one or both variables has approached its upper limit.

Client   A person, group, or system targeted in assessment. "Client" may refer to an individual, outpatient, or inpatient, a person with developmental disabilities, a family, a teacher, a classroom, the administrators of a large bank, or group of substance abusers.

Clinical applicability (of an assessment instrument)   The degree of clinical utility of an assessment instrument across clinical populations, settings, ages, and other sources of individual differences.

Clinical judgment   A prediction or decision regarding a client. Clinical judgments include diagnosis, functional analysis, the prediction of behavior, treatment design, and treatment-outcome evaluation.

Clinical significance/substantive significance   The extent to which an obtained measure or effect (e.g., intervention effect, estimate of shared variance between variables) is important, has practical value, or can guide clinical judgments. The degree to which measures contribute meaningful information. Often contrasted with "statistical significance."

Clinical utility (of an assessment instrument)   The degree to which the results of an assessment instrument enhance the validity of clinical judgments. The clinical utility of an assessment instrument can vary across its applications (e.g., diagnosis, brief screening).

Codes   Rules, usually in the form of definitions, for specifying how observations or measures should be classified or scored.

Coefficient   The numerical factor in an algebraic term (Karush, 1989), most often used as a multiplier.

Composite measure   (see *Aggregated measure*).

Compound stimulus   A stimulus that includes multiple components. Often, each component is capable of serving as a discriminative stimulus, or reinforcer, for different behaviors (Donahoe & Palmer, 1994).

Condition   (see *Domain*).

Conditional probability   The chance that an event will occur, given that some other event has occurred. If A and B are events, the conditional probability of A given B is the probability of A, assuming B holds. If $P(B) \neq 0$, then the conditional probability of P(A/B) of A given B is P(A and B)/P(B) (James & James, 1992; see Schlundt, 1985 for example of clinical application).

Conditioned (conditional) stimulus   A stimulus whose behavior-eliciting properties result from being paired with other eliciting stimuli, usually within a classical-conditioning paradigm (Donahoe & Palmer, 1994).

Confound; confounding variable   A variable that attenuates the effect of another, that attenuates a functional relation, or that makes it difficult to draw inferences about the relations between other variables.

Consensual observer drift   When two or more observers demonstrate similar observer drift over time (Johnson & Bolstad, 1975).

Constant conjunction   An invariable association between two events: Whenever Y occurs, X occurs. The idea that the causal variable must always be present if the effect occurs. Proposed by some as a necessary but insufficient condition for inferring causality, but rejected by many philosophers of science. It is not a condition that is necessary for causal inference in psychopathology (Haynes, 1992).

Construct   A synthetic variable, usually composed of multiple systematically related elements, that is inferred but cannot be directly observed. Similar to a *latent variable*.

Construct-irrelevant test variance   The assessment instruments include dimensions and facets that are irrelevant to the targeted construct (Messick, 1993).

Construct systems (in psychology)   An orderly conceptual system that integrates multiple variables and relations for the purpose of making predictions, explaining behavior, or guiding interventions. Construct systems may vary in level (e.g., neurophysiological vs. psychodynamic) and may have various foci (e.g., behavior disorder vs. treatment construct systems).

Construct underrepresentation   The assessment instrument fails to include important dimensions or facets of the targeted construct (Messick, 1993).

Constructionism   A model of epistemology and perception that holds that mental processes are required in order for an environmental event to be described (Donahoe & Palmer, 1994). Environmental stimuli are necessary but insufficient to understand or describe the environment.

Content validity   (see *Validity, content*).

Context (setting)   A naturally occurring environmental unit, having physical, behavioral, and temporal properties (e.g., family supper, outpatient clinic testing room, a group of strangers drinking wine, a particular classroom). The context often affects responses to stimuli presented to a person within it, often through classical or operant conditioning.

Contextual stimuli (context)   Stimuli and conditions that accompany specific antecedent-response-consequence associations. May involve a physical setting, occurring actions, physiological state, and historical events.

Continuous function   Where the values of a dependent variable are equally associated with the values of another variable throughout the values of both variables.

Continuous measurement   Measurement in which all possible occurrences of the targeted variable can be detected (Johnston & Pennypacker, 1993).

Continuous variable   A variable that can be measured on an interval or ratio scale across a large range of values (Vogt, 1993).

Correlation   A statistic that provides an index of how strongly two variables are associated. A correlation coefficient can range from -1 to $+1$, which indicate perfect inverse and positive relationships, respectively. A correlation of "0" indicates that two variables have no shared variance. Can be Pearson correlations (usually for variables measured on interval or ratio scales), Phi (usually for two dichotomous variables).

Cost-effectiveness (of an assessment instrument)   The cost (e.g., time, financial) of deriving information with an assessment instrument relative to the contribution of that information to a clinical judgment.

Covariation   When two variables vary together. One measure of the common variance between two variables is covariance—the mean of the summed cross products for two variables.

Criterion (predicted variable)   A variable to be explained or predicted from another variable (Pedhazur & Schmelkin, 1991) (see *Ultimate criteria* and *Intermediate criteria*).

Criterion contamination   When both a predictor and criterion instrument contain the same elements. When a predictor contains elements of a criterion. The estimate of shared variance between the two instruments (the predictive relation between the two constructs) is inflated because of shared elements (see *Item contamination*).

Criterion reference test (assessment instrument)   (1) An assessment instrument whose product is interpreted in reference to an established criterion (Silva, 1993). (2) An assessment instrument that yields measurements that are representative of targeted tasks and interpretable in terms of specified performance standards (Kratochwill & Roseby, 1988).

Criterion variance   Disagreement between judges (e.g., diagnosticians) that is attributable to insufficiently precise criteria (Spitzer, Endicott, & Robins, 1975).

Critical event sampling   An assessment strategy where the most important behaviors, contexts, or causal events are selected for measurement. Examples would be assessment only during panic episodes, marital arguments, and at bedtime for an oppositional child.

Critical level (in causal relations)   A *threshold level* in causal relations; when variation in the causal variable is associated with variation in the behavior disorder, only when the value of the causal and dependent variable exceeds a particular level (Haynes, 1992).

Critical period   (see *Sensitive period*).

Cross-lagged correlations   In two time-series, when two variables are correlated, with one variable lagged behind the other.

Cue   A *discriminative stimulus*.

Dependent variable   The variable that may change depending on the value (e.g., occurrence, magnitude) of the independent variable (Johnston & Pennypacker, 1993).

Desynchrony   Two variables have a different time-course and, as a result, show low levels of covariation.

Deterministic functional equation   A functional equation in which the criterion is completely determined by the predictors.

Deviation   A *response set*. The degree to which measures derived from an assessment instrument reflect the respondents tendency to provide unusual or uncommon responses (Anastasi & Urbina, 1997).

Diathesis-stress model (in psychopathology)   A model of behavior disorders that hypothesizes a biologically determined vulnerability to the effects of psychosocial stressors. Genetic and other physiological factors are presumed to affect the chance that a person will manifest schizophrenic symptoms, or other behavior disorders, upon exposure to environmental stressors.

Differential item functioning   When respondents from different groups respond differentially to an item (presuming that they are equal on the trait/construct that the item measures).

Differential reinforcement of incompatible behavior (DRI)   Reinforcement of a behavior that is incompatible with the target behavior. Usually done to reduce the rate of the target behavior (Grant & Evans, 1994).

Differential reinforcement of other behaviors (DRO)   (1) Omission training; reinforcement contingent on the absence of behavior for a period of time (Grant & Evans, 1994). Designed to reduce the rate of a behavior. (2) Differential reinforcement of incompatible behaviors; reinforcement of behavior other than the targeted behavior in order to reduce its occurrence; reinforcement of 0 rate responding.

Dimension (of measurement/assessment/event)   (1) Quantitative attribute of an event, such as the frequency, duration, magnitude, cyclicity, and rate of an event. A fundamental quantity on which psychological/behavioral phenomena can be measured. (2) A homogeneous facet of a construct, such as a "unidimensional" measure of fear. A multidimensional variable has several facets or aspects.

Dimensional measurement   Measurement that describes the amounts of the dimensional quantities of the targeted phenomena (Johnston & Pennypacker, 1993).

Discontinuous function   Where the units of change of one variable, as a function of a second variable, vary according to the values of either variable.

Discriminative stimulus   (1) A stimulus that has come to guide or control responding through being paired with differential reinforcement contingencies. (2) A stimulus that affects responding as a result of individual selection (Donahoe & Palmer, 1994). (3) A stimulus that has been consistently paired with a response contingency (Tryond, 1996).

Discriminative stimulus class   Multiple stimuli that have similar effects on responses; often, the stimuli share physical similarities (Donahue & Palmer, 1994).

Disposition   The heightened conditional probability that a person will emit a class of behaviors in a particular situation, or across time and situations.

Dissimulation   A *response set*. The degree to which measures derived from an assessment instrument reflect the respondent's intent to affect the derived inferences in a particular direction (e.g., an intent to appear healthy or disturbed on a questionnaire measure of psychopathology). Faking.

Dissimulation, negative   When a respondent responds in a way to purposefully appear "bad," "disordered," "distressed," or to exaggerate symptoms on an assessment instrument. Faking bad on an assessment instrument. Malingering.

Dissimulation, positive   When a respondent responds in a way to purposefully appear "good," "healthy," "nondistressed," or to minimize symptoms on an assessment instrument. Faking good on an assessment instrument.

Domain   (1) A quantifiable dimension a variable, sample, or population (e.g., behavior problem, causal variable, or group). Examples of parameters include magnitude, duration, level, latency, frequency, recovery rate, intensity, mean, and standard deviation.

Domain (of a causal relation)   Conditions under which a causal relation, or a particular form or strength of the causal relation, is operational. Domains may involve developmental stages, environmental settings and contexts, physiological states, parameter values, time, persons, or the presence or absence of particular variables.

Duration event   A behavior of homogeneous content whose onset and offset is recorded; its functional properties are associated with its duration as well as its occurrence (see *Event*).

Dynamic   An adjective indicating that the object or functional relation changes across time or as a function of some dimension.

Dynamic relation   A term suggesting that the form or strength of a relation can vary across time or some other parameter.

Ecological validity   The generalizability of findings to groups or populations that are of primary interest.

Ecologically valid observations   Observations that occur in natural settings; observations that occur in settings to which the inferences from the obtained data are generalizable to the group or population of interest.

Effect indicator model   A measurement model in which responses to test items are a function of the amount of the latent trait or construct possessed by the respondent (Bollen & Lennox, 1991).

Effect size   (1) A coefficient of the statistical relation between two variables. It is usually expressed as some form of "proportion of variance accounted for." (2) In treatment outcome research it is a way of expressing the difference between two groups in a metric that can be applied across studies (e.g., difference between means divided by pooled standard deviation) (Kazdin, 1998). (3) The mean difference between the control group and the treatment group [(mean1 − mean2)/SD of control group] or [(mean1 − mean2)/pooled SD] and then adjusted by instrument reliability coefficient.

Effectiveness (of a treatment)   (1) The magnitude of effects of a treatment when applied in typical clinical settings. (2) The degree to which intended effects are achieved (Vogt, 1993).

(3) The performance of a treatment under trial conditions (Ayd, 1995). Often confused with *efficacy*.

Efficacy (of a treatment)   (1) The degree to which changes in clients' behavior can be ascribed to hypothesized active treatment components. Inferences are based on comparisons with control groups (similar to internal validity) (Ayd, 1995; Kazdin, 1998). (2) The power to produce the intended effects. Often confused with *effectiveness*.

Efficiency (of a treatment)   The magnitude of change associated with a treatment relative to the cost (e.g., time, financial) of its delivery. In physics it is the output divided by the input.

Eliciting stimulus   A stimulus that reliably evokes behavior (Donahoe & Palmer, 1994).

Empiricism   In the behavioral sciences, an epistemology that emphasizes the use of observation and systematic experimentation and that deemphasizes theory. In philosophy of science, it is the assumption that only what is observable can be known, contrast to "rationalism" (Blackburn, 1994).

Epistemology   A branch of philosophy and philosophy of science that addresses the theory and methods of acquiring knowledge. The methods and criteria used to determine when something is "known," and sources of errors in the acquisition of knowledge (Blackburn, 1994).

Equilibrium latency   The time required for the effects of a causal variable to stabilize.

Equilibrium state   A condition in which the effects of a causal variable have stabilized.

Equilibrium time   (see *Equilibrium latency*).

Equivalence class   A class of stimuli or responses in which all members respond in a similar manner to the same stimulus. A type of functional stimulus or response class in which all members are similarly affected by selection processes (Donahoe & Palmer, 1994).

Error, systematic   Error in measures that are nonrandom and that occur in a consistent direction.

Error variance   Unexplained variance in a measure or effect.

Establishing operations   Stimuli or events that alter the rates of responses associated with a reinforcer or change the effectiveness of a reinforcer (Creer & Bender, 1993). Antecedent events that strengthen or weaken potential reinforcers. Sometimes referred to as setting events.

Eta squared   An effect size measure or correlation ratio used to describe the amount of variance accounted for in one variable by one or more other variables.

Event   In behavioral observation, a behavior of homogeneous content (Bakeman & Casey, 1995) and usually with an identifiable functional property (see *Duration event*; *Timed event*); sometimes called a *unit*.

Facets   Components that contribute to an overall whole, as in facets of a construct or variable. For example, there are behavior, cognitive, and physiological facets of the construct of depression. The construct of guilt is composed of hindsight bias, violation of personal standards, and beliefs of personal responsibility.

Factor   (1) A group of correlated variables that are presumed to affect another variable. (2) In factor analysis, a cluster of highly correlated variables within a larger group of variables. In mathematics and physiology the term has multiple meanings.

Factor analysis   Several methods of analysis to examine the pattern of covariance among multiple variables. A factor is composed of a cluster of highly intercorrelated variables.

Form (of a causal or noncausal functional relation)   The mathematical function(s) that best expresses the relation between two variables (e.g., log, liner, sine wave, parabolic, quadratic).

Frequency   Rate of recurrence of a periodic phenomena, per unit of time (Darton & Clark, 1994).

Functional analysis   (1) The identification of important, controllable, causal functional relations applicable to specified behaviors for an individual (Haynes & O'Brien, 1990) (see *Functional assessment*). (2) The experimental manipulation of hypothesized controlling variables as a method of determining functional relations.

Functional antecedents (antecedent controlling factors)   Discriminative stimuli; almost immediately before a R; in their presence, the effectiveness of a selected response increases or decreases (Alessi, 1988).

Functional assessment   (1) The identification of the antecedent and consequent events that are temporally contiguous to the target response, and that occasion and maintain it (Sisson & Taylor, 1993); similar to definition for functional analysis. (2) An assessment of functional capabilities; this definition is often used in rehabilitation psychology and neuropsychology.

Functional class (functional stimulus class)   Multiple stimuli that may differ in form but have similar effects.

Functional plateau   A special case of causal discontinuity in which a variable may have no causal relation to another variable (e.g., a behavior disorder) while its values remain within a particular range, but significant causal relations if its values fall below or rise above that range (Haynes, 1992).

Functional relation   A relation that can be expressed as an equation (Vogt, 1993). It does not imply a causal relation. A functional relation exists when two or more variables have shared variance. Some dimension (e.g., rate, magnitude, length, age) of one variable is associated with some dimension of another. In an alternative language, variables are functionally related when they demonstrate a mathematical relation (Haynes, 1992). A mathematically describable relation between two or more variables.

Functional response class   A set of behavior, that may differ in form, under the control of the same contingencies. A set of behaviors that has the same function (e.g., completion of a homework assignment, raising a hand in class, and talking to classmates may obtain teacher attention).

Functional response group (functional response class)   A set of behaviors that may differ in form and other characteristics and that are under the control of the same contingencies (multiple behaviors that have the same function). A set of topographically different dependent variables that have a similar functional relation to an independent variable (Schneider & Morris, 1988) (see *Equivalence class*).

Functional stimulus class   Multiple stimuli that may differ in form but have similar effects.

Functional variable   A variable that demonstrates a mathematical relation with another variable of interest.

Funneling (funnel strategy)   A strategy for assessment in which responses to more generally focused instruments or elements are used to select more specifically focused instruments and elements (e.g., broadly surveying behavior problems in an interview and then following up with assessment of the specific behavior problems reported by a client).

Fuzzy boundary (of a stimulus class)   A stimulus class in which no single element is necessary for its effects (e.g., functional relations, reinforcement effects).

Generalizability   The degree to which data or inferences derived from one sample, setting, or behavior are representative of data or inferences from another sample, setting, or behavior.

Graphic rating scale   (see *Visual analogue scale*).

Habituation   The weakening of an unlearned environment-behavior relation when the environmental event is repeatedly presented without consequence.

Hierarchy   A set of stimuli or responses rank ordered on some dimension.

Homogeneity   The conceptual integrity of a set of assessment instrument (or scale) elements (e.g., questionnaire items, behavior codes). The degree to which elements are similar or uniform. This judgment is often aided by measures of internal consistency (not to be confused with use of the term in statistical analyses).

Idiographic assessment   Assessment pertaining to an individual or individual case. Assessment procedures that are not standardized, and observed relations and results that are not necessarily generalizable, across persons or groups. Sometimes called idiothetic (e.g., Tallent, 1992) and incorrectly labeled "ideographic."

Incremental validity   (see *Validity, incremental*).

Index   A measure that is used to estimate another phenomenon, event, or functional relation.

Indicators   (see *Marker variable*).

Informants   Persons furnishing information about a participant/client; typically the participant and those with frequent contact, such as parents, teachers, spouses.

Instructional variables   Instructions to participants/clients that are given prior to an assessment procedure (e.g., instructions at the beginning of a questionnaire, verbal instructions prior to an interview).

Interactive interventions   An intervention strategy that mediates the effects of a causal variable (e.g., a therapy strategy to mediate the interpersonal and self-concept effects of a client's history of sexual abuse); as opposed to additive interventions that do not involve the same pathways as the causal variable.

Intermediate criterion   An indicator of an ultimate criterion; often more efficiently measured than an ultimate criterion (Pedhazur & Schmelkin, 1991).

Internal consistency   The degree of consistency of the items or elements within an assessment instrument. Can be reflected by split-half reliability, Kuder-Richardson 20 formula, coefficient alpha (Kazdin, 1998).

Interobserver, interrater, interscorer agreement   (1) The extent of agreement between scores (or ratings, diagnoses, behavior rates) obtained from different assessors. Can be indicated by percentage agreement, kappa, or correlation. (2) The extent to which different assessors agree on the scores they provide when assessing (e.g., rating, coding, classifying) a subjects performance (Kazdin, 1998).

Intervening variable   (see *Mediating variable*).

Item contamination   When two assessment instruments contain the same or similar elements. The magnitude of shared variance between the two instruments can overestimate the relation between the two constructs because of the duplicate items (see *Criterion contamination*).

Item discrimination   How well an item or other element of an assessment instrument (e.g., behavior code) discriminates among subjects who differ on the measured construct.

Item response theory   A measurement model that suggests that item difficulty and discrimination determine the probability of a response of a respondent who is at a given level on the targeted construct or trait.

Latency   The time between two events.

Latent causal variable   A causal variable that remains inactive unless triggered by other variables.

Level (of a causal relation)   The number of causal paths that can be subsumed within it or that are summed by it.

Level (of a variable)   The number of variables or paths included in a variable. High-level, less specific, variables can be partioned into many lower-level variables and paths.

Level of inference (specificity)   The number of elements or components subsumed by the variable label (Haynes, 1994). Behavior problems, goals, and causal variables at higher or lower levels (sometimes termed "molar" or "molecular," "higher-order," or "lower-order"). A higher level behavior problem is illustrated by "depression," that can refer to multiple lower-level phenomena such as motor slowness, negative affect, insomnia, and eating disturbances.

Level of measurement   The rules used to assign numbers to observations. Describes the amount of information contained in measurement scales (see *Scale*).

Longitudinal assessment   An assessment strategy that involves repeated measures of participants/subjects over time. Longitudinal assessment can, but need not, be *time-series assessment*.

Magnitude of effect   A measure of the strength of relation between variables, or the magnitude of change across time, or the magnitude of difference between groups. Indices of the magnitude of effect include "r," "R^2" (see *Effect size*).

Malingering   (see *Dissimulation, negative*).

Marker variable   A variable whose value is correlated with another variable of interest or the magnitude of covariance between variables. For example, a parental history of hypertension may serve as a marker variable for an increased probability of developing hypertension (the variable of interest) or a heightened cardiovascular response to laboratory stressors (the relation between environmental stressors and cardiovascular response) (Haynes, 1992).

Measure   (1) A number that represents the variable being measured. The score obtained from an assessment instrument (e.g., blood pressure reading, MMPI scale score, observed rate of behavior). (2) A system of units with which variables can be described (e.g., "ounces" to describe the variable "weight," "rate" to describe the variable "aggression") (James & James, 1992).

Measurement   The assignment of a numerical value to a variable dimension so that relations of the numbers reflect relations among the measured variables.

Measurement error   The part of an obtained measure that does not reflect true variance in the targeted variable.

Measurement invariance   The degree to which a score in one group means the same as the same score in another group.

Measurement/assessment strategy   (1) The procedures used to acquire data. (2) The assessment instruments used to acquire data and the methods in which they are applied. These methods may include time, behavior, and situation sampling parameters.

Mediating/moderator variable (intervening variable)   A variable that explains the relations between other variables. It provides a causal link between other variables (Vogt, 1993). Sometimes confused with *moderator variable*.

Mediating variable (mediator)   (1) A variable that accounts for, or explains, the relation between two other variables; similar to a *causal mechanisms* (Baron & Kenny, 1986; Shadish, 1996). (2) The mechanism through which the independent variable influences the dependent variable; the mediator is affected by the independent variable and affects the dependent variable.

Methodology   (1) The study of methods; the science of methods. (2) Application of the principles of logic and reasoning to scientific inquiry.

Moderator variable   A variable that can influence the strength and/or direction of the relation between two or more other variables (Baron & Kenny, 1986). A variable whose value covaries with (affects) the magnitude of a causal relation (Shadish, 1996).

Momentary event   A brief behavior of homogeneous content; its functional properties are typically associated with its occurrence rather than its duration.

Momentary time sampling   (1) Measuring a variable at a single instant in time. Sometimes referred to as "flash-point" sampling. (2) An observation procedure in which the observer only notes the status of the target behavior at the end of an interval.

Monomethod assessment   Assessment that includes only one method of gathering information. Assessment that involves only self-report, or only psychophysiological measures, is an example of monomethod assessment.

Multicollinearity   When two or more variables are highly correlated. In multiple regression it makes it difficult to separate their independent effects, and in psychological assessment it implies that two measures are tapping the same facets of the same variable.

Multiinformant assessment   Assessment that includes more than one informant, such as the client, parents, teachers, spouse, and staff members.

Multimethod assessment   Assessment that includes more than one method of gathering information, such as self-monitoring, psychophysiological assessment, and interviews.

Multimodal assessment   Assessment that targets more than one response mode, such as thoughts, behavior, physiological responses, and emotions.

Multisource assessment   Assessment that includes multiple sources of information, such as multiple methods, instruments, occasions, situations, and informants.

Negative predictive power   True negative rate/true negative + false negative rate; the proportion of individuals indicated as not having a disorder/behavior who truly do not; sometimes confused with *specificity*.

Nomothetic, assessment strategy   An assessment strategy in which judgments are based on the comparison of measures from the target person with data on the same instrument gathered from other persons, such as the use of normative or comparison groups.

Noncontiguous variables   Causal events that are temporally distant from the target behaviors. Noncontiguous causal variables such as childhood sex abuse and work stress can significantly affect temporally remote behaviors. Although noncontiguous causal variables are often clinically useful, their mechanism of action (e.g., specific social skills deficits of the abused child, attention deficits by a stressed parent) are often the targets of intervention and must be carefully specified.

Norm-referenced test (assessment instrument)   An assessment instrument whose product is interpreted in reference to the products of others from the same assessment instrument (Silva, 1993).

Observer drift   (1) When an observer rates the same event differently over time, in a systematic manner (Foster & Cone, 1986). (2) An unintended change in the accuracy of an observers' performance (Johnston & Pannypecker, 1993). When two or more observers drift in the same manner, it is called "consensual observer drift."

Obtrusive measure   An assessment instrument that affects the behavior of the participant; one that the participant is aware of and that produces *reactive effects*.

Operational definition   (1) The procedures or measures that are used to define a construct. (2) A definition of a construct in terms of the operations used to produce and measure it (Johnston & Pennypacker, 1993).

Original causes   The "first" cause in a sequence of events leading to a causal effect. For example, anoxic birth conditions may be considered an "original cause" of impaired social functioning.

Paradigm   The principles, beliefs, values, hypotheses, and methods advocated in a discipline or its adherents. An assessment paradigm includes beliefs and hypotheses about the relative importance of behavior problems, the causal variables that affect behavior, the mechanisms of causal action, the importance of assessment, and the best methods of obtaining data. It also includes guidelines for deductive and inductive problem solving, decision-making strategies, and data interpretation.

Parameter   (1) Sometimes used to refer to a "domain": A quantifiable dimension, a variable, sample, or population (e.g., behavior problem, causal variable, or group). Examples of parameters include magnitude, duration, level, latency, frequency, recovery rate, intensity, mean and standard deviation. (2) In statistics, a numerical characteristic (e.g., mean, standard deviation) estimated for a population. (3) A quantity that is constant for a particular individual or event, but may vary across individuals and events. (4) Limit or boundary.

Parsimony   (1) Maximizing the ratio of predictor/explanatory elements that provide a particular outcome. Economy of measurement and prediction. Given equal outcome (e.g., valid clinical judgment) the strategy that includes the least measures and variables is best. A principle applied to selecting the number of instruments to use for a given assessment goal, determining the number of variables needed to explain behavior problems, retaining elements of a multielement treatment program, and selecting the number of factors to retain in factor analysis. (2) A principle that emphasizes simplicity in models and explanations (McGuigan, 1990).

Partial function   A causal relation that only partially accounts for behavior. For example, the probability of relapse into schizophrenic behaviors following the cessation of psychotropic medication may be "partial function" of the degree of emotional support received from friends, indicating that other variables also contribute to the probability of relapse.

Participant observation   (1) Observation by a person who is normally part of the client's natural environment (e.g., teachers, staff, parents). (2) In ethnographic research, observation, usually qualitative, by an observer who is not normally part of the client's natural environment. The observer typically joins and participates in the natural environment in order to derive subjective judgments about the environment.

Path coefficient   A coefficient that expresses the strength of relation between two variables; usually expressed as the proportion of shared variance between the variables. Path coefficients may be either obtained or predicted.

Phase-space   The time-course context of a variable. The phase state of a variable is its historical and projected curve at the time of measurement.

Phenomenon (in psychological assessment)   An event that can be described and measured. An aggressive behavior, thought, traumatic life event, pain sensation, guilt feeling, and reprimand are phenomena.

Positive predictive power   (1) Indicates the positive "hit rate" for an assessment instrument score; true positive rate/true positive + false positive rate (e.g., the proportion of individuals identified by an instrument as having a disorder or emitting a behavior who truly have the disorder or emit the behavior). Sometimes confused with *sensitivity*.

Positivism   An epistemological system that stresses the importance of observable scientific facts and the relations among observables; it demeans the use of inferential constructs.

Power (of an assessment instrument)   (1) The predictive accuracy of measures from an assessment instrument. Usually estimated by the proportion of persons it accurately identified with (*sensitivity*) and without (*specificity*) an attribute (such as a diagnosis). (2) The probability of detecting a difference between groups when a difference truly exists (Kazdin, 1998).

Precision (of a measure)   (1) The degree to which a class of measurements approximate the "true" value as estimated through coefficients of internal consistency, temporal stability, and dispersion (Marriott, 1990). (2) The way in which repeated observations conform to themselves (Marriott, 1990).

Predictive efficacy   The degree to which a measure can predict another measure, usually taken at a later time, but a time frame can be implied rather than real (e.g., the degree to which an IQ measure predicts grades).

Predisposition   A "risk" factor. A person has a "predisposition" for a behavior when the probability that the behavior will occur, given a particular condition, is greater for the person than for people on average. Similar to *vulnerability*. Predispositions may be conditional or unconditional.

Premack principle (probability-differential hypothesis)   A higher probability response contingent on a lower probability response will result in an increase in the rate of a lower probability response. A lower probability response contingent on a higher probability response will result in a decrease in the rate of the higher probability response (Timberlake & Farmer-Dougan, 1991).

Psychological assessment   The systematic measurement of a person's behavior and the inferences derived from those measurements. It incorporates measurement strategies (e.g., observation, interviews), measurement targets (e.g., behavior problems, causal and correlated measurements), and the inferences and clinical judgments (e.g., functional analysis, estimates of treatment outcome) affected by the obtained measures.

Psychometry (psychometrics)   The evaluative processes applied to psychological assessment. Psychometrics is concerned with the evaluation of data from assessment instruments and the judgments based on that data. It is the science of psychological measurement.

Psychosocial stressor   An event characterized by social interaction that leads to negative behavioral, cognitive, or physiological consequences. They may include events such as marital arguments, rejection by an important person, and disapproval from a supervisor.

Random responding   A *response set*. The degree to which measures derived from an assessment instrument reflect the respondents tendency to provide random responses.

Range   The highest and lowest values of a variable or data set.

Rate   A relation between (one quantity in) one form of units and (another quantity in) another form of units (Darton & Clark, 1994). A relation between the units of one variable and the units of another variable. Often, rate is the frequency of an event per unit of time.

Rate-of-change   The magnitude of change of a variable across a period of time or across a dimension of another variable.

Ratio   A way of comparing two quantities by considering their quotient (by dividing one into the other) (Darton & Clark, 1994). In a ratio of 3:4, 3 is the "antecedent" and 4 is the "consequent."

Ratio scale   (see *Scale, ratio*).

Reactive effects (of assessment)   The degree to which an assessment instrument modifies the behavior of the target person or others in the target person's environment.

Recidivism   The probability of manifesting a behavior problem following successful treatment.

Recovery (post-stress)   Rate or speed of recovery to prestress levels following termination of a stressor, the degree to which a measure approximates prestress levels following termination of a stressor.

Reference period   Synonymous with base period. It may also refer to the length of time for which data are collected (Marriott, 1990).

Reinforcer   A stimulus that when presented contingent on a response, increases the rate of that response (Timberlake & Farmer-Dougan, 1991).

Reliability   (1) The part of test result that is due to permanent, systematic effects and therefore persists across time and settings (Marriott, 1990). (2) The stability of data yielded by an assessment instrument under constant conditions.

Reliability, alternative-form   The correlation between different forms of the same assessment instrument when all items are presumed to tap the same construct or to be drawn from the same pool.

Reliability, interrater   The degree to which different observers or raters agree on the dimensions (e.g., occurrence, magnitude) of an event or person being measured. Often estimated with Kappa or Intraclass correlation coefficients.

Reliability coefficient   A coefficient that represents the systematic component of a variate as distinct from its error component (Marriott, 1990) (see *internal consistency*).

Remote causal variable (noncontiguous causal variable)   A causal variable that is temporally distant from its effect (e.g., the effect of anoxic birth on grade school performance).

Resistance to extinction   The degree to which a response will continue to be emitted after the reinforcing stimulus has been omitted.

Response class   A collection of individual responses that have common sources of influence in the environment (Johnston & Pennypacker, 1993).

Response mode (response system)   The form, type, or method of behavior. Response modes are organizational categories or a taxonomy of behavior. Response modes can include motor, verbal, cognitive, physiological, and combinations of these, such as emotional.

Response set   Systematic or unsystematic variance in responses to an assessment instrument that are a function of variables other than the assessment instrument content. Can include *social desirability*, *dissimulation*, and *random responding*.

Response set, acquiescence   A tendency to endorse items or respond to questions in an affirmative direction.

Response style   (1) The degree to which measures derived from an assessment instrument reflect the respondents tendency to provide responses in a particular direction regardless of item content (e.g., a tendency to respond in a positive manner to a behavior problem questionnaire). (2) A distortion in a particular direction regardless of item content (Meier, 1994).

Risk factor   A risk factor is a variable whose value is statistically associated (covaries) with a parameter of a behavior disorder. Although the phrase is used inconsistently, a risk factor, but not a marker variable, often implies the operation of a causal relation (e.g.,

Yoshikawa, 1994). Driving without a seatbelt may be considered a risk factor for bodily injury in an accident.

Sampling, behavior   A procedure in which a subset of behaviors are selected for measurement. Behaviors can be selected on the basis of referral questions in clinical assessment, their frequency, their hypothesized functional relations with other behaviors, the predictive efficacy, and their importance to clients and others.

Sampling, event   A procedure in which a subset of events are selected for measurement. Events can be selected randomly, or on the basis of salience, importance, sensitivity to change, or their correlation with criteria of interest.

Sampling, momentary time   A sampling procedure in which observations are conducted briefly, at designated times (e.g., measurement by a staff member of a client's social behavior once at the beginning of each hour during the day).

Sampling, situation   A procedure in which a subset of settings are selected for observation of a person. Settings are usually selected on the basis of their association with a high likelihood that behaviors or functional relations of interest will occur in them.

Sampling, subject   A procedure in which observations are conducted on a subset of persons available for observation. Subjects can be selected randomly, or on the basis of assessment goals (e.g., the most aggressive children in a classroom).

Scale   A set of graduations and figures that calibrate a measurement instrument or obtained measure (Darton & Clark, 1994).

Scale, absolute   Persons or objects are assigned numbers such that all properties of the numbers reflect analogous properties of the attribute (Sarle, 1995).

Scale, interval   When numbers are assigned to persons or objects that are rank ordered on an attribute and the differences between the numbers can be meaningfully interpreted. Involves the use of constant units of measurement and a presumption of equality of intervals or differences (Nunnally & Bernstein, 1994; Pedhazur & Schmelkin, 1991).

Scale, log-interval   Persons or objects are assigned numbers such that ratios between the numbers reflect ratios of the attribute (Sarle, 1995).

Scale, nominal   When numbers are assigned to unordered classes of persons or objects (Pedhazur & Schmelkin, 1991).

Scale, ordinal   When numbers are assigned to persons or objects on the basis of their rank order on an attribute without implying equal differences between ranks (Pedhazur & Schmelkin, 1991).

Scale, ratio   When numbers are assigned to persons or objects on an interval scale that also has a true "0" point (Pedhazur & Schmelkin, 1991). A scale that allows the determination of equality, order, the quality of intervals among data values and the equality of ratios among values (Johnston & Pennypacker, 1993; Nunnally & Bernstein, 1994).

Scale discriminability   The degree to which a measure discriminates among individuals ordered along some continuum, such as depressive severity.

Sensitive period   A period of time (usually a developmental period) in which the effects of a particular environmental stimulus are particularly strong.

Sensitivity   The probability that a person with a particular attribute will manifest a particular behavior. The proportion of positive cause so identified by an assessment instrument (see *Positive predictive power*).

Sensitivity to change   The degree to which measures from an instrument reflect true changes across time in the targeted construct.

Setting events   Temporally distant antecedent events that set the occasion for behavior by influencing the valence of contiguous antecedent or consequent stimuli (see *Establishing operations*).

Shaping   A gradual change in response contingencies to successively reinforce responses that are closer approximations to a criterion response (Donahue & Palmer, 1994).

Shared method variance (common method variance)   The similarity in the procedures used to acquire data; can contribute to the magnitude of correlation between data from different assessment instruments (e.g., both instruments are self-report; both instruments use the same informant; shared items).

Skewness   The degree of asymmetry in the distribution of scores. A positive skew indicates a disproportionate number of low scores.

Slope   A coefficient of rate and direction of change of one variable in relation to another. It often refers to the rate and direction of change of a variable over time.

Social desirability, characteristic an assessment instrument   A *response set*. The degree to which measures derived from an assessment instrument reflect the respondents tendency to provide socially approved or accepted responses.

Specification (of a behavioral and causal variable)   The definition of a behavior or variable in measurable terms. Specification involves determination of the units of analysis (e.g., rate of "interruptions" during observation of dyadic communication), which involves a definition and dimension.

Specificity (of an assessment instrument)   The probability that a person without a particular attribute will be so identified by a particular assessment instrument. The proportion of negative cases so identified by an assessment instrument (see *Negative predictive power*).

Specificity (of a measure or variable)   The degree of molarity or precision of a measure and can refer to the diversity and number of elements subsumed by a measure (*Level of inference*), the degree to which the dimensions or parameters of a variable are specified, the degree to which situational and temporal conditions relevant for the target variable are specified, and the level of specificity of clinical judgments based on obtained measures (Haynes, Nelson, & Blaine, 1999).

Standard deviation   Usually denoted as "SD" particularly when referring to a sample; sometimes as "σ" although this symbol is often used to refer to the standard deviation in the population from which a sample was drawn. The square root of the sum of the deviations around the mean divided by N; $SD = (\Sigma x^2/N)^{1/2}$; the square root of the variance.

Standard error of measurement (standard error of a score)   In classical test theory, the positive square root of the reliability of a test (r_{tt}), times the standard deviation of the test scores (SD_t); $SD_t(1 - r_{tt})^{1/2}$.

Standard score   A measure of the relative standing of a subject among a group, usually derived by transforming raw scores into a z-score (reflecting a person's standing in relation to the mean and standard deviation of the group).

State-phase functions   The time-course of the magnitudes of causal and dependent variables. Similar to state-space functions.

Stimulus class   A range of associated stimuli that exhibit similar effects on responses. Usually refers to a set of antecedent stimuli.

Stimulus generalization   The process by which a range of stimuli, dissimilar in topography to an original selecting stimulus, acquire the ability to demonstrate similar effects on a response (Donahoe & Palmer, 1994).

Suppressed premise   A premise that is in fact necessary for a conclusion to follow, but is not explicitly stated (Blackburn, 1994).

Symptom   (1) Synonymous with "behavior problem." The term as used in this book does not imply that it is a marker of a "disorder" or of an underlying cause. (2) A sign (e.g., behavior, thought, cognitive process) of a "disorder" (Campbell, 1996).

Synchrony (synchronism)   The degree to which two events covary across time or persons. The degree to which the time-course of the two events overlap.

Syndrome   (1) A group of symptoms that characterize a disease or disorder (Krasner, 1992). (2) A group of behaviors that cluster across persons. (3) A group of behaviors that covary across time for a person. (4) A group or pattern of symptoms, affects, thoughts and behaviors that covary across time in many individuals (First et al., 1992).

Synthetic causal model   A multivariate causal model that depicts various causal weights and paths, the directionality of causal relations, and interactions among causal variables. In this sense, "synthetic" means "integrative" (Haynes, 1992).

Systems-functional analysis   A functional analysis that identifies sequences of reciprocal influences of child and parent behavior (Emery et al., 1983).

Target behavior   A response class selected for measurement or modification (Johnston & Pennypacker, 1993).

Task analysis   A procedure where a specific task is broken down into its molecular components. The behaviors necessary to complete an ultimate task are identified.

Taxonomy   (1) An organizational structure or schema for behaviors or other events based on similarities in characteristics, patterns of covariation, or functional relations. (2) The interdisciplinary science of classification.

Temporal contiguity   The degree to which two events (stimuli, responses) are separated in time.

Temporally contiguous   An adjective phrase referring to two events (stimuli, responses) that occur with a short time interval between them.

Temporal stability (test-retest reliability)   The degree of agreement between measures of the same variable acquired at different times. The stability of obtained scores over a specified time; can be reflected by correlations or degree of agreement between scores obtained at different assessment occasions.

Test   An assessment instrument.

Test sensitization   Changes in a participant's response to an intervention as a result of assessment (e.g., when a marital satisfaction test affects a client's response to subsequent marital therapy).

Threshold level   (see *Critical level*).

Time cluster   The pattern of occurrence of a causal or other variable across time. Time clusters may be regular, cyclic, bursts, random, multiharmonic, chaotic, and so forth.

Time-course   (1) The values of a variable dimension as a function of time. (2) The temporally related dimensions of a variable, such as cyclicity, latency, duration, and rate. The time-courses of variables are frequently presented in graphical form with time on the horizontal axis and the value of the variable on the vertical axis (Haynes, Blaine, & Meyer, 1995).

Timed event   In behavioral observation, a behavior of homogeneous content (Bakeman & Casey, 1995) and usually with an identifiable functional property, whose onset is timed. Timed events are characteristics of many observation coding systems.

Time-lag   The difference in time that one observation lags behind another (Marriott, 1990).

Time-lagged correlations   Correlating serial data points at time point I with data points at a subsequent or prior time period. The time lag of the correlations may vary.

Time sampling   An assessment strategy in which an observation period is divided into smaller periods. Usually, the duration and number of samples covary directly with the frequency and inversely with the duration of the observed events.

Time sampling, partial interval/whole interval   A behavioral observation procedure in which an event is counted as occurring if it occurs anytime during a sampling interval ("partial interval") or it occurs during the entire interval ("whole interval").

Time-series assessment   Includes a diverse set of assessment strategies to describe and analyze the time-courses and interrelations of multiple variables. With time-series assessment, behavior problems or hypothesized causal variables are measured frequently (e.g., 30 or more measurements) across time. Measurement occurs at a sufficient rate, and at sufficiently short intervals, to detect serial correlation in the time-series and the dynamic characteristics of measured variables.

Topography (of behavior)   The form of the behavior; its characteristics; often qualitative in nature; often involves descriptions of behavior occurring in space (e.g., specific definition of what a "hit" is).

Transitional period   That interval between two equilibrium states; often, but not necessarily, characterized by increased slope and variability of variables.

Transitional state   The condition of a person (or behavior) between a change in a causal variable and the establishment of an equilibrium state.

Treatment goals, intermediate   Necessary intermediate steps to achieving ultimate treatment goals.

Treatment goals, ultimate   Primary goals of therapy, expected end point of therapy.

Treatment utility   (see *Validity, treatment*).

Trend   A consistent change in values of a variable across time.

Trigger (triggering cause)   A variable that controls the immediate onset of a behavior problem. It usually occurs in close temporal proximity to the behavior problem.

Triggered causal variable   A causal variable that does not appear, is inactive, or is not measurable, unless preceded by another causal variable.

Type I error   The probability that a statistical test has or will yield a significant finding when, in fact, there is no significant relation among the variables being evaluated. Wrongly rejecting a true null hypothesis.

Type II error   The probability that a statistical test has or will yield a nonsignificant finding when, in fact, the variables evaluated are significantly related. Wrongly accepting a false null hypothesis.

Ultimate criterion   That criterion that furnishes the ultimate standard upon which other variables will be judged (Pedhazur & Schmelkin, 1991).

Unit (of analysis)   (1) The standard of measurement of a dimension or response class that is the subject of measurement and inference. Units can vary in type, degree of molarity, and breadth of specificity (Johnston & Pennypacker, 1993). (2) The events that are the object of inference. Units are best selected on the basis of functional utility.

User friendliness   The ease with which an assessment instrument can be administered and the data obtained and interpreted.

Utility   In reference to behavioral utility theory. The joint function of the likelihood that a given alternative actually achieves a particular goal and its value (Nezu & Nezu, 1989).

Utility (of a measure and assessment instrument)   The value of a measure, relative to other measures, for a particular purpose.

Validation (validity assessment)   (1) The process of establishing the validity of data from an assessment instrument (e.g., content validation is the process of establishing the content validity). (2) The process of evaluating the validity of inferences based on the scores from an assessment instrument.

Validity   An integrated evaluative judgment of the degree to which empirical evidence and theoretical rationales support the adequacy and appropriateness of inferences and actions based on the data acquired from an assessment instrument (Messick, 1993). (2) The scientific utility of an assessment instrument; how well it measures what it purports to measure (Nunnally & Bernstein, 1994). (3) The meaning of scores from an assessment instrument (Cronbach & Meehl, 1955; Foster & Cone, 1995). Closest in meaning to "construct validity."

Validity, concurrent   (1) An index of validity obtained when multiple measures of the same construct are administered on the same assessment occasion. (2) The correlation of a measure or criterion at the same point in time (Kazdin, 1998).

Validity, construct   (1) Comprises the evidence and rationales supporting the trustworthiness of assessment instrument data interpretation in terms of explanatory concepts that account for both the obtained data and relations with other variables (Messick, 1993). (2) The degree of validity of inferences about unobserved variables (constructs) based on observed indicators (Pedhazur & Schmelkin, 1991). (3) The extent to which the measure assesses the domain, trait, or characteristic of interest; refers broadly to the evidence bearing on the measure and encompasses all types of validity (Kazdin, 1998).

Validity, content   The degree to which elements of an assessment instrument are relevant to and representative of the targeted construct for a particular assessment purpose (Haynes, Richard, & Kubany, 1995).

Validity, convergent   (1) The degree to which the data from the assessment instrument are coherently related to other measures of the same construct as well as to other variables that it is expected, on theoretical grounds, to be related to (Messick, 1993). (2) The extent of covariance between scores from two assessment instruments that measure the same or related constructs. The correlation between the measures is expected based on the overlap or relation between the constructs (Campbell & Fiske, 1959).

Validity, criterion-referenced (criterion-related validity; criterion validity)   (1) The degree to which measures from an assessment instrument correlate with scores from previously validated instruments that measure the phenomena of interest or with nontest criterion of practical value. (2) Correlation of a measure with some other (validated) criterion. This can encompass concurrent or predictive validity (Kazdin, 1998).

Validity, discriminant (divergent)   (1) The degree to which data from an assessment instrument are not related unduly to other exemplars of other constructs (Messick, 1993). (2) The correlation between measures that are expected not to relate to each other or to assess dissimilar or unrelated constructs (Kazdin, 1998). (3) The degree to which data from an assessment instrument are distinct from measures of dissimilar constructs. Discriminant validity of an instrument is suggested by small or no significant correlation with data from instruments that tap dissimilar constructs (Campbell & Fiske, 1959). Most useful when applied to constructs that should not, but could, account for variance in the primary measure of interest.

Validity, discriminative   The degree to which measures from an assessment instrument can differentiate individuals in groups, formed from independent criteria, known to vary on the measured construct. For example, the ability of a score from a marital inventory to differentiate individuals who are and who are not seeking marital counseling.

Validity, divergent   (se *Validity, discriminant*).

Validity, ecological   Similar to external validity; the degree to which findings from one study are generalizable across populations and settings.

Validity, face   A component of content validity. The degree that respondents or users judge that the items of an assessment instrument are appropriate to the targeted construct and assessment objectives (Anastasi & Urbina, 1997; Nevo, 1985). It is commonly thought to measure the "acceptability" of the assessment instrument to users and administrators (Haynes, Richard, & Kubany, 1995).

Validity, incremental   (1) The degree to which data from an assessment instrument/ process increase the validity of judgments beyond that associated with assessment instruments/ processes currently in use or beyond that associated with alternative assessment instrument/ processes (Sechrest, 1963). (2) The degree to which additional assessment data provide information that is valid and unique from that provided by other measures of the same or similar constructs.

Validity, nomological   How well measures from an assessment instrument represent a theoretical construct. Determined by the relations obtained between the instrument and instruments measuring other, theoretically related, constructs (Cronbach & Meehl, 1955). Similar to "construct validity."

Validity, postdictive   The degree to which scores from an assessment instrument correlate with scores from another validated assessment administered at a previous point in time, or the degree to which scores predict historical events.

Validity, predictive   (1) The degree to which scores from an assessment instrument correlate with scores from another, validated assessment administered at a later point in time. (2) The degree to which scores from an instrument estimate an external criterion (Nunnally & Bernstein, 1994; note that the time frame of prediction is not important in this definition; the "criterion" is the determining factor).

Validity (utility), treatment   The degree to which data from an assessment instrument(s), or from a model of clinical case formulation is associated with increased treatment effectiveness (Hayes, Nelson, & Jarrett, 1987; Silva, 1993). Also termed "treatment utility."

Variable   An attribute that can change or that can be expressed as more than one value (Vogt, 1993) (e.g., sex, blood pressure, sleep-onset latency).

Variance   (1) The sum of the deviations of individual scores from the mean, divided by N; variance $= \Sigma\, x^2/N$, where x^2 = the deviation of a score, squared. The square of the standard deviation of a test; SD^2. (2) The second moment of a frequency distribution taken from the arithmetic mean as the origin. It is a quadratic mean in the sense that it is the mean of the squares of the variations from the arithmetic mean (Marriott, 1990).

Verbal rating scale   A list of adjectives describing different magnitudes of a variable dimension (e.g., "not distressing at all," "moderately distressing," "extremely distressing"). Respondents pick the adjective that best describes their placement on the variable dimension.

Visual analogue scale (VAS) (or graphic rating scale)   A line (e.g., 8–12 cm) whose ends are labeled as the extremes of a variable dimension (e.g., extremely relaxed—extremely tense; no pain—extreme pain). Points along the scale may be denoted with intermediate descriptors (i.e., verbal visual analogue scale) or numbers (numerical visual analogue scale). Respondents usually mark the point along the scale that best describes their placement on the variable dimension. VASs are often scored as a distance from an endpoint.

Vulnerability   The degree to which an individual is susceptible to developing a behavior disorder given the occurrence of particular causal events. A "vulnerable" person is one with a relatively higher probability of developing a disorder when exposed to specific conditions.

Vulnerability factor   A variable that affects the probability of a behavior disorder, given the occurrence of triggering variables. A risk factor.

Weight   The importance of an object in relation to a set of objects to which it belongs (Marriott, 1990).

Weighted average   An average of quantities to which have been attached different weights to reflect their relative importance (Marriott, 1990).

Z-score   The score expressed as a deviation from the sample mean value, in units of the sample standard deviation (Marriott, 1990).

References

Achenbach, T. M. (1997). *Empirically based assessment of child and adolescent psychopathology: Practical applications*. Thousand Oaks, CA: Sage.

Achenbach, T. M., & McConaughy, S. H. (1997). *Empirically based assessment of child and adolescent psychopathology: Practical applications* (2nd ed.). Thousand Oaks, CA: Sage.

Achenbach, T. M., McConaughy, S. H., & Howell, C. T. (1987). Child/adolescent behavioral and emotional problems: Implications of crossinformant correlations for situational specificity. *Psychological Bulletin, 101*, 213–232.

Acierno, R., Hersen, M., & Ammerman, R. T. (1994). Overview of the issues in prescriptive treatment. In M. Hersen & R. T. Ammerman (Eds.), *Handbook of prescriptive treatments for adults*. New York: Plenum.

Acierno, R., Hersen, M., & VanHasselt, V. B. (1998). *Handbook of psychological treatment protocols for children and adolesents*. Mahwah, NJ: Lawrence Earlbaum Associates.

Alder, A. G., & Sher, S. J. (1994). Using growth curve analyses to assess personality change and stability in adulthood. In T. F. Heatherton & J. L. Weinberger (Eds.), *Can personality change* (pp. 149–174). Washington, DC: American Psychological Association.

Alessi, G. (1988). Direct observation methods for emotional/behavior problems. In E. S. Shapiro & T. R. Kratochwill (Eds.), *Behavioral assessment in schools: Conceptual foundations and practical applications* (pp. 14–75). New York: Guilford.

Alessi, G. (1992). Models of proximate and ultimate causation in psychology. *American Psychologist, 47*, 1359–1371.

Alexander, F. G., & Selesnick, S. T. (1966). *The history of psychiatry: An evaluation of psychiatric thought and practice from prehistoric times to the present*. New York: Harper & Row.

Allison, D. B. (Ed.). (1995). *Handbook of assessment methods for eating behaviors and weight-related problems*. Thousand Oaks, CA: Sage.

Allport, G. W. (1937). *Personality: A psychological interpretation*. New York: Holt.

American Psychiatric Association (1994). *Diagnostic and statistical manual of mental disorders*. Washington, DC: American Psychological Association.

Anastasi, A., & Urbina, S. (1997). *Psychological testing*. Englewood Cliffs, NJ: Prentice-Hall.

Anderson, S. A., Vaulx-Smith, P., & Keshavan, M. S. (1994). Schizophrenia. In M. Hersen & R. T. Ammerman (Eds.), *Handbook of prescriptive treatments for adults* (pp. 73–94). New York: Plenum.

Andreassi, J. L. (1995). *Psychophysiology human behavior and physiological response* (3rd ed.). Hillsdale, NJ: Lawrence Erlbaum Associates.

Applegate, W. B., Blass, S., John, P., & Williams, T. F. (1990). Instruments for the functional assessment of older patients. *New England Journal of Medicine, 322*, 1207–1214.

Arkes, H. R. (1981). Impediments to accurate clinical judgement and possible ways to minimize their impact. *Journal of Consulting and Clinical Psychology, 49*, 323–330.

Arrington, R. E. (1939). Time-sampling studies of child behavior. *Psychological Monographs, 51*(2), 3–185.

Ashbaugh, R., & Peck, S. (1998). Treatment of sleep problems in a toddler: A replication of the faded bedtime with response cost protocol. *Journal of Applied Behavior Analysis, 31*, 127–129.

Asher, H. B. (1976). *Causal modeling*. Beverly Hills, CA: Sage.

Asterita, M. F. (1985). *The physiology of stress*. New York: Human Sciences Press.

Ayd, F. J., Jr. (1995). *Lexicon of Psychiatry, Neurology, and the Neurosciences*. Baltimore, MD: Williams & Wilkins.

Azar, B. (1994). Psychology's input leads to better tests. *Monitor, 25*, 1–15.

Bachrach, A. J. (Ed.). (1962). *Experimental foundations of clinical psychology*. New York: Basic Books.

Bakeman, R., & Casey, R. L. (1995). Analyzing family interaction: Taking time into account. *Journal of Family Psychology, 9,* 131–143.

Baker, G. L., & Gollub, J. P. (1990). *Chaotic dynamics: An introduction.* Cambridge, England: Cambridge University Press.

Baltes, P. B., Reese, H. W., & Nesselroade, J. R. (1988). *Introduction to research methods: Life-span developmental psychology.* Hillsdale, NJ: Lawrence Erlbaum.

Bandura, A. (1969). *Principles of behavior modification.* New York: Holt, Rinehart & Winston.

Bandura, A. (1982). The psychology of chance encounters and life paths. *American Psychologist, 37,* 747–755.

Banks, S. M., & Kerns, R. D. (1996). Explaining high rates of depression in chronic pain: A Diathesis-stress framework. *Psychological Bulletin, 119,* 95–110.

Barker, R. G. (1968). *Ecological psychology: Concepts and methods for studying the environment of human behavior.* Stanford, CA: Stanford University Press.

Barlow, D. H., & Hersen, M. (1984). *Single case experimental designs: Strategies for studying behavior change* (2nd ed.). New York: Pergamon.

Barnett, P. A., & Gotlib, I. (1988). Psychosocial functioning and depression: Distinguishing among antecedents, concomitants and consequences. *Psychological Bulletin, 104,* 97–126.

Baron, R. M., & Kenny, D. A. (1986). The moderator-mediator variable distinction in social psychological research: Conceptual, strategic and statistical consideration. *Journal of Personality and Social Psychology, 51,* 1173–1182.

Barrett, B. H., Johnston, J. M., & Pennypacker, H. S. (1986). Behavior: Its units, dimensions, and measurement. In R. O. Nelson & S. C. Hayes (Eds.), *Conceptual foundations of behavioral assessment* (pp. 156–200). New York: Guilford.

Barrios, B. A. (1988). On the changing nature of behavioral assessment. In A. S. Bellack & M. Hersen (Eds.), *Behavioral assessment: A practical handbook* (3rd ed., pp. 3–41). New York: Pergamon.

Barrios, B. A. (1993). Behavioral observation. In T. H. Ollendick & M. Hersen (Eds.), *Handbook of child and adolescent assessment* (pp. 140–164). Boston: Allyn & Bacon.

Batshaw, M. L. (1997). Understanding your chromosomes. In M. L. Batshaw (Ed.), *Children with disabilities* (4th ed., pp. 3–16). Baltimore: Paul H. Brookes.

Beach, S., Sandeen, E., & O'Leary, K. D. (1990). *Depression in marriage.* New York: Guilford.

Beck, J. G., & Zebb, B. J. (1994). Behavioral assessment and treatment of panic disorder: Current status, future directions. *Behavior Therapy, 25,* 581–612.

Beidel, D. C., & Morris, T. L. (1995). Social phobia. In J. S. March (Ed.), *Anxiety disorders in children and adolescents* (pp. 181–211). New York: Guilford.

Bellack, A. S., & Hersen, M. (Eds.). (1988). *Behavioral assessment: A practical handbook* (pp. 3–41). New York: Pergamon.

Bellack, A. S., & Hersen, M. (Eds.). (1993). *Handbook of behavior therapy in the psychiatric setting.* New York: Plenum.

Bellack, A. S., & Hersen, M. (Eds.). (1998). *Behavioral assessment: A practical handbook* (pp. 3–41). Boston: Allyn & Bacon.

Bellack, A. S., & Mueser, K. T. (1990). Schizophrenia. In A. S. Bellack, M. Hersen, A. E. Kazdin (Eds.), *International handbook of behavior modification and therapy* (2nd ed., pp. 353–366). New York: Plenum.

Bellack, A. S., Mueser, K. T., Gingerich, S., & Agresta, J. (1997). *Social skills training for schizophrenia—A step-by-step guide.* New York: Guilford.

Bennett, K., & Cavanaugh, R. A. (1998). Effects of immediate self-correction, delayed self-correction, and no correction on the acquisition and maintenance of multiplication facts by a fourth-grade student with learning disabilities. *Journal of Applied Behavior Analysis, 31,* 303–306.

Bentall, R. P., Haddock, G., & Slade, P. D. (1994). Cognitive behavior therapy for persistent auditory hallucinations: From theory to therapy. *Behavior Therapy, 25,* 51–66.

Black, L., & Novaco, R. W. (1993). Treatment of anger with a developmentally handicapped man. In R. A. Wells & V. J. Giannetti (Eds.), *Casebook of the brief psychotherapies* (pp. 143–158). New York: Plenum.

Blackburn, S. (1994). *The Oxford dictionary of philosophy.* New York: Oxford University Press.

Blalock, H. M. (1964). *Causal inferences in nonexperimental research.* Chapel Hill, NC: University of North Carolina Press.

Blanchard, E. B. (1993). Irritable bowel syndrome. In R. J. Gatchel & E. B. Blanchard (Eds.), *Psychophysiological disorders, research and clinical applications* (pp. 23–61). Washington, DC: American Psychological Association.

Blanchard, E. B., Hickling, E. J., Taylor, A. E., Loos, W. R., & Gerardi, R. J. (1994). The psychophysiology of motor vehicle accident related posttraumatic stress disorder. *Behavior Therapy, 25,* 453–467.

Block, N. (1993). Troubles with functionalism. In A. I. Goldman (Ed.), *Readings in philosophy and cognitive science* (pp. 231–254). Cambridge, MA: MIT Press.

Bollen, K., & Lennox, R. (1991). Conventional wisdom on measurement: A structural equation perspective. *Psychological Bulletin, 110*, 305–314.

Bootzin, R. R., Manber, R., Perlis, M. L., Salvio, M.-A., & Wyatt, J. K. (1993). Sleep disorders. In P. B. Sutker & H. E. Adams (Eds.), *Comprehensive handbook of psychopathology* (2nd ed., pp. 531–562). New York: Plenum.

Boring, E. G. (1957). *A history of experimental psychology.* New York: Appleton-Century-Crofts.

Bornstcin, M. H. (Ed.). (1987). *Sensitive periods in development: Interdisciplinary perspectives.* Hillsdale, NJ: Erlbaum.

Botella, C., Banos, R. M., Perpina, C., Villa, H., Alcaniz, M., & Rey, A. (1998). Virtual reality treatment of claustrophobia: A case report. *Behavior Research and Therapy, 36*, 239–246.

Bott, H. (1928). Observations of play activity in nursery school. *Genetic Psychology Monographs, 4*, 44–88.

Boutelle, K. N. (1998). The use of exposure with response prevention in a male anorexic. *Journal of Behavior Therapy and Experimental Psychiatry, 29*, 79–84.

Boyd, R. D., & DeVault, M. V. (1966). The observation and recording of behavior. *Review of Educational Research, 36*, 529–551.

Bramlett, R. K., & Barnett, D. W. (1993). The development of a direct observation code for use in preschool settings. *School Psychology Review, 22*, 49–62.

Breen, M. J., & Fiedler, C. R. (Eds.). (1996). *Behavioral approach to assessment of youth with emotional/behavioral disorders—A handbook for school-based practitioners.* Austin, TX: PRO-ED.

Brewer, M. B., & Crano, W. D. (1994). *Social psychology.* St. Paul: West Publishing.

Briggs, J., & Peat, F. D. (1989). *Turbulent mirror: An illustrated guide to chaos theory and the science of wholeness.* New York: Harper & Row.

Brown, E. J., Turovsky, J., Heimberg, R. G., Juster, H. R., Brown, T. A., & Barlow, D. H. (1997). Validation of the social interaction anxiety scale and the social phobia scale across the anxiety disorders. *Psychological Assessment, 9*, 21–27.

Brunk, M., Henggeler, S. W., & Whelan, J. P. (1987). Comparison of multisystematic therapy and parent training in the brief treatment of child abuse and neglect. *Journal of Consulting and Clinical Psychology, 55*, 171–178.

Brussell, E. E. (1988). *Webster's New World Dictionary of quotable definitions* (2nd ed.). Englewood Cliffs, NJ: Prentice-Hall.

Bunge, M. (1959). *Causality: The place of the causal principle in modern science.* Cambridge, MA: Harvard University Press.

Butcher, J. N. (Ed.). (1995). *Clinical personality assessment: Practical approaches.* New York: Oxford University Press.

Butcher, J. N., Narikiyo, T., & Vitousek, K. B. (1992). Understanding abnormal behavior in cultural context. In P. B. Stuker & H. E. Adams (Eds.). *Comprehensive handbook of psychopathology* (pp. 83–108). New York: Plenum.

Byerly, H. C. (1973). *A primer of logic.* New York: Harper & Row.

Cacioppo, J. T., & Tassinary, L. G. (1990). *Principles and psychophysiology: Physical, social, and inferential elements.* New York: Cambridge University Press.

Çambel, A. B. (1993). *Applied chaos theory: A paradigm for complexity.* Boston: Academic Press.

Campbell, D. T., & Fiske, D. (1959). Convergent and discriminant validation by the multitrait-multimethod matrix. *Psychological Bulletin, 56*, 81–105.

Campbell, R. J. (1996). *Psychiatric dictionary.* New York: Oxford University Press.

Cantor, N. (1990). From thought to behavior: "Having" and "doing" in the study of personality and cognition. *American Psychologist, 45*, 735–750.

Cardillo, J. E. (1994). Goal-setting, follow-up, and goal monitoring. In T. J. Kiresuk, A. Smith, & J. E. Cardillo (Eds.), *Goal attainment scaling: Applications, theory and measurement* (pp. 39–60). Hillsdale, NJ: Lawrence Erlbaum Associates.

Cardillo, J. E., & Choate, R. O. (1994). Illustrations of goal setting. In T. J. Kiresuk, A. Smith, & J. E. Cardillo (Eds.), *Goal attainment scaling: Applications, theory and measurement* (pp. 15–37). Hillsdale, NJ: Lawrence Erlbaum Associates.

Cardillo, J. E., & Smith, A. S. (1994). Reliability of goal attainment scores. In T. J. Kiresuk, A. Smith, & J. E. Cardillo (Eds.), *Goal attainment scaling: Applications, theory, and measurement.* Hillsdale, NJ: Lawrence Erlbaum Associates.

Carey, M. P., Lantinga, L. J., & Krauss, D. J. (1994). Male erective disorder. In M. Hersen & R. T. Ammerman (Eds.), *Handbook of prescriptive treatments for adults* (pp. 347–367). New York: Plenum.

Carr, E. G., Robinson, S., & Palumbo, L. R. (1990). The wrong issue; aversive versus nonaversive treatment; the right issue: functional versus nonfunctional treatment. In A. C. Repp, & S. Nirbhay (Eds.), *Perspectives on the use of nonaversive and aversive interventions for persons with developmental disabilities* (pp. 361–379). Sycamore, IL: Sycamore Publishing.

Cascio, W. F. (1991). *Applied psychology in personnel management* (4th ed.). Englewood Cliffs, NJ: Prentice-Hall.

Cattell, R. B., & Johnson, R. C. (1986). *Functional psychological testing.* New York: Brunner/Mazel.

Chadwick, P. D. J., Lowe, C. F., Horne, P. J., & Higson, P. J. (1994). Modifying delusions: The role of empirical testing. *Behavior Therapy, 25,* 35–49.

Chamberlain, P., Patterson, G. R., Reid, J. B., Kavanagh, K., & Forgatch, M. S. (1984). Observation of client resistance. *Behavior Therapy, 15,* 144–155.

Chapman, L. J., & Chapman, J. P. (1969). Illusory correlation as an obstacle to the use of valid psychodiagnostic signs. *Journal of Abnormal Psychology, 74,* 271–280.

Chapman, S., Fisher, W., Piazza, C. C., & Kurtz, P. F. (1993). Functional assessment and treatment of life-threatening drug ingestion in a dually diagnosed youth. *Journal of Applied Behavioral Analysis, 26,* 255–256.

Chorpita, B. F., Albano, A. M., Heimberg, R. G., & Barlow, D. H. (1996). Systematic replication of the prescriptive treatment of school refusal behavior in a single subject. *Journal of Behavior Therapy and Experimental Psychiatry, 27,* 1–10.

Ciminero, A. R. (1986). Behavioral assessment: An overview. In A. R. Ciminero, K. S. Calhoun, & H. E. Adams (Eds.), *Handbook of behavior assessment* (2nd ed., pp. 446–495). New York: John Wiley & Sons.

Clark, L. A., Watson, D., & Reynolds, S. (1995). Diagnosis and classification of psychopathology: Challenges to the current system and future directions. In J. T. Spence, J. M. Darley, & D. J. Foss (Eds.), *Annual review of psychology, 46* (pp. 121–153). Palo Alto, CA: Annual Reviews.

Clement, P. W. (1996). Evaluation in clinical practice. *Clinical Psychology—Science and Practice, 3,* 146–159.

Cloninger, C. R., Bohman, M., & Sigvardsson, S. (1981). Inheritance of alcohol abuse: Cross-fostering analysis of adopted men. *Archives of General Psychiatry, 38,* 861–868.

Collins, L. M., & Horn, J. L. (1991). *Best methods for the analysis of change.* Washington, DC: American Psychological Association.

Cone, J. D. (1979). Confounded comparisons in triple response mode assessment research. *Behavioral Assessment, 11,* 85–95.

Cone, J. D. (1982). Validity of direct observation assessment procedures. *New Directions for Methodology of Social and Behavioral Science, 14,* 67–79.

Cone, J. D. (1986). Idiographic, nomothetic and related perspectives in behavioral assessment. In R. O. Nelson & S. C. Hayes (Eds.), *Conceptual foundations of behavioral assessment* (pp. 111–128). New York: Guilford.

Cone, J. D. (1988). Psychometric considerations and the multiple models of behavioral assessment. In A. S. Bellack & M. Hersen (Eds.), *Behavioral assessment: A practical handbook* (3rd ed., pp. 42–66). Elmsford, NY: Pergamon.

Cone, J. (1998). Psychometric considerations: Concepts, contents, and methods. In A. S. Bellack & M. Hersen (Eds.), *Behavioral assessment—A practical handbook* (4th ed., pp. 22–46). Boston, MA: Allyn & Bacon.

Cook, T. D., & Campbell, D. T. (1979). *Quasi-experimentation: Design and analysis issues for field settings.* Chicago: Rand McNally.

Copeland, A. L., Brandon, T. H., & Quinn, E. P. (1995). The Smoking Consequences Questionnaire—Adult: Measurement of smoking outcome expectancies of experienced smokers. *Psychological Assessment, 7,* 484–494.

Cordon, I. M., Lutzker, J. R., Bigelow, K. M., & Doctor, R. M. (1998). Evaluating Spanish protocols for teaching bonding, home safety, and health care skills to a mother reported for child abuse. *Journal of Behavior Therapy and Experimental Psychiatry, 29,* 41–54.

Corsini, R. J. (1987). *The concise encyclopedia of psychology.* New York: John Wiley & Sons.

Costa, P. T., Jr., & McCrae, R. R. (1994). Set like plaster? Evidence for the stability of adult personality. In T. F. Heatheron & J. L. Weinberger (Eds.), *Can personality change* (pp. 21–40). Washington, DC: American Psychological Association.

Costello, C. G. (Ed.). (1993). *Basic issues in psychopathology* (pp. 1–18). New York: Guilford.

Coyne, J. C., & Downey, G. (1991). Social factors and psychopathology: Stress, social support, and coping processes. In M. R. Rosenzweig & L. W. Porter (Eds.), *Annual review of psychology, 42* (pp. 401–426). Palo Alto, CA: Annual Reviews.

Craske, M. G. (1993). Assessment and treatment of panic disorder and agoraphobia. In A. S. Bellack & M. Hersen (Eds.), *Handbook of behavior therapy in the psychiatric setting* (pp. 229–249). New York: Plenum.

Craske, M. G., Rapee, R. M., & Barlow, D. H. (1992). Cognitive-behavioral treatment of panic disorder, agoraphobia, and generalized anxiety disorder. In S. M. Turner, K. S. Calhoun, & H. E. Adams (Eds.), *Handbook of clinical behavior therapy* (2nd ed., pp. 39–66). New York: John Wiley & Sons.

Craske, M. G., & Walkar, S. V. (1994). Panic disorder. In M. Hersen & R. T. Ammerman (Eds.), *Handbook of prescriptive treatments for adults* (pp. 135–155). New York: Plenum.

Creer, T. L., & Bender, B. G. (1993). Asthma. In R. J. Gatchel & E. B. Blanchard (Eds.), *Psychophysiological disorders, research and clinical applications* (pp. 151–204). Washington, DC: American Psychological Association.

Crewe, N. M., & Dijkers, M. (1995). Functional assessment. In L. A. Cushman & M. J. Scherer (Eds.), *Psychological assessment in medical rehabilitation* (pp. 101–144). Washington, DC: American Psychological Association.

Cronbach, L. (1960). *Essentials of psychological testing* (2nd ed.). New York: Harper & Brothers.

Cronbach, L. J., & Meehl, P. E. (1955). Construct validity in psychological tests. *Psychological Bulletin, 52,* 281–302.

Cushman, L., & Scherer, M. (Eds.). (1996). *Psychological assessment in medical rehabilitation* (pp. 199–236). Washington, DC: American Psychological Association.

Cuvo, A. J., Lerch, L. J., Leurquin, D. A., Gaffaney, T. J., & Poppen, R. L. (1998). Response allocation to concurrent fixed-ration reinforcement schedules with work requirements by adults with mental retardation and typical preschool children. *Journal of Applied Behavior Analysis, 31,* 43–63.

Cvitanovic, P. (Ed.). (1984). *Universality of chaos.* Bristol: Adam Hilger.

Darton, M., & Clark, J. (1994). *The Macmillan dictionary of measurement.* New York: Macmillan.

Davison, G. C., & Neale, J. M. (1990). *Abnormal psychology.* New York: John Wiley & Sons.

Dawes, R. M., Faust, D., & Meehl, P. E. (1989). Clinical versus actuarial judgment. *Science, 243,* 1668–1673.

de Beurs, E., Van Dyck, R., van Balkom, A. J., Lange, A., & Koele, P. (1994). Assessing the clinical significance of outcome in agoraphobia research: A comparison of two approaches. *Behavior Therapy, 25,* 147–158.

Derby, K. M., Wacker, D. P., Sasso, G., Steege, M., Northup, J., Cigrand, K., & Asmus, J. (1992). Brief functional analysis techniques to evaluate aberrant behavior in an outpatient setting: A summary of 79 cases. *Journal of Applied Behavior Analysis, 25,* 713–721.

DeVellis, R. F. (1991). *Scale development theory and applications.* Beverly Hills, CA: Sage.

Diamond, S., & Dalessio, D. J. (Eds.). (1992). *The practicing physicians' approach to headache.* Baltimore: Williams & Wilkins.

Dixon, M. R., Hayes, L. J., Binder, L. M., Manthey, S., Sigman, C., & Zdanowski, D. M. (1998). Using a self-control training procedure to increase appropriate behavior. *Journal of Applied Behavior Analysis, 31,* 203–210.

Donahoe, J. W., & Palmer, D. C. (1994). *Learning and complex behavior.* Boston: Allyn & Bacon.

Dumas, J. E. (1987). Interact—A computer-based coding and data management system to assess family interactions. In R. J. Priz (Ed.), *Advances in behavioral assessment of children* (Vol. 3, pp. 177–202). Greenwich, CT: JAI Press.

Dumas, J. E., & Serketich, W. J. (1994). Maternal depressive symptomatology and child maladjustment: A comparison of three process models. *Behavior Therapy, 25,* 161–181.

Dumont, F., & Lecomte, C. (1987). Inferential processes in clinical work: Inquire into logical errors that affect diagnostic judgments. *Professional Psychology: Research and Practice, 18,* 433–438.

Durand, V. M. (1990). *Severe behavior problems: A functional communication training approach.* New York: Guilford.

Durand, V. M., & Carr, E. G. (1991). Functional communication training to reduce challenging behavior: Maintenance and application in new settings. *Journal of Applied Behavior Analyses, 24,* 251–264.

Durand, V. M., & Crimmins, D. B. (1988). Identifying variables maintaining self–injurious behavior. *Journal of Autism and Developmental Disorders, 18,* 99–117.

Dwyer, C. A. (1996). Cut scores and testing: Statistics, judgment, truth, and error. *Psychological Assessment, 8,* 360–362.

Ebel, R. L., & Frisbie, D. A. (1991). *Essentials of educational measurement* (5th ed.). Englewood Cliffs, NJ: Prentice-Hall.

Edelbrock, C. (1988). Informant reports. In E. S. Shapiro & T. R. Kratochwill (Eds.), *Behavioral assessment in schools: Conceptual foundations and practical applications* (pp. 351–383). New York: Guilford.

Eells, T. (Ed.). (1997). *Handbook of psychotherapy case formulation.* New York: Guilford.

Eifert, G. H., Evans, I. M., & McKendrick, V. G. (1990). Matching treatments to client problems not diagnostic labels: A case for paradigmatic behavior therapy. *Journal of Behavior Therapy and Experimental Psychiatry, 21,* 163–172.

Einhorn, H. J. (1988). Diagnosis and causality in clinical and statistical prediction. In D. C. Turk & P. Salovey (Eds.), *Reasoning, inference and judgment in clinical psychology* (pp. 51–70). New York: Free Press.

Eisen, A. R., & Silverman, W. K. (1998). Prescriptive treatment for generalized anxiety disorder in children. *Behavior Therapy, 29,* 105–121.

Elliot, A. J., Miltenberger, R. G., Kaster-Bundgaard, J., & Lumley, V. (1996). A national survey of assessment and therapy techniques used by behavior therapists. *Cognitive and Behavioral Practice, 3,* 107–125.

Elstein, A. S. (1988). Cognitive processes in clinical inference and decision making. In D. C. Turk & P. Salovey (Eds.), *Reasoning, inference, and judgment in clinical psychology* (pp. 17–50). New York: Free Press.

Emery, R. E., Binkoff, J. A., Houts, A. C., & Carr, E. G. (1983). Children as independent variables: Some clinical implications of child-effects. *Behavior Therapy, 14,* 398–412.

Ervin, R. A., DuPaul, G. J., Kern, L., & Friman, P. C. (1998). Classroom-based functional and adjunctive assessments: Proactive approaches to intervention selection for adolescents with attention deficit hyperactivity disorder. *Journal of Applied Behavior Analysis, 31,* 65–78.

Esar, E. (1968). *20,000 quips and quotes.* New York: Barnes & Noble.

Evans, I. M. (1986). Response structure and the triple-response-mode concept. In R. O. Nelson & S. C. Hayes (Eds.), *Conceptual foundations of behavioral assessment* (pp. 131–155). New York: Guilford.

Evans, I. (1993a). Constructional perspectives in clinical assessment. *Psychological Assessment, 5,* 264–272.

Evans, I. M. (1993b). Dynamic response relationships: The challenge for behavioral assessment. *European Journal of Psychological Assessment, 9,* 206–212.

Eysenck, H. J., & Martin, I. (Eds.). (1987). *Theoretical foundations of behavior therapy* (pp. 331–351). New York: Plenum.

Fahrenberg, J., & Myrtek, M. (Eds.) (1996). *Ambulatory assessment—Computer-assisted psychological and psychophysiological methods in monitoring and field studies.* Kirkland, WA: H & H Publishers.

Farmer-Dougan, V. (1998) A disequilibrium analysis of incidental teaching: Determining reinforcement effects. *Behavior Modification, 22,* 78–95.

Farrell, S. P., Hains, A. A., & Davies, W. H. (1998). Cognitive behavioral interventions for sexually abused children exhibiting PTSD symptomatology. *Behavior Therapy, 29,* 241–255.

Fayers, P. M., & Hand, D. J. (1997). Factor analysis, causal indicators and quality of life. *Quality of Life Research, 6,* 139–150.

Feigl, H., & Brodbeck, M. (1953). *Readings in the philosophy of science.* New York: Appleton-Century-Crofts.

Felton, J. L., & Nelson, R. O. (1984). Inter-assessor agreement on hypothesized controlling variables and treatment proposals. *Behavioral Assessment, 6,* 199–208.

Finch, Jr., A. J., & Belter, R. W. (1993). Projective techniques. In T. H. Ollendick & M. Hersen (Eds.), *Handbook of child and adolescent assessment* (pp. 224–236). Boston: Allyn & Bacon.

Finch, Jr., A. J., & McIntosh, J. A. (1990). Assessment of anxieties and fears in children. In A. M. La Greca (Ed.), *Through the eyes of the child: Obtaining self-reports from children and adolescents* (pp. 234–258). Boston: Allyn & Bacon.

First, M. B., Frances, A., Widiger, T. A., Pincus, H. A., & Davis, W. W. (1992). DSM-IV and behavioral assessment. *Behavioral Assessment, 14,* 297–306.

Fletcher, K. E., Fischer, M., Barkley, R. A., & Smallish, L. (1996). A sequential analysis of the mother–adolescent interactions of ADHD, ADJD/ODD, and normal teenagers during neutral and conflict discussions. *Journal of Abnormal Child Psychology, 24,* 271–297.

Floyd, F., Haynes, S. N., & Kelly, S. (1997). Marital assessment: A dynamic and functional analytic and perspective. In W. K. Halford & H. J. Markman (Eds.), *Clinical handbook of marriage and couples intervention* (pp. 349–378). New York: Guilford.

Forehand, R., & McMahon, R. J. (1981). *Helping the noncompliant child: A clinician's guide to parent training.* New York: Guilford.

Foreyt, J. P., & McGavin, J. K. (1989). Anorexia nervosa and bulimia nervosa. In E. J. Mash & R. A. Barkley (Eds.), *Treatment of childhood disorders* (pp. 529–558). New York: Guilford.

Forsyth, J. P., & Eifert, G. H. (1998). Phobic anxiety and panic: An integrative behavioral account of their origin and treatment. In J. J. Plaud & G. H. Eifert (Eds.), *From behavior theory to behavior therapy* (pp. 38–67). Boston: Allyn & Bacon.

Foster, S. L., Bell-Dolan, D. J., & Burge, D. A. (1988). Behavioral observation. In A. S. Bellack & M. Hersen (Eds.), *Behavioral assessment: A practical handbook* (3rd ed., pp. 119–160). Elmsford, NY: Pergamon.

Foster, S. L., & Cone, J. D. (1995). Validity issues in clinical assessment. *Psychological Assessment, 7,* 248–260.

Foxx, R. M., McMorrow, M. J., Davis, L. A., & Bittle, R. G. (1988). Replacing a chronic schizophrenic man's delusional speech with stimulus appropriate responses. *Journal of Behavior Therapy and Experimental Psychiatry, 19,* 43–50.

Frame, C. L., & Matson, J. L. (Eds.). (1987). *Handbook of assessment in childhood psychopathology applied issues in differential diagnosis and treatment evaluation.* New York: Plenum.

Frame, C. L., Robinson, S. L., & Cuddy, E. (1992). Behavioral treatment of childhood depression. In S. M. Turner, K. S. Calhoun, & H. E. Adams (Eds.), *Handbook of clinical behavior therapy* (2nd ed., pp. 245–258). New York: John Wiley & Sons.

Franks, C. M. (Ed.). (1969). *Behavioral therapy: Appraisal and status.* New York: McGraw-Hill.

Gannon, L. R., & Haynes, S. N. (1987). Cognitive-physiological discordance as an etiological factor in psychophysiologic disorders. *Advances in Behavior Research and Therapy, 8,* 223–236.

Garb, H. N. (1989). Clinical judgement, clinical training, and professional experience. *Psychological Bulletin, 105,* 387–396.

Garb, H. N. (Ed.). (1998). *Studying the clinician—Judgment research and psychological assessment.* Washington, DC: American Psychological Association.

Gatchel, R. J., & Blanchard, E. B. (1993). *Psychophysiological disorders, research and clinical applications.* Washington, DC: American Psychological Association.

Geisinger, K. F. (1987). Psychometry. In R. Corsini (Ed.), *Concise encyclopedia of psychology* (pp. 925–926). New York: John Wiley & Sons.

George, M. S., Huggins, T., McDermut, W., Parekh, P. I., Rubinow, D., & Post, R. M. (1998). Abnormal facial emotion recognition in depression: Serial testing in an ultra-rapid-cycling patient. *Behavior Modification, 22,* 192–204.

Gesell, A. (1925). *The mental growth of the pre-school child.* New York: Macmillan.

Gettinger, M., & Kratochwill, T. R. (1987). Behavioral assessment. In C. L. Frame & J. L. Matson (Eds.), *Handbook of assessment in childhood psychopathology applied issues in differential diagnosis and treatment evaluation* (pp. 131–161). New York: Plenum.

Glass, C. (1993). A little more about cognitive assessment. *Journal of Counseling and Development, 71,* 546–548.

Glass, C. R., & Arnkoff, D. B. (1989). Behavioral assessment of phobia. *Clinical Psychology Review, 9,* 75–90.

Goldfried, M. R., & Kent, R. N. (1972). Traditional versus behavioral assessment: A comparison of methodological and theoretical assumptions. *Psychological Bulletin, 77,* 409–420.

Goldman, M. S., Brown, S. A., Christiansen, B. A., & Smith, G. T. (1991). Alcoholism and memory: Broadening the scope of alcohol expectancy research. *Psychological Bulletin, 110,* 137–146.

Goldstein, A., & Hersen, M. (Eds.). (1999). *Handbook of psychological assessment* (3rd ed.). Boston: Allyn & Bacon.

Goldstein, W. M., & Hogarth, R. M. (Eds.). (1997). *Research on judgement and decision making: Currents, connections, and controversies.* New York: Cambridge University Press.

Goodenough, F. L. (1928). Measuring behavior traits by means of repeated short samples. *Journal of Juvenile Research, 12,* 230–235.

Gottman, J. M. (1995). *The analysis of change.* Mahwah, NJ: Lawrence Erlbaum Associates.

Gottman, J. M. (1996). *The analysis of change.* Hillsdale, NJ: Lawrence Erlbaum Associates.

Gottman, J. M. (1998). Psychology and the study of marital processes. *Annual review of psychology, 49* (pp. 169–197). Palo Alto, CA: Annual Reviews.

Gottman, J. M., & Roy, A. K. (1990). *Sequential analysis: A guide for behavioral researchers.* New York: Cambridge University Press.

Grant, L., & Evans, A. (1994). *Principles of behavior analysis.* New York: HarperCollins.

Greenberg, L. S. (1995). The use of observational coding in family therapy research: Comment on Alexander et al. (1995). *Journal of Family Psychology, 9,* 366–370.

Greenwood, C., Carta, J. J., Kamps, D., Terry, B., & Delaquardi, J. (1994). Development and validation of standard classroom observation systems for school practitioners: Ecobehavioral assessment systems software (EBASS). *Exceptional Children, 61,* 197–210.

Groden, G. (1989). A guide for conducting a comprehensive behavioral analysis of a target behavior. *Journal of Behavior Therapy and Experimental Psychiatry, 20,* 163–170.

Groth-Marnat, G. (1997). *Handbook of psychological assessment* (3rd ed.). New York: John Wiley & Sons.

Guevremont, D. C., & Spiegler, M. D. (1990, November). What do behavior therapists really do? A survey of the clinical practice of AABT members. Paper presented at the 24th Annual Convention of the Association for Advancement of Behavior Therapy, San Francisco, CA.

Gutting, G. (Ed.). (1980). *Paradigms and revolutions.* Notre Dame, IN: University of Notre Dame Press.

Haaga, D. A. F., et al. (1994). Mode-specific impact of relaxation training for hypertensive men with Type A behavior pattern. *Behavior Therapy, 25,* 209–223.

Haccou, P., & Meelis, E. (1992). *Statistical analysis of behavioural data—An approach based on time-structured models.* New York: Oxford University Press.

Halford, W. K., & Markman, H. J. (Eds.). (1997). *Clinical handbook of marriage and couples intervention.* New York: Guilford.

Halford, W. K., Sanders, M. R., & Behrens, B. C. (1994). Self-regulation in behavioral couples' therapy. *Behavior Therapy, 25,* 431–452.

Hamilton, M., & Shapiro, C. M. (1990). Depression. In D. F. Peck & C. M. Shapiro (Eds.), *Measuring human problems: A practical guide* (pp. 25–65). New York: John Wiley & Sons.

Handel, R. W., Ben–Porath, Y. S., & Watt, M. (1998). Computerized adaptive testing with the MMPI–2: A clinical trial. *Psychological Assessment.*

Hanley, G. P., Piazza, C. C., Keeney, K. M., Blakeley-Smith, A. B., & Worsdell, A. S. (1998). Effects of wrist weights on self-injurious and adaptive behavior. *Journal of Applied Behavior Analysis, 31,* 307–310.

Harris, F. C., & Lahey, B. B. (1982). Subject reactivity in direct observational assessment: A review and critical analysis. *Clinical Psychology Review, 2,* 523–538.

Harris, T. A., Peterson, S. L., Filliben, T. L., Glassberg, M., & Favell, J. E. (1998). Evaluating a more cost-effective alternative to providing in-home feedback to parents: The use of spousal feedback. *Journal of Applied Behavior Analysis, 31,* 131–134.

Harrop, A., Foulkes, C., & Daniels, M. (1989). Observer agreement calculations: The role of primary data in reducing obfuscation. *British Journal of Psychology*, *80*, 181–189.

Harter, S., Alexander, P. C., & Neimeyer, R. A. (1988). Long-term effects of incestuous child abuse in college women: Social adjustment, social cognition, and family characteristics. *Journal of Consulting and Clinical Psychology*, *56*, 5–8.

Hartmann, D. P. (Ed.). (1982). *Using observers to study behavior*. San Francisco: Jossey-Bass.

Hartmann, D., Gottman, J., Jones, R., Gardner, W., Kazdin, A., & Vaught, R. (1980). Interrupted time-series analysis and its application to behavioral data. *Journal of Applied Behavior Analysis*, *13*, 543–559.

Hartmann, D. P., Roper, B. L., & Bradford, D. C. (1979). Some relationships between behavioral and traditional assessment. *Journal of Behavior Assessment*, *1*, 3–21.

Hartmann, D. P., & Wood, D. D. (1990). Observational methods. In A. S. Bellack, M. Hersen, A. E. Kazdin (Eds.), *International handbook of behavior modification and therapy* (2nd ed., pp. 107–138). New York: Plenum.

Hatch, J. P. (1993). Headache. In R. J. Gatchel & E. B. Blanchard (Eds.), *Psychophysiological disorders, research and clinical applications* (pp. 111–150). Washington, DC: American Psychological Association.

Hawkins, R. P. (1986). Selection of target behaviors. In R. O. Nelson & S. C. Hayes (Eds.), *Conceptual foundations of behavioral assessment* (pp. 311–385). New York: Guilford.

Hayes, S. C., & Follette, W. C. (1992). Can functional analysis provide a substitute for syndromal classification? *Behavioral Assessment*, *14*, 345–365.

Hayes, S. C., Follette, V. M., Dawes, R. M., & Grady, K. E. (Eds.). (1995). *Scientific standards of psychological practice: Issues and recommendations*. Reno, NV: Context Press.

Hayes, S. L., Nelson, R. O., & Jarret, R. B. (1987). The treatment utility of assessment: A functional approach to evaluate assessment quality. *American Psychologist*, *42*, 963–974.

Haynes, S. N. (1978). *Principles of behavioral assessment*. New York: Gardner.

Haynes, S. N. (1986a). A behavioral model of paranoid behaviors. *Behavior Therapy*, *17*, 266–287.

Haynes, S. N. (1986b). The design of intervention programs. In R. O. Nelson & S. Hayes (Eds.), *Conceptual foundations of behavioral assessment* (pp. 386–429). New York: Guilford.

Haynes, S. N. (1992). *Models of causality in psychopathology: Toward synthetic, dynamic and nonlinear models of causality in psychopathology*. Boston: Allyn & Bacon.

Haynes, S. N. (1993). Treatment implications of psychological assessment. *Psychological Assessment*, *5*, 251–253.

Haynes, S. N. (1994). Clinical judgment and the design of behavioral intervention programs: Estimating the magnitudes of intervention effects. *Psicologia Conductual*, *2*, 165–184.

Haynes, S. N. (1998a). The assessment-treatment relationship and functional analysis in behavior therapy. *European Journal of Psychological Assessment*, *14*(1), 26–34.

Haynes, S. N. (1998b). The principles and practice of behavioral assessment with adults. In A. P. Goldstein & M. Hersen (Eds.), *Comprehensive clinical psychology: Assessment*, Vol. 4. Amsterdam: Elsevier Science.

Haynes, S. N. (1999). The behavioral assessment of adult disorders. In A. Goldstein and M. Hersen (Eds.), *Handbook of psychological assessment* (3rd ed.). New York: Pergamon.

Haynes, S. N., Blaine, D., & Meyer, K. (1995). Dynamical models for psychological assessment: Phase-space functions. *Psychological Assessment*, *7*, 17–24.

Haynes, S. N., Falkin, S., & Sexton-Radek, K. (1989). Psychophysiological measurement in behavior therapy. In G. Turpin (Ed.), *Handbook of clinical psychophysiology* (pp. 175–214). London: John Wiley.

Haynes, S. N., & Horn, W. F. (1982). Reactive effects of behavioral observation. *Behavioral Assessment*, *4*, 369–385.

Haynes, S. N., & Jensen, B. J. (1979). The interview as a behavioral assessment instrument. *Behavioral Assessment*, *1*, 97–106.

Haynes, S. N., Leisen, M. B., & Blaine, D. D. (1997). Functional analytic clinical case models and clinical decision-making. *Psychological Assessment*, *9*, 334–348.

Haynes, S. N., Nelson, K. & Blaine, D. C. (1998). Psychometric foundations of assessment research. In J. N. Butcher, G. N. Holmbeck, & P. C. Kendall. *Handbook of research methods in clinical psychology* (2nd ed., pp. 125–154). New York: John Wiley & Sons.

Haynes, S. N. & O'Brien, W. H. (1990). The functional analysis in behavior therapy. *Clinical Psychology Review*, *10*, 649–668.

Haynes, S. N., Richard, D. C. S., & Kubany, E. (1995). Content validity in psychological assessment. A functional approach to concepts and methods. *Psychological Assessment*, *7*, 238–247.

Haynes, S. N., Richard, D., O'Brien, W. H., & Grant, C. (1999). *Clinical case modeling*. Washington, DC: American Psychological Association.

Haynes, S. N., Spain, H., & Oliveira, J. (1993). Identifying causal relationships in clinical assessment. *Psychological Assessment*, *5*, 281–291.

Haynes, S. N., & Uchigakiuchi, P. (1993). Incorporating personality trait measures in behavioral assessment: Nuts in a fruitcake or raisins in a mai tai? *Behavior Modification, 17,* 72–92.

Haynes, S. N., Uchigakiuchi, P., Meyer, K., Orimoto, L., Blaine, D., and O'Brien, W. H. (1993). Functional analytic causal models and the design of treatment programs: Concepts and clinical applications with childhood behavior problems. *European Journal of Psychological Assessment, 9,* 189–205.

Haynes, S. N., & Waialae, K. (1994). Psychometric foundations of behavioral assessment. In R. Fernández-Ballestros (Ed.), *Evaluacion conductual hoy: (Behavioral assessment today).* Madrid: Ediciones Piramide.

Hazelett, R. L., & Haynes, S. N. (1992). Fibromyalgia: A time-series analysis of the stressor-physical symptom association. *Journal of Behavioral Medicine, 15,* 541–558.

Heatherton, T. F., & Weinberger, J. L. (Eds.). (1994). *Can personality change.* Washington, DC: American Psychological Association.

Heiby, E. M. (1995a). Assessment of behavioral chaos with a focus on transitions in depression. *Psychological Assessment, 7,* 10–16.

Heiby, E. M. (1995b). Chaos theory, nonlinear dynamic models, and psychological assessment. *Psychological Assessment, 7,* 5–9.

Heller, M. C., Sobel, M., & Tanaka, M. J. (1996). A functional analysis of verbal interactions of drug-exposed children and their mothers: The utility of sequential analysis. *Journal of Clinical Psychology, 52,* 687–697.

Hersen, M., & Ammerman, R. T. (Eds.). (1994). *Handbook of prescriptive treatments for adults.* New York: Plenum.

Hersen, M., & Bellack, A. S. (Eds.). (1998). *Behavioral assessment: A practical handbook* (4th ed.). Boston: Allyn & Bacon.

Hersen, M. & Bellack, A. S. (Eds.). (1998). *Dictionary of behavioral assessment techniques.* New York: Pergamon.

Heyman, R. E., Weiss, R. L., & Eddy, J. M. (1995). Marital interaction coding system: Revision and empirical evaluation. *Behavior Research and Therapy, 33,* 737–746.

Hillbrand, M., & Waite, B. M. (1994). The everyday experience of an institutionalized sex offender: An idiographic application of the experience sampling methods. *Archives of Sexual Behavior, 23,* 453–463.

Hillson, J. M. C., & Kuiper, N. A. (1994). A stress and coping model of child maltreatment. *Clinical Psychology Review, 14,* 261–285.

Hodges, K., & Cools, J. N. (1990). Structured diagnostic interviews. In A. M. La Greca (Ed.), *Through the eyes of the child: Obtaining self-reports from children and adolescents* (pp. 85–108). Boston: Allyn & Bacon.

Hohlstein, L. A., Smith, G. T., & Atlas, J. G. (1995). An application of expectancy theory to eating disorders: Development and validation of measures of eating and dieting. *Psychological Assessment, 10,* 49–58.

Hollandsworth, J. G. (1986). *Physiology and behavior therapy: Conceptual guidelines for the therapist.* New York: Plenum.

Hops, H., Davis, B., & Longoria, N. (1995). Methodological issues in direct observation: Illustrations with the living in familial environments (LIFE) coding system. *Journal of Clinical Child Psychology, 24,* 193–203.

Horner, R. H. (1994). Functional assessment: Contributions and future directions. *Journal of Applied Behavior Analysis, 27,* 401–404.

Hume, D. (1740). *A treatise of human nature.* New York: Dutton (1911).

Hutt, S. J., & Hutt, C. (1970). *Direct observation and measurement of behavior.* Springfield, IL: Charles C. Thomas.

Hyland, M. (1981). *Introduction to theoretical psychology.* Baltimore: University Park Press.

Imber, S. D., et al. (1990). Mode-specific effects among three treatments for depression. *Journal of Consulting and Clinical Psychology, 58,* 352–359.

Iwata, B. A., Pace, G. M., Dorsey, M. F., Zarcone, J. R., Vollmer, B., & Smith, J. (1994). The function of self injurious behavior: An experimental-epidemiological analysis. *Journal of Applied Behavior Analysis, 27,* 215–240.

Jacobson, N. (1985). The role of observational measures in behavior therapy outcome research. *Behavioral Assessment, 7,* 297–308.

Jacobson, N. S., & Revenstorf, D. (1988). Statistics for assessing the clinical significance of psychotherapy techniques: Issues, problems and new developments. *Behavioral Assessment, 10,* 133–145.

Jacobson, N. S., & Truax, P. (1991). Clinical significance: A statistical approach to defining meaningful change in psychotherapy research. *Journal of Consulting and Clinical Psychology, 59,* 12–19.

James, L. R., Mulaik, S. A., & Brett, J. M. (1982). *Causal analysis: Assumptions, models and data.* Beverly Hills, CA: Sage.

James, R. C., & James, G. (1992). *Mathematics dictionary* (5th ed.). New York: Van Nostrand Reinhold.

James, W. (1893). *Psychology.* New York: Henry Holt.

Jensen, M. P., & Karoly, P. (1992). Self-report scales and procedures for assessing pain in adults. In D. C. Turk & R. Melzack (Eds.), *Handbook of pain assessment* (pp. 135–151). New York: Guilford.

Johnson, S. M., & Bolstad, O. D. (1975). Reactivity to home observation: A comparison of audio recorded behavior with observers present or absent. *Journal of Applied Behavior Analysis, 8,* 181–185.

Johnston, J. M., & Pennypacker, H. S. (1993). *Strategies and tactics of behavioral research* (2nd ed.). Hillsdale, NJ: Lawrence Erlbaum.

Kail, R. V., & Wickes-Nelson, R. (1993). *Developmental psychology.* New York: Prentice-Hall.

Kamphaus, R. W., & Frick, P. J. (1996). *Clinical assessment of child and adolescent personality and behavior.* Boston: Allyn & Bacon.

Kanfer, F. H. (1985). Target selection for clinical change programs. *Behavioral Assessment, 7,* 7–20.

Kanfer, F. H., & Grimm, L. G. (1980). Managing clinical change: A process model of therapy. *Behavior Modification, 4,* 419–444.

Kanfer, F. H., & Schefft, B. K. (1988). *Guiding the process of therapeutic change.* Champaign, IL: Research Press.

Kareken, D. A., & Williams, J. M. (1994). Human judgment and estimation of premorbid intellectual function. *Psychological Assessment, 6,* 83–91.

Karush, W. (1962). *Webster's new world dictionary of mathematics.* New York: Prentice-Hall Trade.

Kazdin, A. E. (1978). *History of behavior modification.* Baltimore: University Park Press.

Kazdin, A. E. (1985). Selection of target behaviors: The relationship of the treatment focus to clinical dysfunction. *Behavioral Assessment, 7,* 33–48.

Kazdin, A. E. (1998). *Research design in clinical psychology* (3rd ed.). Boston: Allyn & Bacon.

Kazdin, A. E., & Kagan, J. (1994). Models of dysfunction in developmental psychopathology. *Clinical Psychology: Science and Practice, 1,* 35–52.

Kearney, C. A., & Silverman, W. K. (1990). A preliminary analysis of a functional model of assessment and treatment for school refusal behavior. *Behavior Modification, 14,* 340–366.

Kelly, S., Green, G., & Sidman, M. (1998). Visual identity matching and auditory-visual matching: A procedural note. *Journal of Applied Behavior Analysis, 31,* 237–243.

Kendrick, D. T., & Funder, D. C. (1988). Profiting from controversy, lessons from the person-situation debate. *American Psychologist, 43,* 23–34.

Kennedy, C. H., & Souza, G. (1995). Functional analysis and treatment of eye poking. *Journal of Applied Behavioral Analysis, 28,* 27–37.

Kenny, D. A., & Kashy, D. A. (1992). Analysis of the multitrait-multimethod matrix by confirmatory factor analysis. *Psychological Bulletin, 112,* 165–172.

Kern, J. M. (1991). An evaluation of a novel role-play methodology: The standardized idiographic approach. *Behavior Therapy, 22,* 13–29.

Kerwin, M. E., Ahearn, W. H., Eicher, P. S., & Swearingin, W. (1998). The relationship between food refusal and self-injurious behavior: A case study. *Journal of Behavior Therapy and Experimental Psychiatry, 29,* 67–77.

Kessler, R. C. (1997). The effects of stressful life events on depression. In J. T. Spence, J. M. Darley, & D. J. Foss (Eds.), *Annual review of psychology, 48* (pp. 191–214). Palo Alto, CA: Annual Reviews.

Kinder, B. N. (1997). Eating disorders. In S. M. Turner & M. Hersen (Eds.), *Adult psychopathology and diagnosis* (3rd ed., pp. 465–482). New York: John Wiley & Sons.

Kiresuk, T. J., Smith, A., & Cardillo, J. E. (Eds.). (1994). *Goal attainment scaling: Applications, theory, and measurement.* Hillsdale, NJ: Lawrence Erlbaum Associates.

Kleinmuntz, B. (1990). Why we still use our heads instead of formulas: Toward an integrative approach. *Psychological Bulletin, 107,* 296–310.

Koerner, K., & Linehan, M. M. (1997). Case formulation in dialectical behavior therapy. In T. D. Eells (Ed.), *Handbook of psychotherapy case formulation* (pp. 340–367). New York: Guilford.

Kohlenberg, R. J., & Tsai, M. (1991). *Functional analytic psychotherapy—Creating intense and curative therapeutic relationships.* New York: Plenum.

Kraaimaat, F. W., Brons, M. R., Greenen, R., & Bijlsma, J. W. J. (1995). The effect of cognitive behavior therapy in patients with rheumatiod arthritis. *Behavior Research and Therapy, 33,* 487–495.

Kraemer, H. C. (1992). *Evaluating medical tests—Objective and quantitative guidelines.* Beverly Hills, CA: Sage.

Krantz, P. J., & McClannahan, L. E. (1998). Social interaction skills for children with autism: A script-fading procedure for beginning readers. *Journal of Applied Behavior Analysis, 31,* 191–202.

Krasner, L. (1992). The concepts of syndrome and functional analysis: Compatible or incompatible. *Behavioral Assessment, 14,* 307–321.

Krasner, L., & Ullmann, L. P. (Eds.). (1965). *Research in behavior modification.* New York: Holt, Rinehart, & Winston.

Kratochwill, T. R., & Levin, J. R. (1992). *Single-case research design and analysis: New directions for psychology and education.* Hillsdale, NJ: Lawrence Erlbaum Associates.

Kratochwill, T. R., & Plunge, M. (1992). DSM-III-R, treatment validity, and functional analysis: Further considerations for school psychologists. *School Psychology Quarterly, 7,* 227–232.

Kratochwill, T. R., & Roseby, V. (1988). Psychoeducational assessment. In: P. Karoly, et al. (Eds.), *Handbook of child health assessment: Biopsychosocial perspectives* (pp. 173–226). New York: John Wiley & Sons.

Kratochwill, T. R., & Shapiro, E. S. (1988). Introduction: Conceptual foundations of behavioral assessment. In E. S. Shapiro & T. R. Kratochwill (Eds.), *Behavioral assessment in schools: Conceptual foundations and practical applications* (pp. 1–13). New York: Guilford.

Krejbeil, D., & Lewis, P. T. (1994). An observation emphasis in undergraduate psychology laboratories. *Teaching of Psychology, 21*, 45–48.

Kuhn, T. S. (1970). *The structure of scientific revolutions* (2nd ed). Chicago: University of Chicago Press.

La Greca, A. M. (1990). *Through the eyes of the child.* New York: Allyn & Bacon.

Lalli, J. S., & Kates, K. (1998). The effect of reinforcer preference on functional analysis outcomes. *Journal of Applied Behavior Analysis, 31*, 79–90.

Lambert, M. J. (1994). Use of psychological tests for outcome assessment. In M. E. Maruish et al. (Eds.), *The use of psychological testing for treatment planning and outcome assessment* (pp. 75–97). Hillsdale, NJ: Lawrence Erlbaum Associates.

Lane, S. D., & Critchfield, T. S. (1998). Classification of vowels and consonants by individuals with moderate mental retardation: Development of arbitrary relations via match-to-sample training with compound stimuli. *Journal of Applied Behavior Analysis, 31*, 21–41.

Lang, P. J. (1995). The emotion probe: Studies of motivation and attention. *American Psychologist, 50*, 519–525.

Lanyon, R. I., & Lanyon, B. J. (1976). Behavioural assessment and decision-making: The design of strategies for therapeutic behaviour change. In M. P. Feldman & A. Broadhurst (Eds.), *Theoretical and experimental bases of the behaviour therapies* (pp. 289–329). London: John Wiley & Sons.

Last, C. G., Strauss, C. C., & Francis, G. (1987). Comorbidity among childhood anxiety disorders. *Journal of Nervous and Mental Disease, 175*, 426–430.

Laties, V. G., & Mace, F. C. (1993). Taking stock: The first 25 years of the journal of applied behavior analysis. *Journal of Applied Behavior Analysis, 26*, 513–525.

Lazarus, R. S. (1993). From psychological stress to the emotions: A history of changing outlooks. In L. W. Porter & M. R. Rosenzweig (Eds.), *Annual review of psychology, 44* (pp. 1–21). Palo Alto, CA: Annual Reviews.

Leary, M. R. (1991). Social anxiety, shyness, and related constructs. In J. P. Robinson, P. R. Shaver, & L. S. Wrightsman (Eds.), *Measures of personality and social psychological attitudes* (Vol. 1 in Measures of Social Psychological Attitudes Series, pp. 161–194). San Diego, CA: Academic Press.

Lees, M. C., & Neufeld, R. W. J. (1994). Matching the limits of clinical inference to the limits of quantitative methods: A formal appeal to practice what we consistently preach. *Canadian Psychology, 35*, 268–282.

Lehman, A. F. (1996). Quality of life interview (QOLI). In L. I. Sederer & B. Dickey (Eds.), *Outcomes assessment in clinical practice* (pp. 117–119). Baltimore: Williams & Wilkins.

Lennox, D. B., Miltenberger, R. G., Spengler, P., & Erfanian, N. (1988). Decelerative treatment practices with persons who have mental retardation: A review of five years of the literature. *American Journal of Mental Retardation, 92*, 492–501.

Lerner, R. G., & Trigg, G. L. (1991). *Encyclopedia of physics* (2nd ed.). New York: VCH Publishers.

Liberman, R. P., Kopelowicz, A., & Young, A. S. (1994). Biobehavioral treatment and rehabilitation of schizophrenia. *Behavior Therapy, 25*, 89–107.

Lichstein, K. L., & Riedel, B. W. (1994). Behavioral assessment and treatment of insomnia: A review with an emphasis on clinical application. *Behavior Therapy, 25*, 659–688.

Lilienfeld, S. O., Waldman, I. D., & Israel, A. C. (1994). A critical examination of the use of the term and concept of "comorbidity" in psychopathology research. *Clinical Psychology: Science and Practice, 1*, 71–83.

Linehan, M. M. (1993). *Cognitive-behavioral treatment of borderline personality disorder.* New York: Guilford.

Linn, R. L. (1993). *Educational measurement* (3rd ed.). Phoenix: American Council on Education/Oryx Press.

Linscott, J., & DiGiuseppe, R. (1998). Cognitive assessment. In A. S. Bellack & M. Hersen (Eds.), *Behavioral assessment—A practical handbook* (4th ed., pp. 104–125). Boston: Allyn & Bacon.

Locke, J. (1690). *An essay concerning human understanding.* London: Routledge.

Loehlin, J. C. (1998). *Latent variable models—An introduction to factor, path, and structural analysis* (3rd ed.). Mahwah, NJ: Lawrence Erlbaum Associates.

Lovejoy, M. C. (1991). Maternal depression: Effects on social cognition and behavior in parent–child interactions. *Journal of Abnormal Child Psychology, 19*, 693–706.

Luborsky, L. (1984). *Principles of psychoanalytic psychotherapy: A manual for supportive-expressive (SE) treatment.* New York: Basic Books.

Magill, F. N., & McGreal, I. P. (1961). *Masterpieces of world philosophy.* New York: Harper & Row Publishers.

Maisto, S. A., McKay, J. R., & Connors, G. J. (1990). Self-report issues in substance abuse: State of the art and future directions. *Behavioral Assessment, 12*, 117–134.

Maloney, M. P., & Ward, M. P. (1976). *Psychological assessment: A conceptual approach.* New York: Oxford University Press.

Mann, J., Ten Have, T., Plunkett, J. W., & Meisels, S. J. (1991). Time sampling: A methodological critique. *Child Development, 62,* 227–241.

March, J. S. (ed.). (1995). *Anxiety disorders in children and adolescents* (pp. 3–34). New York: Guilford.

Marcus, L. M., & Schopler, E. (1993). Pervasive developmental disorders. In Ollendick, T. H., & Hersen, M. (Eds.), *Handbook of child and adolescent assessment* (pp. 346–363). Boston: Allyn & Bacon.

Margolin, G. (1981). Practical applications of behavioral marital assessment. In E. E. Filsinger & R. A. Lewis (Eds.), *Assessing marriage: New behavioral approaches.* Beverly Hills, CA: Sage.

Margolin, G., Talovie, S., & Weinstein, C. D. (1983). Areas of change questionnaire: A practical approach to marital assessment. *Journal of Consulting and Clinical Psychology, 51,* 920–931.

Marriott, F. H. C. (1990). *A dictionary of statistical terms.* New York: Wiley.

Marsella, A. J., & Kameoka, V. (1989). Ethnocultural issues in the assessment of psychopathology. In S. Wetzler (Ed.), *Measuring mental illness: Psychometric assessment for clinicians.* Washington, DC: American Psychiatric Association.

Martin, G., & Pear, J. (1996). *Behavior modification: What it is and how to do it* (5th ed.). Englewood Cliffs, NJ: Prentice-Hall.

Maruish, M. E. (Ed.). (1994). *The use of psychological testing for treatment planning and outcome assessment.* Hillsdale, NJ: Lawrence Erlbaum Associates.

Mash, E. J., & Barkley, R. A. (1989). *Treatment of childhood disorders.* New York: Guilford.

Mash, E. J., & Hunsley, J. (1990). Behavioral assessment: A contemporary approach. In A. S. Bellack, M. Hersen, & A. E. Kazdin (Eds.), *International handbook of behavior modification and therapy* (2nd ed., pp. 87–106). New York: Plenum.

Mash, E. J., & Hunsley, J. (1993). Assessment considerations in the identification of failing psychotherapy: Bringing the negatives out of the darkroom. *Psychological Assessment, 5,* 292–301.

Mash, E. J., & Terdal, L. G. (1988). Behavioral assessment of child and family disturbance. In E. J. Mash & L. G. Terdal (Eds.), *Behavioral assessment of childhood disorders* (pp. 3–65). New York: Guilford.

Mash, E. J., & Terdal, L. G. (1997a). Assessment of child and family disturbance: A behavioral-systems approach. In E. J. Mash & L. G. Terdal (Eds.), *Assessment of childhood disorders* (3rd ed., pp. 3–68). New York: Guilford.

Mash, E. J., & Terdal, L. G. (Eds.). (1997b). *Assessment of childhood disorders* (3rd ed.). New York: Guilford.

Matarazzo, J. D., & Wiens, A. N. (1972). *The interview: Research on its anatomy and structure.* Chicago: Aldine-Atherton.

Matthysse, S. (1993). Genetics and the problem of causality in abnormal psychology. In P. B. Sutker & H. E. Adams (Eds.), *Comprehensive handbook of psychopathology* (2nd ed., pp. 47–56). New York: Plenum.

Matyas, T. A., & Greenwood, K. M. (1990). Visual analysis of single-case time series: Effects of variability, serial dependence, and magnitude of intervention effect. *Journal of Applied Behavior Analysis, 23,* 341–351.

McAllister, W. R., & McAllister, D. E. (1995). Two-factor fear theory: Implications for understanding anxiety-based clinical phenomena. In W. O'Donohue & L. Krasner (Eds.), *Theories of behavior therapy—Exploring behavior change* (pp. 145–172). Washington, DC: American Psychological Association.

McCann, B. S. (1987). The behavioral management of hypertension. In M. Hersen, R. M. Eisler, & P. M. Miller (Eds.), *Progress in behavior modification, 21* (pp. 191–229). Newbury Park, CA: Sage.

McCleary, R., & Hay, R. (1980). *Applied time series analysis for the social sciences.* Beverly Hills, CA: Sage.

McComas, J. J., Wacker, D. P., & Cooper, L. J. (1998). Increasing compliance with medical procedures: Application of the high-probability request procedure to a toddler. *Journal of Applied Behavior Analysis, 31,* 287–290.

McConaghy, N. (1998). Assessment of sexual dysfunction and deviation. In A. S. Bellack & M. Hersen (Eds.), *Behavioral assessment—A practical handbook* (4th ed., pp. 315–341). Boston: Allyn & Bacon.

McFall, R. M. (1982). A review and reformulation of the concept of social skills. *Behavioral Assessment, 4,* 1–33.

McFall, R. M. (1986). Theory and method in assessment: The vital link. *Behavioral Assessment, 8,* 3–10.

McFall, R. M., & McDonel, E. (1986). The continuing search for units of analysis in psychology: Beyond persons, situations and their interactions. In R. O. Nelson & S. C. Hayes (Eds.), *Conceptual foundations of behavioral assessment* (pp. 201–241). New York: Guilford.

McFall, R. M., & Townsend, J. T. (1998). Foundation of psychological assessment: Implications for cognitive assessment in clinical science. *Psychological Assessment, 10,* 316–330.

McGlynn, F. D., & Rose, M. P. (1998). Assessment of anxiety and fear. In A. S. Bellack & M. Hersen (Eds.), *Behavioral assessment—A practical handbook* (4th ed., pp. 179–209). Boston: Allyn & Bacon.

McGuigan, F. J. (1990). *Experimental psychology: Methods of research.* New York: Prentice Hall.

McNeil, D. W., Ries, B. J., & Turk, C. L. (1995). Behavioral assessment: Self-report, physiology, and overt behavior. In R. G. Heimberg, M. R. Liebowitz, D. A. Hope, & F. R. Schneier (Eds.), *Social phobia: Diagnosis, assessment and treatment.* New York: Guilford.

McReynolds, P. (1986). History of assessment in clinical and educational settings. In R. O. Nelson & S. C. Hayes (Eds.), *Conceptual foundations of behavioral assessment* (pp. 42–80). New York: Guilford.

McReynolds, P. (Ed.). (1968). *Advances in psychological assessment* (Vol. 1). San Francisco: Jossey-Bass.

Meehl, P. (1986). The causes and effects of my disturbing little book. *Journal of Personality Assessment, 50,* 370–375.

Meehl, P. E. (1954). *Clinical vs. statistical prediction: A theoretical analysis and review of the evidence.* Minneapolis: University of Minnesota Press.

Meier, S. T. (1994). *The chronic crisis in psychological measurement and assessment: A historical survey.* San Diego, CA: Academic Press.

Mellers, B. A., Schwartz, A., & Cooke, A. D. J. (1998). Judgment and decision making. *Annual Review of Psychology, 49* (pp. 447–477). Palo Alto, CA: Annual Reviews.

Merskey, H., & Spear, P. G. (1964). The reliability of the pressure algometer. *British Journal of Social Clinical Psychology, 3,* 130–136.

Messick, S. (1991). Psychology and methodology of response styles. In R. E. Snow, D. E. Wiley, et al. (Eds.), *Improving inquiry in social science: A volume in honor of Lee J. Cronbach* (pp. 161–200). Hillsdale, NJ: Lawrence Erlbaum Associates.

Messick, S. (1993). Validity. In R. L. Linn (Ed.), *Educational measurement* (3rd ed., pp. 13–103). Phoenix, AZ: Oryx Press.

Messick, S. (1994). Foundations of validity: Meaning and consequences in psychological assessment. *European Journal of Psychological Assessment, 10,* 1–9.

Messick, S. (1995). Validation of inferences from persons' responses and performances as scientific inquiry into score meaning. *American Psychologist, 50,* 741–749.

Metalsky, G. I., Laird, R. S., Heck, P. M., & Joiner, Jr., T. E. (1995). Attribution theory: Clinical applications. In W. O'Donohue & L. Krasner (Eds.), *Theories of behavior therapy—Exploring behavior change* (pp. 385–414). Washington, DC: American Psychological Association.

Michael, J. (1993). Establishing operations. *The Behavior Analyst, 16,* 191–206.

Michelson, L. (1986). Treatment consonance and response profiles in agoraphobia: The role of individual differences in cognitive, behavioral, and physiological treatments. *Behaviour Research and Therapy, 24,* 264–275.

Michelson, L., Mavissakalian, M., Marchione, K., Ulrich, R. F., Marchione, N., & Testa, S. (1990). Psychophysiological outcome of cognitive, behavioral and psychophysiologically based treatments of agoraphobia. *Behavior Research and Therapy, 28,* 127–139.

Mill, J. S. (1967). *A system of logic ratiocinative and inductive.* London: Longmans (from 1843 original edition).

Miller, T. W. (Ed.). (1996). *Theory and assessment of stressful life events.* Madison, CT: International Universities Press.

Miltenberger, R. G., Long, E. S., Rapp, J. T., Lumley, V., & Elliott, A. J. (1998). Evaluating the function of hair pulling: A preliminary investigation. *Behavior Therapy, 29,* 211–219.

Milton, S. B., Scaglione, C., Flanagan, T., Cox, J. L., et al. (1991). Functional evaluation of adolescent students with traumatic brain injury. *Journal of Head Trauma Rehabilitation, 6,* 35–46.

Mohr, D. C. (1995). Negative outcome in psychotherapy: A critical review. *Clinical Psychology: Science and Practice, 2,* 1–27.

Morin, C. M. (1993). *Insomnia: Psychological assessment and management.* New York: Guilford.

Morin, C. M., & Edinger, J. D. (1997). Sleep disorders: Evaluation and diagnosis: In S. M. Turner & M. Hersen (Eds.), *Adult psychopathology and diagnosis* (3rd ed., pp. 483–507). New York: John Wiley & Sons.

Morris, E. K. (1988). Contextualism: The world view of behavior analysis. *Journal of Experimental Child Psychology, 46,* 289–323.

Moxley, R. A. (1992). From mechanistic to functional behaviorism. *American Psychologist, 47,* 1300–1311.

Mueser, K. T. (1997). Schizophrenia. In S. M. Turner & M. Hersen (Eds.), *Adult psychopathology and diagnosis* (3rd ed., pp. 203–299). New York: John Wiley & Sons.

Muran, J. C., & Segal, Z. V. (1992). The development of an idiographic measure of self-schemas: An illustration of the construction and use of self-scenarios. *Psychotherapy, 29,* 524–535.

Murphy, K. R., & Cleveland, J. N. (1995). *Understanding performance appraisal: Social, organizational, and goal based perspectives.* Thousand Oaks, CA: Sage.

Murphy, K. R., & Davidshofer, C. O. (1994). *Psychological testing: Principles and applications* (3rd ed.). Englewood Cliffs, NJ: Prentice-Hall.

Nagel, E. (1961). *The structure of science.* New York: Harcourt, Brace and World.

Nathan, P. E. (1993). Alcoholism: Psychopathology, etiology, and treatment. In P. B. Sutker & H. E. Adams (Eds.), *Comprehensive handbook of psychopathology* (pp. 471–476). New York: Plenum.

Nay, W. F. (1979). *Multimethod clinical assessment.* New York: Gardner Press.

Nelson, R. O. (1983). Behavioral assessment: Past, present, and future. *Behavioral Assessment, 5,* 195–206.

Nelson, R. O., & Hayes, S. C. (1986). The nature of behavioral assessment. In R. O. Nelson & S. C. Hayes (Eds.), *Conceptual foundations of behavioral assessment* (pp. 1–41). New York: Guilford.

Nelson-Gray, R. O. (1996). Treatment outcome measures: Nomothetic or idiographic? *Clinical Psychology: Science and Practice, 3,* 164–167.

Newman, M. G., Hofmann, S. G., Trabert, W., Roth, W. T., & Taylor, C. B. (1994). Does behavioral treatment of social phobia lead to cognitive changes? *Behavior Therapy, 25,* 503–517.

Newsom, C., & Hovanitz, C. A. (1997). Autistic disorder. In E. J. Mash & L. G. Terdal (Eds.), *Assessment of childhood disorders* (3rd ed., pp. 408–452). New York: Guilford.

Nevo, B. (1985). Face validity revisited. *Journal of Educational Measurement, 22,* 287–293.

Nezu, A. M. & Nezu, C. M. (1993). Identifying and selecting target problems for clinical interventions: A problem-solving model. *Psychological Assessment, 5,* 254–263.

Nezu, A., Nezu, C., Friedman, S. H., & Haynes, S. N. (1997). Case formulation in behavior therapy: Problem-solving and functional analytic strategies. In T. D. Eells (Ed.), *Handbook of psychotherapy case formulation.* New York: Guilford (pp. 368–401).

Nezu, A. M., & Nezu, C. M. (1989). *Clinical decision making in behavior therapy: A problem solving perspective.* Champaign, IL: Research Press.

Nezu, A. M., & Nezu, C. M. (1993). Identifying and selecting target problems for clinical interventions: A problem-solving model. *Psychological Assessment, 5,* 254–263.

Niccols, G. A. (1994). Fetal alcohol syndrome: Implications for psychologists. *Clinical Psychology Review, 14,* 91–111.

Nietzel, M. T., & Trull, T. (1988). Meta-analytic approaches to social comparisons: A method for measuring clinical significance. *Behavioral Assessment, 10,* 159–169.

Nunnally, J. C., & Bernstein, I. H. (1994). *Psychometric theory.* New York: McGraw-Hill.

O'Brien, W. H. (1995). Inaccuracies in the estimation of functional relationships using self-monitoring data. *Journal of Behavior Therapy and Experimental Psychiatry, 26,* 351–357.

O'Brien, W. H., & Haynes, S. N. (1995a). A functional analytic approach to the conceptualization, assessment and treatment of a child with frequent migraine headaches. *In Session, 1,* 65–80.

O'Brien, W. O., & Haynes, S. N. (1995b). Behavioral assessment. In L. Heiden & M. Hersen (Eds.), *Introduction to clinical psychology* (pp. 106–139). New York: Plenum.

O'Brien, W. O., & Haynes, S. N. (1993). Behavioral assessment in psychiatric settings. In M. Hersen & A. S. Bellack (Eds.), *Behavior therapy in psychiatric settings.* New York: Pergamon Press.

O'Brien, W. H., & Haynes, S. N. (1997). Functional analysis. In Gualberto Buela-Casal (Ed.), *Handbook of psychological assessment.* Madrid: Sigma.

O'Donohue, W. T., & Krasner, L. (1995). *Theories of behavior therapy: Exploring behavior change.* Washington, DC: American Psychological Association.

Ogles, B. M., Lambert, M. J., & Masters, K. S. (1996). *Assessing outcome in clinical practice.* Boston: Allyn & Bacon.

Okazaki, S., & Sue, S. (1995). Methodological issues in assessment research with ethnic minorities. *Psychological Assessment, 7,* 367–375.

O'Leary, K. D. (1987). *Assessment of marital discord.* Hillsdale, NJ: Lawrence Erlbaum Associates.

O'Leary, K. D., Vivian, D., & Malone, J. (1992). Assessment of physical aggression against women in marriage: The need for multimodal assessment. *Behavioral Assessment, 14,* 5–14.

Ollendick, T. H., & Hersen, M. (1993a). Child and adolescent behavioral assessment. In T. H. Ollendick & M. Hersen (Eds.), *Handbook of child and adolescent assessment* (pp. 3–14). Boston: Allyn & Bacon.

Ollendick, T. H., & Hersen, M. (Eds.) (1993b). *Handbook of child and adolescent assessment.* Boston: Allyn & Bacon.

Ost, L. G., Jerremalm, A., & Johansson, J. (1981). Individual response patterns and the effects of different behavior methods in the treatment of social phobia. *Behaviour Research and Therapy, 20,* 445–460.

Pantalon, M. V., & Motta, R. W. (1998). Effectiveness of anxiety management training in the treatment of post-traumatic stress disorder: A preliminary report. *Journal of Behavior Therapy and Experimental Psychiatry, 29,* 21–29.

Parten, M. B. (1932). Social participation among preschool children. *Journal of Abnormal and Social Psychology, 27,* 243–269.

Patterson, G. R. (1993). Orderly change in a stable world: The antisocial trait as a chimera. *Journal of Consulting and Clinical Psychology, 61,* 911–919.

Patterson, G. R., Dishion, T. J., & Chamberlain, P. (1993). Outcomes and methodological issues relating to treatment of antisocial children. In T. R. Giles (Ed.), *Handbook of effective psychotherapy* (pp. 43–88). New York: Plenum.

Patterson, G. R., & Forgatch, M. S. (1995). Predicting future clinical adjustment from treatment outcome and process variables. *Psychological Assessment, 7,* 275–285.

Paul, G. L. (1986). *The time sample behavioral checklist: Observational assessment instrumentation for service and research.* Champaign, IL: Research Press.

Pedhazur, E. J., & Schmelkin, L. P. (1991). *Measurement, design, and analysis: An integrated approach* (student ed.). Hillsdale, NJ: Lawrence Erlbaum Associates.

Peine, H. A., Darvish, R., Blakelock, H., Osborne, J. G., & Jenson, W. R. (1998). Non-aversive reduction of cigarette smoking in two adult men in a residential setting. *Journal of Behavior Therapy and Experimental Psychiatry, 29*, 55–65.

Peitgen, H.-O., Jürgens, H., & Saupe, D. (1992). *Chaos and fractals: New frontiers of science.* New York: Springer-Verlag.

Persons, J. B. (1989). *Cognitive therapy in practice: A case formulation approach.* New York: Norton.

Persons, J. B. (1991). Psychotherapy outcome studies do not accurately represent current models of psychotherapy: A proposed remedy. *American Psychologist, 46*, 99–106.

Persons, J. B., & Bertagnolli, A. (1994). Cognitive-behavioural treatment of multiple-problem patients: Application to personality disorders. *Clinical Psychology and Psychotherapy, 1*, 279–285.

Persons, J. B., & Fresco, D. M. (1998). Assessment of depression. In A. S. Bellack & M. Hersen (Eds.), *Behavioral assessment—A practical handbook* (4th ed., pp. 210–231). Boston: Allyn & Bacon.

Persons, J. B., Mooney, K. A., & Padesky, C. A. (1995). Interrater reliability of cognitive-behavioral case formulations. *Cognitive Therapy and Research, 19*, 21–34.

Persons, J. B., & Tompkins, M. A. (1997). Cognitive-behavioral case formulation. In T. D. Eells (Ed.), *Handbook of psychotherapy case formulation* (pp. 314–339). New York: Guilford.

Pervin, L. A. (1984). Idiographic approaches to personality. In N. S. Endler & J. M. Hunt (Eds.), *Personality and the behavior disorders* (pp. 261–282). New York: John Wiley & Sons.

Phelps, L., & McClintock, K. (1994). Papa and peers: A biosocial approach to conduct disorder. *Journal of Psychopathology and Behavioral Assessment, 16*, 53–67.

Piazza, C. C., Fisher, W. W., Hanley, G. P., LeBlanc, L. A., Worsdell, A. S., Lindauer, S. E., & Keeney, K. M. (1998). Treatment of pica through multiple analyses of its reinforcing functions. *Journal of Applied Behavior Analysis, 31*, 165–189.

Pierce, W. D., & Epling, W. F. (1999). *Behavior analysis and learning.* Upper Saddle River, NJ: Prentice-Hall.

Piotrowski, C., & Keller, J. W. (1984). Attitudes toward clinical assessment by members of the AABT. *Psychological Reports, 55*, 831–838.

Piotrowski, C., & Lubin, B. (1990). Assessment practices of health psychologists: Survey of APA division 38 clinicians. *Professional Psychology: Research and Practice, 21*, 99–106.

Piotrowski, C., & Zalewski, C. (1993). Training in psychodiagnostic testing in APA-approved PsyD and PhD clinical psychology programs. *Journal of Personality Assessment, 61*, 394–405.

Pitman, R. K., Orr, S. P., Forgue, D. F., Altman, B., de Jong, J. B., & Herz, L. R. (1990). Psychophysiologic responses to combat imagery of Vietnam veterans with posttraumatic stress disorder versus other anxiety disorders. *Journal of Abnormal Psychology, 99*, 49–54.

Plaud, J. J., & Eifert, G. H. (Eds.). (1998). *From behavior theory to behavior therapy.* Boston: Allyn & Bacon.

Popper, K. R. (1959). *The logic of scientific discovery* (Die Logik der Forschung). New York: Basic Books, 1959 (originally published in 1935).

Quera, V. (1990). A generalized technique to estimate frequency and duration in time sampling. *Behavioral Assessment, 12*, 409–424.

Rachlin, H. (1970). *Introduction to modern behaviorism.* San Francisco: Freeman.

Rachman, S. J., & Hodgson, R. S. (1974). Synchrony and desynchrony in fear and avoidance. *Behaviour Research and Therapy, 12*, 311–318.

Rapee, R. M., & Barlow, D. H. (1993). Generalized anxiety disorder, panic disorder, and the phobias. In P. B. Sutker & H. E. Adams (Eds.), *Comprehensive handbook of psychopathology* (2nd ed., pp. 109–128). New York: Plenum.

Rapp, J. T., Miltenberger, R. G., Long, E. S., Elliott, A. J., & Lumley, V. A. (1998). Simplified habit reversal treatment for chronic hair pulling in three adolescents: A clinical replication with direct observation. *Journal of Applied Behavior Analysis, 31*, 299–302.

Regier, D. A., Farmer, M. E., Rae, D. S., Locke, B. Z., Keith, S. J., Judd, L. L., & Goodwin, F. K. (1990). Comorbidity of mental disorders with alcohol and other drug abuse. *Journal of the American Medical Association, 264*, 2511–2518.

Rehm, L. P., LePage, J. P., & Bailey, S. (1994). Unipolar depression. In M. Hersen & R. T. Ammerman (Eds.), *Handbook of prescriptive treatments for adults* (pp. 95–117). New York: Plenum.

Reid, D. H., Parsons, M. A., & Green, C. A. (1998). Identifying work preferences among individuals with severe multiple disabilities prior to beginning supported work. *Journal of Applied Behavior Analysis, 31*, 281–285.

Repp, A. C., Karsh, K. G., Munk, D., & Dahlquist, C. M. (1995). Hypothesis-based interventions: A theory of clinical decision making. In W. O'Donohue & L. Krasner (Eds.), *Theories of behavior therapy* (pp. 585–608). Washington, DC: American Psychological Association.

Riedel, B. W., & Lichstein, K. L. (1994). *Handbook of prescriptive treatments for adults.* New York: Plenum.

Rosen, R. C., Brondolo, E., & Kostis, J. B. (1993). Nonpharmacological treatment of essential hypertension: Research and clinical applications. In R. J. Gatchel & E. B. Blanchard (Eds.), *Psychophysiological disorders, research and clinical applications* (pp. 63–110). Washington, DC: American Psychological Association.

Russo, D. C. (1990). A requiem for the passing of the three-term contingency. *Behavior Therapy, 21*, 153–165.

Russo, D. C., Hamada, R. S., & Marques, D. (1988). Linking assessment and treatment in pediatric health psychology. In P. Karoly (Ed.), *Handbook of child health assessment* (pp. 30–50). New York: John Wiley & Sons.

Rust, J., & Golombok, S. (1989). *Modern psychometrics: The science of psychological assessment.* New York: Routledge.

Rychtarik, R. G., & McGillicuddy, N. B. (1998). Assessment of appetitive disorders: Status of empirical methods in alcohol, tobacco, and other drug use. In A. S. Bellack & M. Hersen (Eds.), *Behavioral assessment—A practical handbook* (4th ed., pp. 271–292). Boston: Allyn & Bacon.

Salmon, W. C. (1984). *Scientific explanation and the causal structure of the world.* Princeton, NJ: Princeton University Press.

Samelson, F. (1981). Struggle for scientific authority: The reception of Watons's behaviorism, 1913–1920. *Journal of the History of the Behavioral Sciences, 17*, 399–425.

Saper, Z., & Brasfield, C. R. (1998). Two-phase treatment of panic disorder and posttraumatic stress disorder with associated personality features resulting from childhood abuse: Case study. *Journal of Behavior Therapy and Experimental Psychiatry, 29*, 171–178.

Sarle, W. S. (1995). *Measurement theory: Frequently asked questions. Dieesminations of the International Statistical Applications Institute* (4th ed., pp. 61–66). Wichita, KS: ACG Press, URL: ftp://ftp.sas.com/pub/neural/measurement.faq

Saris, W. E., & Strankhorst, L. H. (1984). *Causal modeling in nonexperimental research: An introduction to the LISREL approach.* Amsterdam: Sociometric Research Foundation.

Sarwer, D. B., & Sayers, S. L. (1998). Behavioral interviewing. In A. S. Bellack & M. Hersen (Eds.), *Behavioral assessment—A practical handbook* (4th ed., pp. 63–78). Boston: Allyn & Bacon.

Sasso, G. M., Reimers, T. M., Cooper, L. J., Wacker, D., Berg, W., Steege, M., Kelly, L., & Allaire, A. (1992). Use of descriptive and experimental analysis to identify the functional properties of aberrant behavior in school settings. *Journal of Applied Behavior Analysis, 25*, 809–821.

Sattler, J. M. (1988). *Assessment of children.* San Diego, CA: Jerome M. Sattler, Publisher.

Schill, M. T., Kratochwill, T. R., & Gardner, W. I. (1996). Conducting a functional analysis of behavior. In M. J. Breen & C. R. Fiedler (Eds.), *Behavioral approach to assessment of youth with emotional/behavioral disorders—A handbook for school-based practitioners* (pp. 83–180). Austin, TX: PRO-ED.

Schlundt, D. G. (1985). An observational methodology for functional analysis. *Bulletin for the Society of Psychologists in Addictive Behaviors, 4*, 234–249.

Schlundt, D. G., Johnson, W. G., & Jarrel, M. P. (1986). A sequential analysis of environmental, behavioral, and affective variables predictive of vomiting in bulimia nervosa. *Behavioral Assessment, 8*, 253–269.

Schmidt, N. B. (1994). The schema questionnaire and the schema avoidance questionnaire. *The Behavior Therapist, 17*, 90–92.

Schneider, S. M., & Morris, E. K. (1988). Comments on quanta in the analysis of stimulus control. *Psychological Record, 38*, 501–514.

Schoggen, P. (1989). *Behavior settings: A revision and extension of Roger G. Barker's ecological psychology.* Stanford, CA: Stanford University Press.

Schreibman, L., Charlop, M. H., & Kurtz, P. F. (1992). Behavioral treatment for children with autism. In S. M. Turner, K. S. Calhoun, & H. E. Adams (Eds.), *Handbook of clinical behavior therapy* (2nd ed., pp. 337–351). New York: John Wiley & Sons.

Schulte, D. (1992). Criteria of treatment selection in behaviour therapy. *European Journal of Psychological Assessment, 8*, 157–162.

Schulte, D., Kuenzel, R., Pepping, G., & Schulte-Bahrenberg, T. (1992). Tailor-made versus standardized therapy of phobic patients. *Advances in Behaviour Research and Therapy, 14*, 67–92.

Sederer, L. I., Dickey, B., & Eisen, S. V. (1997). Assessing outcomes in clinical practice. *Psychiatric Quarterly, 68*, 311–325.

Shadish, W. R. (1996). Meta-analysis and the exploration of causal mediating processes: A primer of examples, methods, and issues. *Psychological Methods, 1*, 47–65.

Shalev, A. Y., Orr, S. P., & Pittman, R. K. (1993). Psychophysiologic assessment of traumatic imagery in Israeli civilian patients with post-traumatic stress disorder. *American Journal of Psychiatry, 150*, 620–624.

Shapiro, E. W., & Kratochwill, T. R. (Eds.). (1988). *Behavioral assessment in schools, Conceptual foundations and practical applications.* New York: Guilford.

Shiffman, S. (1993). Assessing smoking patterns and motives. *Journal of Consulting and Clinical Psychology, 61,* 732–742.

Sidman, M. (1960). *Tactics of scientific research.* New York: Basic Books.

Silva, F. (1993). *Psychometric foundations and behavioral assessment.* Newbury Park, CA: Sage.

Silverman, W. K., & Kurtines, W. M. (1996). *Anxiety and phobic disorders: A pragmatic approach.* New York: Plenum.

Singh, N. N., Deitz, D. D., Epstein, M. H., & Singh, J. (1991). Social behavior of students who are seriously emotionally disturbed: A quantitative analysis of intervention studies. *Behavior Modification, 15,* 74–94.

Sisson, L. A., & Taylor, J. C. (1993). Parent training. In A. S. Bellack & M. Hersen (Eds.), *Handbook of behavior therapy in the psychiatric setting* (pp. 555–574). New York: Plenum.

Skinner, B. F. (1945). The operational analysis of psychological terms. *Psychological Review, 52,* 270–277.

Smith, A. (1994). Introduction and overview. In T. J. Kiresuk, A. Smith, & J. E. Cardillo (Eds.), *Goal attainment scaling: Applications, theory and measurement* (pp. 1–14). Hillsdale, NJ: Lawrence Erlbaum Associates.

Smith, A., & Cardillo, J. E. (1994). Perspectives on validity. In T. J. Kiresuk, A. Smith, & J. E. Cardillo (Eds.), *Goal attainment scaling: Applications, theory, and measurement* (pp. 243–272). Hillsdale, NJ: Lawrence Erlbaum Associates.

Smith, G. T. (1994). Psychological expectancy as mediator of vulnerability to alcoholism. *Annals of the New York Academy of Sciences, 708,* 165–171.

Smith, G. T., & McCarthy, D. M. (1995). Methodological considerations in the refinement of clinical assessment instruments. *Psychological Assessment, 7,* 300–308.

Snaith, R. P., & Turpin, G. (1990). Clinical anxiety states. In D. F. Peck & C. M. Shapiro (Eds.), *Measuring human problems: A practical guide* (pp. 67–89). New York: John Wiley & Sons.

Sobell, L. C., Breslin, F. C., & Sobell, M. B. (1997). Substance-related disorders: Alcohol. In S. M. Turner & M. Hersen (Eds.), *Adult psychopathology and diagnosis* (3rd ed., pp. 128–158). New York: John Wiley & Sons.

Sobell, L. C., Toneatto, T., & Sobell, M. B. (1994). Behavioral assessment and treatment planning for alcohol, tobacco, and other drug problems: Current states with an emphasis on clinical applications. *Behavior Therapy, 25,* 533–580.

Spengler, P. M., Strohmer, D. C., Dixon, D. N., & Shivy, V. A. (1995). A scientist-practitioner model of psychological assessment: Implications for training, practice, and research. *The Counseling Psychologist, 23,* 506–534.

Spitzer, R. L., Endicott, J., & Robins, E. (1975). Clinical criteria for psychiatric diagnosis and DSM-III. *American Journal of Psychiatry, 132,* 1187–1192.

Staats, A. W. (1986). Behaviorism with a personality: The paradigmatic behavioral assessment approach. In R. O. Nelson & S. C. Hayes (Eds.), *Conceptual foundations of behavioral assessment* (pp. 226–241). New York: Guilford.

Staats, A. W. (1995). Paradigmatic behaviorism and paradigmatic behavior therapy. In W. O'Donohue & L. Krasner (Eds.), *Theories of behavior therapy–Exploring behavior change* (pp. 659–694). Washington, DC: American Psychological Association.

Stein, M. B. (Ed.). (1995). *Social phobia: Clinical and research perspectives.* Washington, DC: American Psychiatric Press.

Stoolmiller, M., Duncan, T., Bank, L., & Patterson, G. R. (1993). Some problems and solutions in the study of change: Significant patterns in client resistance. *Journal of Consulting and Clinical Psychology, 61,* 920–928.

Stromer, R., MacKay, H. A., McVay, A. A., & Fowlder, T. (1998). Written lists as mediating stimuli in the matching-to-sample performances of individuals with mental retardation. *Journal of Applied Behavior Analysis, 31,* 1–19.

Strosahl, K. D., & Linehan, M. M. (1986). Basic issues in behavioral assessment. In A. R. Ciminero, K. S. Calhoun, & H. E. Adams (Eds.), *Handbook of behavioral assessment* (2nd ed., pp. 12–46). New York: John Wiley & Sons.

Suen, H. K. (1988). Agreement, reliability, accuracy and validity: Toward a clarification. *Behavioral Assessment, 10,* 343–366.

Suen, H. K., & Ary, D. (1989). *Analyzing quantitative behavioral data.* Hillsdale, NJ: Lawrence Erlbaum Associates.

Sutker, P. B., & Adams, H. E. (Eds.). (1993). *Comprehensive handbook of psychopathology* (2nd ed.). New York: Plenum.

Suzuki, L. A., Meller, P. J., & Ponterotto, J. G. (Eds.). (1996). *Handbook of multicultural assessment: Clinical, psychological, and educational applications.* San Francisco: Jossey-Bass.

Swan, G. E., & MacDonald, M. L. (1997). Behavior therapy in practice: A national survey of behavior therapists. *Behavior Therapy, 9,* 799–807.

Tallent, N. (1992). *The practice of psychological assessment.* Englewood Cliffs, NJ: Prentice-Hall.

Taylor, J. C., & Carr, E. G. (1992). Severe problem behaviors related to social interaction. I. Attention seeking and social avoidance. *Behavior Modification, 16,* 305–335.

Thompson, R. H., Fisher, W. W., Piazza, C. C., & Kuhn, D. E. (1998). The evaluation and treatment of aggression maintained by attention and automatic reinforcement. *Journal of Applied Behavior Analysis, 31,* 103–116.

Timberlake, W. (1995). Reconceptualizing reinforcement: A causal-system approach to reinforcement and behavior change. In W. O'Donohue & L. Krasner (Eds.), *Theories of behavior therapy–Exploring behavior change* (pp. 59–96). Washington, DC: American Psychological Association.

Timberlak, W. & Farmer-Dougan, V. A. (1991). Reinforcement in applied settings: Figuring out ahead of time what will work. *Psychological Bulletin, 110,* 379–391.

Tingey, R., Lambert, M., Burlingame, G., & Hansen, N. (1996). Assessing clinical significance: Proposed extensions to method. *Psychotherapy Research, 6,* 109–123.

Tomarken, A. J. (1995). A psychometric perspective on psychophysiological measures. *Psychological Assessment, 7,* 387–395.

Torgrud, L. J., & Holborn, S. W. (1992). Developing externally valid role-play for assessment of social skills: A behavior analytic perspective. *Behavioral Assessment, 14,* 245–277.

Tryon, W. W. (1976). Models of behavior disorder: A formal analysis based on Woods' taxonomy of instrumental conditioning. *American Psychologist, 31,* 509–518.

Tryon, W. W. (1998). Behavioral observation. In A. S. Bellack & M. Hersen (Eds.), *Behavioral assessment—A practical handbook* (4th ed., pp. 79–103). Boston: Allyn & Bacon.

Turk, D. C., & Melzack, R. (Eds.). (1992). *Handbook of pain assessment.* New York: Appleton-Century-Crofts.

Turk, D. C., & Salovey, P. (Eds.). (1988). *Reasoning, inference, and judgment in clinical psychology.* New York: Free Press.

Turkat, I. (1986). The behavioral interview. In A. Ciminero, K. S. Calhoun, & H. E. Adams (Eds.), *Handbook of behavioral assessment* (pp. 109–149). New York: John Wiley & Sons.

Turner, R. M. (1994). Borderline, narcissistic, and histrionic personality disorders. In M. Hersen & R. T. Ammerman (Eds.), *Handbook of prescriptive treatments for adults* (pp. 393–420). New York: Plenum.

Turner, S. M., Calhoun, K. S., & Adams, H. E. (1992). *Handbook of clinical behavior therapy.* New York: John Wiley & Sons.

Turner, S. M., & Hersen, M. (Eds.). (1997). *Adult psychopathology and diagnosis* (3rd ed., pp. 483–507). New York: John Wiley & Sons.

Turpin, G. (Ed.). (1989). *Handbook of clinical psychophysiology.* London: John Wiley & Sons.

Ullmann, L. P., & Krasner, L. (1965). *Case studies in behavior modification.* New York: Holt, Rinehart & Winston.

Ulrich, R., Stachnik, T., & Mabry, J. (Eds.). (1966). *Control of human behavior.* Glenview, IL: Scott, Foresman.

United States, Office of Strategic Services. (1948). *Assessment of men: Selection of personnel for the office of strategic services.* New York: Rinehart.

Vallacher, R., & Nowak, A. (Eds.). (1994). *Dynamical systems in social psychology.* San Diego, CA: Academic Press.

Vance, H. B. (Ed.). (1998). *Psychological assessment of children* (2nd ed.). New York: John Wiley & Sons.

Van Houten, R., & Axelrod, S. (Eds.). (1993). *Behavior analysis and treatment* (pp. 102–125). New York: Plenum.

Voeltz, L. M., & Evans, I. M. (1982). The assessment of behavioral interrelationships in child behavior therapy. *Behavioral Assessment, 4,* 131–165.

Vogt, W. P. (1993). *Dictionary of statistics and methodology: A nontechnical guide for the social sciences.* Thousand Oaks, CA: Sage.

Wahler, R. G., & Hann, D. M. (1986). A behavioral systems perspective in childhood psychopathology: Expanding the three-term operant contingency. In N. A. Krasnegor, J. D. Arasteh, & M. F. Cataldo (Eds.), *Child health behavior: A behavioral pediatrics perspective* (pp. 146–167). New York: John Wiley & Sons.

Wainer, H., & Braun, H. I. (Eds.). (1988). *Test validity.* Hillsdale, NJ: Lawrence Erlbaum Associates.

Walitzer, K. S., & Connors, G. J. (1994). Psychoactive substance use disorders. In M. Hersen & R. T. Ammerman (Eds.), *Handbook of prescriptive treatments for adults* (pp. 53–71). New York: Plenum.

Wallace, C. J. (1986). Functional assessment in rehabilitation. *Schizophrenia Bulletin, 12,* 604–630.

Walsh, W. B., & Betz, N. (1995). *Tests and assessment* (3rd ed.). New York: Prentice-Hall.

Watkins, Jr., Campbell, V. L., & McGregor, P. (1990). What types of psychological tests do behavioral (and other) counseling psychologists use? *The Behavior Therapist, 13,* 115–117.

Watson, D. L. & Tharp, R. G. (1997). *Self-directed behavior: Self-modification for personal adjustment* (7th ed.). Pacific Grove, CA: Brooks/Cole.

Weems, C. F. (1998). The evaluation of heart rate biofeedback using a multi-element design. *Journal of Behavior Therapy and Experimental Psychiatry, 29,* 157–162.

Wei, W. S. (1990). *Time series analysis: Univariate and multivariate methods.* Redwood City, CA: Addison-Wesley.

Weiner, I. B. (1994). Rorschach assessment. In Maruish, M. E. (Ed.), *The use of psychological testing for treatment planning and outcome assessment* (pp. 249–278). Hillsdale, NJ: Lawrence Erlbaum Associates.

Weiss, R. L., & Heyman, R. E. (1990). Observation of marital interaction. in F. D. Fincham & T. N. Bradury (Eds.), *The psychology of marriage: Basic issues and applications* (pp. 87–117). New York: Guilford.

Weiss, R. L., & Perry, B. A. (1983). The spouse observation checklist: Development and clinical applications. In E. E. Filsinger (Ed.), *Marriage and family assessment: A sourcebook for family therapy* (pp. 65–84). Beverly Hills, CA: Sage.

Weist, M. D., Finney, J. W., & Ollendick, T. H. (1992). Cognitive biases in child behavior therapy. *The Behavior Therapist*.

Werle, M. A., Murphy, T. B., & Budd, K. S. (1998). Broadening the parameters of investigation in treating young children's chronic food refusal. *Behavior Therapy, 29*, 87–105.

Whittal, M. L., Goetsch, V. L., & Eifert, G. H. (1996). Introduction of a dynamic, idiographic model for identifying panic. *Journal of Anxiety Disorders, 10*, 129–144.

Wicks-Nelson, R., & Israel, A. C. (1997). *Behavior disorders of childhood*. Upper Saddle River, NJ: Prentice-Hall.

Widiger, T. A. (1997). Mental disorders as discrete clinical conditions: Dimensional versus categorical classification. In S. M. Turner & M. Hersen (Eds.), *Adult psychopathology and diagnosis* (3rd ed., pp. 3–23). New York: John Wiley & Sons.

Wiggins, J. S. (1973). *Personality and prediction: Principles of personality assessment*. Reading, MA: Addison-Wesley.

Williams, K. E., Chambless, D. L., & Steketee, G. (1998). Behavioral treatment of obsessive-compulsive disorder in African Americans: Clinical issues. *Journal of Behavior Therapy and Experimental Psychiatry, 29*, 163–170.

Williamson, D. A., Womble, L. G., & Zucker, N. L. (1998). Cognitive behavior therapy for eating disorders. In T. S. Watson & F. M. Gresham, (Eds.), *Handbook of child behavior therapy* (pp. 335–356). New York: Plenum.

Wilson, J. P., & Keane, T. M. (Eds.). (1997). *Assessing psychological trauma and PTSD*. New York: Guilford.

Wincze, J. P., & Carey, M. P. (1991). *Sexual dysfunctions: Guide for assessment and treatment*. New York: Guilford.

Wolfe, D. A., & McEachran, A. (1997). Child physical abuse and neglect. In E. J. Mash & L. G. Terdal (Eds.), *Assessment of childhood disorders* (3rd ed., pp. 523–568). New York: Guilford.

Wolpe, J. (1958). *Psychotherapy by reciprocal inhibition*. Stanford, CA: Stanford University Press.

Wolpe, J. (1995). Reciprocal inhibition: Major agent of behavior change. In W. O'Donohue & L. Krasner (Eds.), *Theories of behavior therapy–Exploring behavior change* (pp. 23–58). Washington, DC: American Psychological Association.

Woods, D. W., & Wright, Jr., L. W. (1998). Dismantling simplified regulated breathing: A case of a bilingual stutterer. *Journal of Behavior Therapy and Experimental Psychiatry, 29*, 179–186.

Woods, P. J. (1974). A taxonomy of instrumental conditioning. *American Psychologist, 29*, 584–597.

Wright, J. C., & Mischel, W. (1987). A conditional approach to dispositional constructs: The local predictability of social behavior. *Journal of Personality and Social Psychology, 53*, 1159–1177.

Yoshikawa, H. (1994). Prevention as cumulative protection: Effects of early family support and education on chronic delinquency and its risks. *Psychological Bulletin, 115*, 28–54.

Zanolli, K., & Daggett, J. (1998). The effects of reinforcement rate on the spontaneous social initiations of socially withdrawn preschoolers. *Journal of Applied Behavior Analysis, 31*, 117–125.

Author Index

Acaniz, M., 246
Achenbach, T. M., 91, 92, 148
Acierno, R., 53
Adams, H. E., 49, 166, 175, 266
Ahearn, W. H., 248
Alder, S. J., 212
Alexander, F. G., 17, 178
Alessi, G., 144, 146, 186, 187, 292
Allison, D. B., 184
American Psychiatric Association
    8, 129, 151, 152, 153, 163
Ammerman, R.T., 53, 150
Anastasi, A., 21, 200, 293, 299, 315
Anderson, S. A., 38,70
Andreassi, J. L., 210
Applegate, W. B., 42
Arkes, H. R., 49, 50, 51, 252
Arnkoff, D. B., 148
Arrington, R. E., 19
Ary, D., 20, 93, 103, 107, 193,
    209, 210, 226, 228, 238, 255,
    258, 259
Ashbaugh, R., 246
Asher, H. B., 160
Asterita, M. F., 178
Atlas, J. G., 168
Axelrod, S., 13
Ayd, F. J., 301
Azar, B., 135

Bachrach, A. J., 19, 20
Bailey, S., 81, 91
Bakeman, R., 155, 301, 313
Baker, G. L., 98
Baltes, P. B., 19, 98
Bandura, A., 20, 166
Banks, S. M., 75
Banos, R. M., 246
Barker, R. G., 19
Barkley, R. A., 49, 155
Barlow, D. H., 19, 93, 110, 153,
    255, 266

Barnett, P. A., 152, 229
Baron, R. M., 176, 305
Barret, B. H., 15, 132, 136, 139
Barrios, B. A., 15, 62, 83, 93, 226,
    229, 231
Batshaw, M. L., 123
Beach, S., 144
Beck, J. G., 112, 142
Behrens, B. C., 37, 118
Beidel, D. C., 20, 183
Bell-Dolan, D. J., 226, 229
Bellack, A. S., 15, 16, 32, 34, 49,
    68, 80, 97, 107, 266
Belter, R. W., 13
Bender, B. G., 80, 153, 155, 301
Bennet, K., 246
Bental, R. P., 179
Bernstein, I. H., 310, 314, 316
Bertagnolli, A., 143, 146
Betz, N., 5
Bigelow, K. M., 246
Bijlsma, J. W., 70
Binder, L. M., 246
Blackburn, S., 89, 110, 310
Blaine, D. D., 16, 57, 97, 98, 132,
    150, 206, 274, 282, 283, 292,
    313
Blakely-Smith, A. B., 247
Blakelock, H., 249
Blalock, H. M., 160, 164
Blanchard, E. B., 16, 20, 34, 37,
    70, 116, 121, 122, 143, 148,
    154, 166
Blass, S., 42
Bloom, M., 68
Bohman, M., 169
Bollen, K., 295
Bolstad, O. D., 297
Bootzin, R. R., 20
Boring, E. G., 42, 163
Bornstein, M. H., 15, 168
Botella, C., 246

Bott, H., 19
Boutelle, K. N., 246
Boyd, R. D., 19
Bradford, D, C., 15, 16
Bramlett, R. K., 229
Brasfield, C. R., 249
Breen, M. J., 292
Breslin, F. C., 175
Brett, J. M., 160, 164
Brewer, M. B., 36
Briggs, J., 17
Brondolo, E., 168
Bronowski, J., 90
Brons, M. R., 70
Brown, E. J., 91, 166
Brunk, M., 178
Brussell, E. E., 90
Budd, K. S., 37, 250
Bunge, M., 160, 163
Burge, D. A., 226, 229
Burlingame, G., 56
Butcher, J. N., 13, 82, 112, 165,
    183

Cacioppo, J. T., 20, 98, 210
Calhoun, S., 49, 266
Cantor, N., 80
Cambell, A. B., 98, 102, 107
Campbell, R. J., 110, 312
Campbell, D. T., 31, 160, 205, 251,
    255, 256, 257, 315
Cardillo, J. E., 118, 119, 121, 124,
    126
Carey, M. P., 70, 148
Carr, E. G., 16, 73, 244
Casey, R. L., 301, 313
Cascio, W. F., 63
Cattell, R.B., 31
Cavenaugh, R. A., 246
Chadwick, P. D. J., 116
Chamberlain, P., 36
Chambless, D. L., 250

337

Subject Index